Radiology of the
Ear, Nose and Throat

Radiology of the Ear, Nose and Throat

Galdino E. Valvassori, Guy D. Potter,
William N. Hanafee, Barbara L. Carter,
Richard A. Buckingham

878 Illustrations

1982

W. B. Saunders Company, Philadelphia · Toronto
Georg Thieme Verlag, Stuttgart

Galdino E. Valvassori, M. D.
Professor of Radiology
and Otolaryngology,
Abraham Lincoln School of Medicine
University of Illinois
55 East Washington Street
Chicago, Illinois 60602, USA

Guy D. Potter, M. D.
Associate Director of Radiology
Roosevelt Hospital
St. Luke's-Roosevelt Hospital Center
428 West 59th Street
New York, New York 10019, USA

William N. Hanafee, M. D.
Dept. of Radiological Sciences
The Center for The Health Sciences
Los Angeles, California 90024, USA

Barbara L. Carter, M. D.
Chief of ENT Radiology and
C. T. Body Scanning
New England Medical Center Hospital
171 Harrison Ave.
Boston, Massachusetts 02111, USA

Richard A. Buckingham, M. D.
Clinical Professor of Otolaryngology
Abraham Lincoln School of Medicine
University of Illinois
Chicago, Illinois 60612
Otologist, Resurrection Hospital
Chicago, Illinois 60631, USA

Important Note:

Medicine is an ever-changing science. Research and clinical experience are continually broadening our knowledge, in particular our knowledge of proper treatment and drug therapy. Insofar as this book mentions any dosage or application, readers may rest assured that the authors, editors and publishers have made every effort to ensure that such references are strictly in accordance with the state of knowledge at the time of production of the book. Nevertheless, every user is requested to carefully examine the manufacturers' leaflets accompanying each drug to check on his own responsibility whether the dosage schedules recommended therein or the contraindications stated by the manufacturers differ from the statements made in the present book. Such examination is particularly important with drugs which are either rarely used or have been newly released on the market.

Some of the product names, patents and registered designs referred to in this book are in fact registered trademarks or proprietary names even though specific reference to this fact is not always made in the text. Therefore, the appearance of a name without designation as proprietary is not to be construed as a representation by the publisher that it is in the public domain.

© 1982 Georg Thieme Verlag, P.O. Box 732,
D-7000 Stuttgart 1, FRG
Typesetting: Appl, Wemding (Linotron 303)
Printed by K. Grammlich, Pliezhausen, West Germany
ISBN 0-7216-8952-3 (Saunders)
ISBN 3-13-592301-0 (Thieme)
LC 81-48515

Preface

The radiographic evaluation of the head and neck has undergone revolutionary changes in the past few years due to the introduction and refinement of computerized tomography (CT).

The increased complexity and variety of methods available for head and neck imaging require a new conceptual approach for the selection and utilization of these techniques which we present here.

Today the clinician, radiologist, otolaryngologist, head and neck surgeon or general surgeon treating the head and neck, is faced with an array of techniques from which he must select the method which will best determine the type and extent of pathology for the least cost and least radiation exposure to the patient.

The present methods available are: conventional radiography, linear and multidirectional tomography, CT with and without enhancement, angiography, laryngography, sialography, opaque and pneumocysternography, digital fluororadiography and dynamic CT blood flow studies. Older techniques are gradually being supplanted by newer ones, and the technique selected will, in specific cases, depend on the availability of more modern equipment. Especially in the field of CT newer generations of scanners become available almost every year.

Sophisticated equipment, no matter how advanced, cannot replace good clinical judgement and close cooperation between clinician and radiologist. It is imperative for the clinician to provide the radiologist with an exact description of the clinical picture. The radiologist must be made aware of the significance of the various clinical findings and laboratory studies which make the x-ray study necessary. Further, the radiologist must be cognizant of the significance of radiologic findings in relation to selection of therapy. The radiographic findings may determine the operability of certain lesions and the type of surgical approach.

We have divided the book into anatomical areas. The radiographic techniques for each area are discussed and evaluated so that the reader may select the best procedure to be used in the study of his patient depending on the location of the lesion and the available equipment.

We want to thank Doctor Günther Hauff, Herr Achim Menge, and Herr Gert Krüger of the Georg Thieme Verlag, Stuttgart, for their encouragement in the production of this book.

The Authors

Contents

Part I
Radiology of the Temporal Bone
Galdino E. Valvassori and Richard A. Buckingham

Chapter 1   Conventional Radiography   3
  Introduction   3
  Law Projection   4
  Schüller Projection   5
  Owen Projection   6
  Chausse III Projection   7
  Transorbital Projection   8
  Stenvers Projection   9
  Towne Projection   10
  Basal View   11

Chapter 2   Tomography of the Temporal Bone .   12
  Multidirectional Tomography of the Normal
  Temporal Bone   13
  Computerized Tomography of the Normal
  Temporal Bone   26

Chapter 3   Congenital Abnormalities of the Tem-
poral Bone   31
  Embryology   32
  Anomalies of the Sound Conducting System . .   34
  Anomalies of the Facial Nerve   37
  Anomalies of the Inner Ear   38
  Vestibular Aqueduct and Semicircular Canals .   40
  Anomalies of the Internal Auditory Canal . . .   40
  Anomalies of the Cochlear Aqueduct   40
  Congenital Obliterative Labyrinthitis   41
  Congenital Cerebrospinal Fluid Otorrhea . . .   41
  Congenital Vascular Anomalies   42

Chapter 4   Temporal Bone Trauma   46
  Classification   46
  Clinical Findings   46
  Radiographic Technique   47
  Tomography   47
  Radiographic Findings in Longitudinal Frac-
  tures   48
  Radiographic Findings in Transverse Frac-
  tures   50
  Direct Mastoid Fractures   50
  Ossicular Dislocation   52
  Projectile Missiles   53

Chapter 5   Acute Otitis Media and Mastoiditis .   54
  Radiographic Technique   54
  Radiographic Findings   54
  Differential Diagnosis   54
  Malignant External Otitis   55

Chapter 6   Chronic Otitis Media and Mastoiditis   57
  Otoscopic Findings   57
  Radiographic Findings   57

Variations of Mastoid Pneumatization   58
The Middle Ear   59
Cholesterol Granuloma   59
Tympanosclerosis   60
Chronic Granulomatous Disorders   60

Chapter 7   Cholesteatoma of the Middle Ear and
Mastoid   61
  Acquired Cholesteatoma of the Middle Ear and
  Mastoid   61
  Clinical and Otoscopic Findings   61
  Radiographic Techniques   62
  Classifications and Radiographic Findings . . .   62
  Diagnosis of Cholesteatoma – Erosion of Bony
  Structures   62
  Soft Tissue Lesions   62
  Patterns of Radiographic Findings   63
  Pars Flaccida Cholesteatoma   63
  Epitympanic Retracion Pockets   65
  Pars Tensa Cholesteatomas   65
  Combined Pars Flaccida and Pars Tensa Choles-
  teatomas   67
  Total Perforation   67
  Evaluation of the Extent of Cholesteatoma . .   67
  Complications   68
  Congenital Cholesteatoma   71
  Computerized Tomography   73
  Cholesteatoma of the External Auditory
  Canal   74

Chapter 8   Postoperative Radiology of the Mas-
toid   75
  Simple and Radical Mastoidectomy   75
  Tympanoplasty   75
  Radiographic Findings   75
  Postoperative Pathology   76
  Ossicles   76
  Soft Tissue Changes   76
  Meningocele and Meningoencephalocele . . .   76
  Stenosis of the External Auditory Canal   76

Chapter 9   Benign Tumors   78
  Exostoses   78
  Osteoma   78
  Adenoma   78
  Hemangioma   78
  Meningioma   80
  Neuromas of the Cranial Nerves V, IX, X,
  XII   82
  Eosinophilic Granuloma   84
  Glomus Tumors   85
  Radiographic Findings   86

Jugular Venography   87
Arteriography   87
Computerized Tomography   89
Malignant Tumors   90
Carcinoma   90
Sarcoma   90

Chapter 10 Internal Auditory Canal and Acoustic Neuroma   95
Normal Internal Auditory Canal   96
Abnormal Internal Auditory Canal   98
Radiographic Visualization of Acoustic Neuromas   100
Pathology in Cisternography   105
Selection of Diagnostic Procedures   106

Chapter 11 Otosclerosis and Bony Dystrophies .   108
Otosclerosis   108

Paget's Disease   114
Osteogenesis Imperfecta   116
Osteopetrosis   116
Fibrous Dysplasia   116
Craniometaphyseal Dysplasia   116

Chapter 12 Radiography of the Facial Canal . .   118
Congenital Anomalies   118
Inflammatory Conditions and Cholesteatoma .   119
Traumatic Facial Nerve Lesions   120
Neuromas of the Facial Nerve   122

Chapter 13 Vestibular Aqueduct Abnormalities   124
Abnormal Aqueducts   124

Chapter 14 Computerized Tomographic Evaluation of Vertebrobasilar Vascular Insufficiency . .   126

Part II
Radiology of the Paranasal Sinuses and Facial Bones
Guy D. Potter

Chapter 1 Radiographic Anatomy on Routine Views   130
Caldwell View (Inclined Posteroanterior) . . .   130
Waters View   134
Base View (Submentovertical or Axial)   137
Lateral View   140
Optic Canal (Rhese) View   142

Chapter 2 Normal Tomographic Anatomy . . .   143
Coronal Tomographic Projection   143
Lateral Tomographic Projection   153
Axial Tomographic Projection   159

Chapter 3 Maxillofacial Trauma   166
General Considerations   166
Zygomatic Arch Fractures   168
Maxillary Sinus (Antrum) Fractures   169
Blowout Fractures   170
Trimalar Fracture   173
LeFort Fractures   174
Ethmoid Sinus Fractures   178
Frontal Sinus Fractures   179
Sphenoid Sinus Fractures   179

Chapter 4 Inflammatory Disease of the Paranasal Sinuses   181
Radiographic Diagnosis of Sinusitis   181

Spurious Opacification of the Maxillary Sinus   181
Spurious Opacification of the Frontal Sinus . .   182
Spurious Opacification of the Ethmoid Sinus .   183
Use of the Lateral View in Diagnosing Opacification   183
Unilateral Opacification of the Sphenoid Sinus   183
Evaluation of the Ethmoid Sinus   183
Acute and Chronic Sinusitis   184
Inflammatory Masses of the Paranasal Sinuses   185
Mucocele   188
Other Complications of Sinusitis   190
Granulomatous Sinusitides   191

Chapter 5 Tumors of the Nasal Fossa and Paranasal Sinuses   193
Maxillary Sinus Destruction   193
Ethmoid Sinus Destruction   199
Frontal Sinus Destruction   201
Sphenoid Sinus Destruction   201
Differential Diagnosis of Bone Destruction . .   202
Destruction of the Hard Palate   206
Carcinoma of the Nasopharynx   207

Part III
Computed Tomography
Barbara L. Carter

Chapter 1   Introduction 212
  Method 213
  Technical Considerations 214
  Radiation Exposure 215

Chapter 2   Orbit 216
  Normal Anatomy 216
  Abnormal 218

Chapter 3   Skull Base 220
  Normal Anatomy 220
  Abnormal 220

Chapter 4   Infratemporal Fossa 222
  Normal Anatomy 222
  Abnormal 225

Chapter 5   Nasopharynx, Nasal Cavity, and
Paranasal Sinuses 227
  Normal Anatomy 227
  Abnormal 229

Chapter 6   Oropharynx and Mandible 236
  Normal Anatomy 236
  Abnormal 237

Chapter 7   Conclusions 239

Part IV
Radiography of the Pharynx and Larynx
William N. Hanafee

Chapter 1   Pharynx 242
  Introduction 242
  Pharynx 242
  Normal Radiographic Anatomy 245
  CT Examination of the Nasopharynx 246
  Disease Processes 249
  Functional Disorders 250
  Trauma 251
  Infections 251
  Tumors 254
  Nasopharyngeal Tumor-Malignant 260

Chapter 2   Larynx 267
  Introduction 267
  Larynx-Radiologic Techniques 269
  Pathologic Conditions 280
  Trauma 282
  Inflammatory Lesions 288
  Miscellaneous Disorders 290
  Laryngeal Tumors 290
  Piriform Sinus Tumors 306
  Summary 308

Part V
Sialography
William N. Hanafee

Anatomy 312
Technique 315
Infection 319
Benign Tumors 325

Location of Tumors by Roentgen Technique . 328
Malignant Tumors 332

Index 339

Part I

Radiology of the Temporal Bone

Galdino E. Valvassori and Richard A. Buckingham

Chapter 1 Conventional Radiography

Introduction

Conventional radiography is of value in screening the entire temporal bone, and in determining the status of pneumatization of the mastoid and petrous pyramid. This method permits evaluation of the size and extent of relatively large lesions that arise in or extend from adjacent structures into the temporal bone. Smaller pathological processes are not visualized by this technique, and tomography is needed.

There are eight conventional projections which we use for evaluation of the temporal bone. Five projections demonstrate the mastoid and middle ear. The Law, Schüller, and Owen are lateral or modified lateral views. The Chausse III and Towne projections are modified frontal views.

Three projections expose the petrous pyramids and inner ear. The transorbital is a frontal view, the Stenvers an oblique view, and the basal a horizontal view.

To obtain consistant satisfactory conventional radiographs of the temporal bone, we use a head unit. The table top and cassette holder are small so that the patient's shoulder can fit underneath. This allows a good approximation of the patient's head to the film. A transparent table top enables the technician to center the area of interest properly, since both entrance and exit points of the x-ray beam are visible. The unit should have a tube with a small 0.3 mm focal spot for increased definition. A slow to average speed screen-film combination gives the best results.

A small port size reduces scatter radiation. When the port exceeds 7.5 cm in diameter a fixed or moving grid will control scatter. To use the small port effectively, the technician must be properly trained in the basic anatomy of the skull and temporal bone so that he can position the patient's head accurately and correctly.

The lateral projections are essential for the study of the mastoid and the mastoid pneumatization. To avoid superimposition of the two ears the x-ray beam is directed obliquely. The degree of angulation is inversely proportional to the distance between the structures we wish to avoid superimposing.

The 15° angulation of the Law view frees one mastoid from superimposition by the contralateral mastoid. An increase of angulation to 30° in the Schüller projection eliminates superimposition and separates the external auditory canal and middle ear from the ipsilateral petrous pyramid.

To interpret correctly mastoid pneumatization, the radiologist and otologist must be aware of the great variation in the extent of pneumatization, the size of the air cells and the size of the mastoid.

It is important to remember that the air cells of the mastoid may appear on the conventional projections to be smaller than they actually are. This appearance is caused by the superimposition of several layers of cells on the single plane of the radiograph. Thus a large superficial mastoid air cell will appear to be septated due to septa of smaller underlying cells which are projected through the image of the larger cell.

There are four stages or degrees of pneumatization of the mastoid:

1. Pneumatization of the antrum only. In these temporal bones the antrum exists as a single, large, smooth-walled air cell without scalloping of its margin by any smaller air cells. The physician should not confuse a single large antral air cell with a cholesteatoma. In cholesteatoma, the antrum will be cloudy and there will be destruction in the middle ear, since most cholesteatomas have their origin in the middle ear. Tomography is necessary to make this differential.
2. The antrum and a few small periantral and perifacial cells are the only areas of mastoid pneumatization.
3. The antrum and the entire mastoid process are well pneumatized.
4. The pneumatization of the antrum and mastoid process may extend into the squamous and zygomatic portions of the temporal bone and even into the occipital bone.

Law Projection

The Law projection is used to study the mastoid, the extent of the pneumatization and the condition of the air cells, Figures 1.1 and 1.2.

To obtain this projection, the midsagittal plane of the skull is parallel to the film plane, and there is a 15° cephalocaudad angulation of the x-ray beam. In a variation of this projection, the face is rotated 15° toward the film.

Interpretation

When the mastoid is well pneumatized, the Law view demonstrates the extent of the air cells into the mastoid process, the temporal squama, the zygomatic arch and the occipital bone.

The internal and external auditory canals are superimposed and are surrounded by the dense bone of the petrous pyramid and otic capsule. The superior petrous ridge crosses the mandibular condyle anteriorly.

A sharp radiodense verticle line, the sinus plate, crosses the mastoid air cells posterior to the labyrinthine density. If the mastoid is well pneumatized, this sinus plate line separates the superficial air cells from the deeper air cells of the mastoid and of the petrous pyramid.

If the mastoid is poorly pneumatized, there are no cells posterior to the sinus plate.

The vertical line of the sinus plate merges postero-superiorly with another similarly dense horizontal or oblique line. This dense line is the superior dural plate formed by the superior margin of the base of the pyramid in the region of the tegmen of the antrum. The sharp angle at the junction of the sinus and dural plates is the angle of Citelli.

Indication

The Law view is useful for the study of pathologic processes involving the mastoid air cells and the sinus plate. However, since this projection does not give information about the external auditory canal or the middle ear cavity, we omit it and use the Schüller projection.

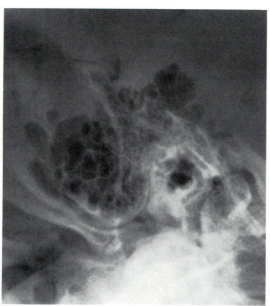

Fig. 1.1   Law projection

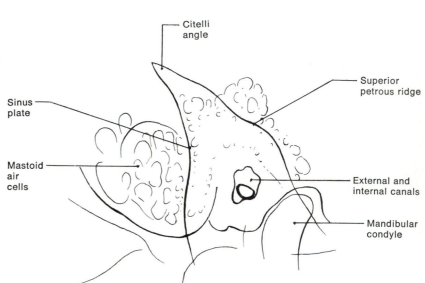

Fig. 1.2   Diagram of Law projection

Schüller Projection

The Schüller projection is another lateral view of the mastoid, Figures 1.3 and 1.4.

In this projection, the sagittal plane of the head lies parallel to the table top, and the x-ray beam is rotated 30° cephalocaudad.

Interpretation

The extent of the pneumatization of the mastoid, the distribution and degree of aeration of the air cells, and the status of the trabecular pattern are revealed in the Schüller projection.

This view projects the internal auditory canal below the external auditory canal. The superior petrous ridge crosses the radiolucency of the external auditory canal and extends forward to reach the neck of the mandibular condyle.

As in the Law projection, the sinus and dural plate form sharply defined lines which merge posterosuperiorly at the angle of Citelli.

The Schüller projection exposes the upper portion of the external auditory canal, the epitympanum, and when the middle ear is aerated, portions of the incus and malleus.

Indication

We use this projection to determine the extent and degree of pneumatization of the mastoid and the condition of the air cells. The Schüller projection also supplies basic information about the size of the external auditory canal, and the relation of the external auditory canal to the sinus plate.

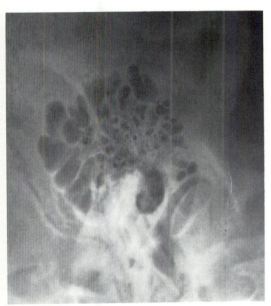

Fig. 1.3   Schüller projection

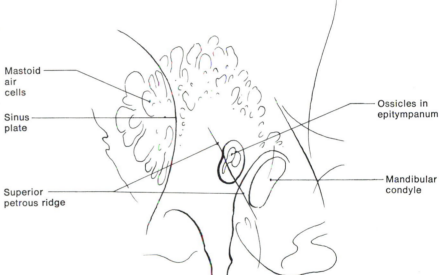

Mastoid air cells

Sinus plate

Superior petrous ridge

Ossicles in epitympanum

Mandibular condyle

Fig. 1.4   Diagram of Schüller projection

Owen Projection

The Owen projection is a modification of the Mayer projection, Figures 1.5 and 1.6. We prefer the Owen projection because there is less distortion of the anatomical structures.

In the Owen projection the sagittal plane of the head first lies parallel to the x-ray film. Then the face is rotated 30° away from the film. The x-ray beam extends in a 30° to 40° cephalocaudad angle.

In the Schüller view, the petrous pyramid obscures the lower half of the lumen of the external auditory canal and middle ear. In the Owen projection the combination of 30° rotation of the face and the 30° to 40° cephalocaudad angulation move the projection of the pyramid downward and posteriorly.

The upper portion of the middle ear and epitympanum are now superimposed on the external auditory canal and appear as a well defined oval radiolucency.

The angulation of the x-ray beam may vary from 30° to 40° depending on the anatomical relationship of the superior petrous ridge to the superimposed external auditory canal.

If the superior petrous ridge in the Schüller projection crosses the midportion of the external auditory canal, an angulation of the x-ray beam of 35° is sufficient. If the petrous ridge in the Schüller view lies superior to the lumen of the external auditory canal, 40° angulation of the beam will be necessary. If, in the Schüller view, the petrous ridge lies below the lumen of the external auditory canal, a 30° angulation of the beam will result in a good Owen projection.

Interpretation

The Owen view exposes the mastoid air cells adequately, but distorts them due to the angulation of head and x-ray beam. The Owen view exposes the sinus and dural plates but not as well as the Schüller.

The epitympanum and ossicles are discernible when the external auditory canal is sufficiently large and normally angulated. When the middle ear is aerated, the Owen view exposes the malleus head. The superimposition of the posterior wall of the external canal partially obstructs the view of the body of the incus.

The aditus and antrum extend posteriorly from the epitympanum from which they are separated by a bony contour formed by the posterior portion of the lateral epitympanic wall.

Indications and Limitations

We use the Owen projection to visualize the external auditory canal, the epitympanum, portions of the ossicles, and the mastoid air cells.

The effectiveness of the Owen view in visualizing the middle ear and epitympanum is limited if the external auditory canal is absent or stenosed, since absence of the external canal results in a bony mass obstructing the view of the middle ear and epitympanum.

Further, to recognize the ossicles, the middle ear must be aerated so that a clear air-bone interface exists between the ossicles and the middle ear space. In chronic infections of the middle ear and mastoid, the middle ear and epitympanum are filled with granulation tissue or cholesteatoma which obscure the ossicles.

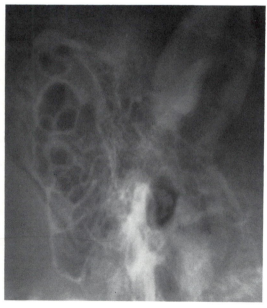

Fig. 1.5   Owen projection

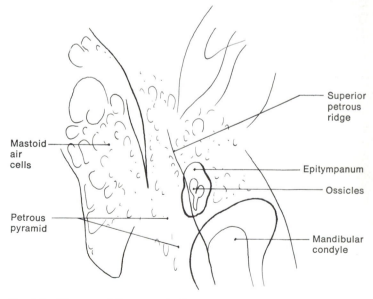

Fig. 1.6   Diagram of Owen projection

Chausse III Projection

The Chausse III projection is a frontal view of the mastoid and middle ear cavity, Figures 1.7 and 1.8. The projection allows satisfactory visualization of the epitympanum, the aditus, the mastoid antrum, and especially the anterior two-thirds of the lateral epitympanic wall.

As seen in horizontal sections, Figures 2.1–2.4 the lateral epitympanic wall forms and angle of 10° to 15° open anteriorly with sagittal plane of the skull. At the aditus the lateral epitympanic wall turns laterally to become the lateral wall of the mastoid antrum.

The Chausse III projection is complementary to the Owen view, since the Chausse III shows the anterior portion of the lateral epitympanic wall while the Owen view shows the posterior and aditus portions.

To obtain a Chausse III view the head is positioned with the occiput on the table top, the chin flexed on the chest, and the head is rotated 10° to 15° to the opposite side of the ear being examined. In a satisfactory Chausse III projection, the superior petrous ridge should form a continuous line with the superior orbital rim, and the lateral wall of the orbit cross the lateral one-third of the internal auditory canal.

Interpretation

The vestibule and horizontal semicircular canal are the basic landmarks and are used to identify other structures. The horizontal semicircular canal bulges laterally into the radiolucency of the mastoid antrum. Inferolateral to the horizontal semicircular canal there is a triangular bony mass made up medially by the malleus head and neck, and superolaterally by a portion of the incus body. Lateral to the ossicles there is a sharply outlined and dense oblique line formed by the anterior portion of the lateral epitympanic wall. This line joins the superior wall of the external auditory canal to form a sharp spur, the scutum.

The mastoid antrum lies above the epitympanum. The antrum is separated from the epitympanum by a narrow radiolucent space, the aditus. The aditus is limited medially by the bulge of the horizontal semicircular canal and laterally by the epitympanic wall. The promontory forms the medial wall of the middle ear cavity. The internal auditory canal lies medial to the vestibule.

Indications

The Chausse III is the most reliable conventional projection for the study of the middle ear. With the Chausse III projection middle ear structures are well seen in aerated middle ears but obscured in middle ears clouded by disease. In sclerotic mastoids the superimposed dense mastoid bone obscures the middle ear and causes an apparent clouding.

The Chausse III is complementary to the lateral mastoid projections. We use it to study chronic otitis media and cholesteatomas, especially cholesteatomas with perforations of the pars flaccida of the tympanic membrane.

The Chausse III is the best of the conventional projections for visualization of fistulas of the horizontal semicircular canal.

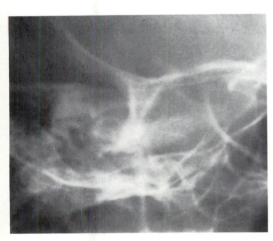

Fig. 1.7   Chausse III projection

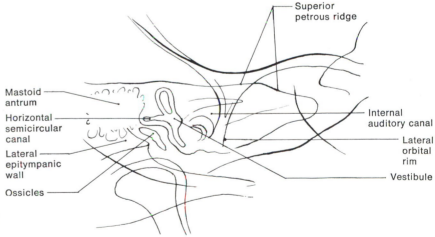

Fig. 1.8   Diagram of Chausse III projection

Petrous Pyramid Projections

Transorbital Projection

The transorbital projection is one of the conventional radiographic views which we use to expose the inner ear structures, Figures 1.9 and 1.10.

This projection is satisfactory for the study of the internal auditory canal which is exposed in its full length. This projection also visualizes the cochlea, the vestibule and the semicircular canals.

The main disadvantage of the transorbital projection is that large air cells in the petrous pyramid can obscure the contour of the internal auditory canal and may even create false contours. The transorbital view is therefore of greatest value in the study of the internal auditory canal in poorly pneumatized pyramids.

The occiput is placed on the x-ray film to magnify the orbital contour. The chin is flexed slightly so that the orbitomeatal line is perpendicular to the film plane. The x-ray beam is directed at a right angle to the film. For better details each side should be radiographed separately, and the x-ray beam centered over each eye. In a proper transorbital view the superior petrous ridge should be projected 1 cm below the superior orbital rim.

Interpretation

The internal auditory canal forms a well defined radiolucency within the surrounding density of the pyramid. The vestibule lies at the lateral end of the internal canal. The semilunar lip of the posterior wall of the internal auditory canal forms the medial boundary of the canal. The radiolucent oval-shaped area medial to this lip represents the groove for the seventh and eighth cranial nerves on the longer anterior wall of the canal.

The cochlea appears below and is partially superimposed on the fundus of the internal canal. The petrous apex is obscured by superimposition of the medial orbital wall and paranasal sinuses.

Indication

The transorbital view is mandatory in the study of possible acoustic neuromas, since it allows study of the shape and size of the internal auditory canal and of the length of the posterior wall. This view also provides a general survey of the status of the cochlea, vestibule, and semicircular canals.

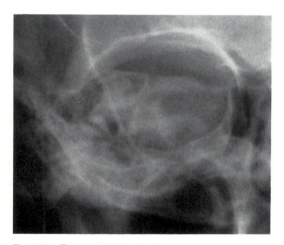

Fig. 1.9   Transorbital projection

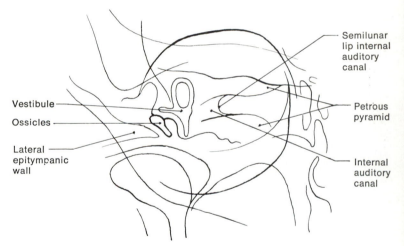

Fig. 1.10   Diagram of Transorbital projection

Stenvers Projection

The Stenvers projection is the best view for the study of the petrous apex, the porus of the internal auditory canal, the vestibule, the semicircular canals, and the mastoid process air cells, Figures 1.11 and 1.12.

In highly pneumatized temporal bones, petrous air cells obscure the contour of the internal auditory canal, and, as in the transorbital view, may cause false contours of the canal.

To obtain the Stenvers projection, the patient faces the x-ray film with the head slightly flexed. The head is rotated 45° toward the opposite side of the ear being examined. This position places the long axis of the petrous pyramid parallel to the film. The x-ray beam is angled 15° caudad.

Interpretation

The Stenvers view projects the mastoid process air cells laterally where they are free of superimposition. The external auditory canal and middle ear cavity are poorly visualized. The vestibule and horizontal semicircular canals are well outlined lateral to the foreshortened internal auditory canal. The porus of the internal auditory canal forms an oval-shaped radiolucency medial to the semilunar lip of the posterior wall of the internal auditory canal. The petrous apex is seen in its entire contour. Under the pyramid the hypoglossal canal is often seen on end above the condyle of the occipital bone.

Indication

The Stenvers view is useful in the study of all pathological processes which involve the petrous pyramid and apex such as petrositis and tumors of various types.

The Stenvers projection cannot be used by itself for the study of the internal auditory canal, since the rotation of the pyramid foreshortens and distorts the contour of the canal.

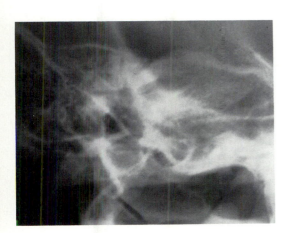

Fig. 1.11   Stenvers projection

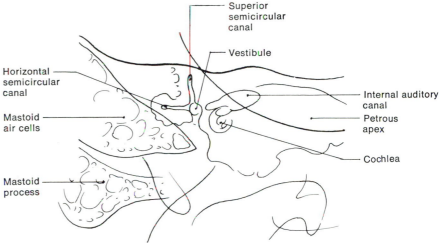

Fig. 1.12   Diagram of Stenvers projection

Towne and Basal Views

The Towne and basal projections are two views useful for the study of the overall contour of the temporal bone at an angle different from the previously discussed projections. Both projections are useful for visualizing lesions that extend from the temporal bone into adjacent structures or from adjacent structures into the temporal bone.

Towne Projection

(Chamberlain-Towne, Worms and Bretton, Superorbital Projection of Lysholen)

In the Towne projection the mastoid air cells of both sides are well seen and can be easily compared because of the simultaneous exposure, Figures 1.13 and 1.14. The epitympanic space and ossicles are poorly visualized. This projection exposes the internal auditory canal and labyrinth fairly well. A problem with the interpretation of the internal auditory canals arises in pneumatic and in sclerotic petrous apices. In pneumatic apices the air cells may confuse the contour of the internal auditory canals, while sclerotic apices may partially obliterate the view of the canals.

The Towne view is obtained with the patient's occiput on the x-ray film. The orbitomeatal line lies perpendicular to the film. The x-ray beam is directed 30° caudad.

Because of the angulation, the posterior aspect of the temporal bone and the occipital bone are well visualized.

Interpretation

In the Towne projection, the mastoid air cells lie at each lateral aspect of the radiograph. If the mastoids are not well pneumatized, the contours of the external auditory canals are visible above the temporomandibular joints. The superior petrous ridges and the posterior cells of the mastoid and petrous pyramid form the superior contour of the temporal bones, while the anterior cells are projected inferiorly.

The dense bone of the labyrinth lies medial to the mastoid air cells. The cochlea is projected inferior to the internal auditory canal which forms a radiolucent channel extending toward the petrous ridge.

The perilabyrinthine cells are usually well seen. The jugular fossa may be recognizable inferior to these cells.

Indication

The main indication for the Towne view is inflammation of the mastoid and petrous air cells.

This view is also useful for the study of the internal auditory canals in acoustic neuroma. With large glomus jugulare tumors, erosion of the jugular fossa and posteroinferior aspects of the petrous pyramid may be recognizable.

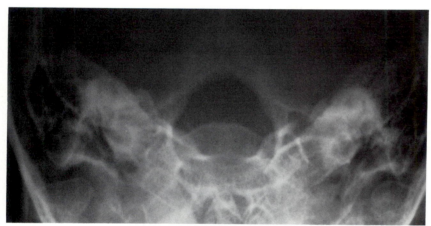

Fig. 1.**13**   Towne projection

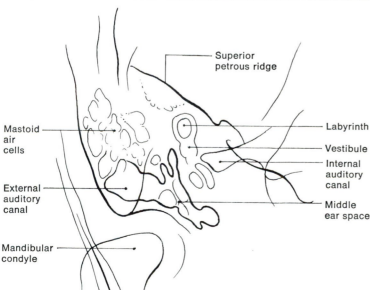

Fig. 1.**14**   Diagram of Towne projection

Basal View

The basal projection adds to the three-dimensional view of the temporal bone, Figures 1.15 and 1.16. This view is particularly useful for the study of the petrous pyramid and apex, the anterior foramen lacerum and, in a modified form, the jugular fossa.

At times, the basal view helps to visualize lesions of the external auditory canal, the middle ear, especially the eustachian tube portion, and the ossicles.

In this projection the mastoids and the pyramids are relatively far from the film and their images are somewhat distorted and unsharp. In adults the middle ear cavity, epitympanum and ossicles are usually obscured by superimposition of the mastoid air cells. Inner ear structures may be identified, but the definition is too poor for detailed study.

The basal projection is obtained with a submental vertex direction of the x-ray beam. The patient's head is overextended until the basal plane of Virchow, a plane from the tragus to the inferior orbital rim, is parallel to the plane of the film.

In the modified basal view the patient's head is less extended so that the basal plane forms an angle, open anteriorly, of 20° to 30° with the film plane.

Interpretation

The mastoid air cells form the lateral portion of each temporal bone.

The middle ear cavity and ossicles are occasionally seen medial to the external auditory canal. The anterior eustachian portion of the middle ear is usually seen as a triangular area of radiolucency directed anteromedially toward the foramen ovale.

The labyrinth forms a dense area in the middle of the petrous pyramid. In a pneumatized pyramid the internal auditory canal is usually not recognizable because of superimposition of the air cells. In a sclerotic petrous bone, the internal auditory canal is obscured by the dense surrounding bone. The petrous apex is well outlined by the radiolucency of the foramen lacerum.

In the standard basal view the jugular fossa is obscured by the superimposition of the overhanging lip of the occipital bone which forms the posteroinferior margin of the jugular fossa.

In the modified basal view, the rotation of the base of the skull exposes the full outline of the jugular fossa and adjacent posteroinferior aspect of the temporal bone. The hypoglossal canal is often visible in this projection.

Indication

The basal view is indicated for evaluation of basal skull fractures, for glomus jugulare tumors and other tumors occurring in the jugular fossa region.

This view is particularly useful to demonstrate extension into the temporal bone from lesions arising outside the bone such as nasopharyngeal carcinoma. Lesions such as carcinoma and malignant external otitis which extend from the temporal bone into adjacent structures are also clearly seen.

The basal view is helpful in the evaluation of the middle ear in atresia of the external auditory canal when tomography is not available.

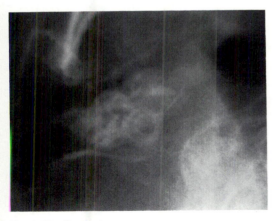

Fig. 1.15   Basal view

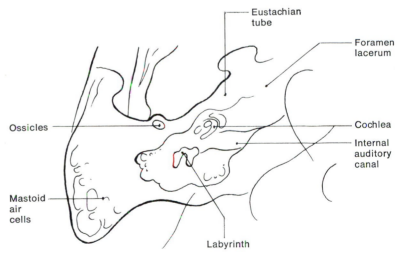

Fig. 1.16   Diagram of basal view

Chapter 2   Tomography of the Temporal Bone

The ear is an extremely complex organ with many minute anatomical structures lying in close relationship to one another in a small portion of the temporal bone. Tomography, both multidirectional and computerized, CT, is the best method for study of the temporal bone. In this book when we use the term tomography we refer to multidirectional techniques. Computerized tomography or CT is mentioned when this technique is used.

Conventional radiography produces a composite on a single plane of the tridimensional temporal bone where each point on the film is a summation of all the points crossed by the x-ray beams traveling through the skull and temporal bone. Conventional radiographs result in a confusing superimposition where larger and denser structures obscure smaller, less dense structures.

Multidirectional tomography yields thin 1–2 mm thick, serial sections through the temporal bone which allow recognition of the minute structures within the bone, free of superimposition. This technique has been used for the study of the temporal bone since 1960.

The recent refinements of CT permit spatial resolution of $0.1 mm^3$, and the displayed picture element or pixel has been reduced to $0.25 \times 0.25 \times 1.5$ mm. A slice thickness of 1.5 mm has been obtained by narrowing the collimator of the x-ray beam and the aperture of each detector. As a result of this improvement ossicles, oval window and facial nerve canal can now be clearly seen in serial sections.

The use of CT in the study of intratemporal bone pathology is, at present, only beginning. The advantages of CT over multidirectional tomography are that CT produces higher contrast images and better differentiation of soft tissue structures and pathology from fluids.

A problem with CT at present is that only horizontal and coronal sections can be obtained. Sagittal and oblique sections are obtained by reconstruction by the computer of the data collected in the horizontal plane. However, these images, today, are not as good as the direct images. Their reconstruction will improve in the future as the equipment improves.

The application of this reconstructive technique in the future will permit a study limited to a single horizontal projection from which reconstruction in various planes can be obtained with reduction of radiation exposure to the patient.

Computerized tomography is performed first without and then following intravenous infusion or bolus injection of a suitable radio-opaque material. In extracranial, nonvascular lesions infusion is not necessary, since there is no differential enhancement of the lesion. Whenever there is any suspicion of intracranial involvement, the double study with and without infusion should be done. Injection of air or contrast material in the subarachnoid space will be discussed in Chapter 10, Acoustic Neuromas.

We find today that cost is the limiting factor in the selection of technique for the study of temporal bone pathology. Since CT equipment costs four times as much as multidirectional tomographic units, we use multidirectional technique except in selected cases. We are continuing our evaluations of these two techniques.

In this chapter we shall present multidirectional and computerized tomography of normal temporal bones in various projections. The illustrations demonstrate how tomography isolates and exposes the fine anatomical structures of the normal temporal bone.

Multidirectional Tomography of the Normal Temporal Bone

Tomographic sections were taken of isolated normal cadaver temporal bones with a Philips polytome which has a hypocycloidal motion. The temporal bones were then sectioned in 2 mm thick sections and photographed. A microradiograph using soft x-rays of each tissue section was obtained. The tissue sections, corresponding tomographs, and microradiography are presented together for comparison.

We will show six projections commonly used for the study of the temporal bone:

1. Horizontal or basal, Figures 2.1–2.8
2. Coronal or frontal, Figures 2.9–2.16
3. Semiaxial or 20° coronal oblique, Figures 2.17–2.24
4. Axial or Poschl, Figures 2.25–2.32
5. Sagittal or lateral, Figures 2.33–2.40
6. Longitudinal or Stenvers, Figures 2.41–2.48.

Horizontal Projection

The patient lies supine with his back elevated from the table. The head is overextended and the vertex touches the table top.

This projection is satisfactory for the study of the temporal bone but is not used routinely because it is quite uncomfortable for the patient to maintain this hyperextended position for the length of time needed to complete the study.

The horizontal projection is used to study fractures, tumors of the temporal and adjacent bones and occasionally for congenital malformations.

Coronal Projection

The patient is positioned supine or prone with the plane from the tragus to the outer canthus perpendicular to the film. This projection is easy to obtain and to reproduce and is satisfactory for the study of all three portions of the ear.

Semiaxial Projection

The semiaxial projection is mainly used to visualize the medial or labyrinthine wall of the middle ear cavity.

The patient lies supine with the head rotated 20° toward the side being examined. Rotation of the head brings the medial or labyrinthine wall of the middle ear perpendicular to the film and sectioning plane. The horizontal tomogram (Fig. 2.7) shows that the labyrinthine wall of the middle ear forms a 15° to 25° angle with the sagittal plane crossing the middle ear cavity.

The semiaxial projection is mandatory for evaluation of the oval window, the promontory, the horizontal semicircular canal, and the tympanic portion of the facial canal. This projection also exposes to good advantage the lumen of the middle ear cavity, the ossicles, the floor of the hypotympanum, and the lateral epitympanic wall. We use this projection to study otosclerosis, cholesteatoma, facial nerve paralysis, and glomus tumors.

Axial Projection

The axial projection is used to study the vestibular aqueduct and the cochlear capsule.

The patient lies supine with the head rotated 45° toward the side being examined. The long axis of the petrous pyramid lies perpendicular to the film plane.

We use the axial projection in combination with the sagittal to study the vestibular aqueducts. The axial projection exposes the entire long axis of the aqueduct.

The section at the level of the long axis of the modiolus presents a good cross section of the cochlear coils. Axial tomographs expose the incus and the posterosuperior wall of the external auditory canal.

Sagittal Projection

The sagittal projection is complementary to the coronal, since it shows the anterior to posterior relationships of the structures seen in the lateral to medial relationships in the coronal projection.

The sagittal projection is useful in the study of the mastoid, the external auditory canal, the ossicles, the vertical portion of the facial canal, the semicircular canals, the internal auditory meatus, and the vestibular aqueduct.

The sagittal projection follows the plane of the surgical approaches to the middle ear and mastoid and is especially helpful to the otologic surgeon.

The patient lies prone with the shoulder of the side to be studied slightly elevated. The head is rotated until the sagittal plane of the skull is parallel to the film plane.

Longitudinal or Stenvers Projection

The longitudinal projection is useful for evaluation of the apical portion of the petrous pyramid and the carotid canal. This projection visualizes well the round window, the posterior semicircular canal, the cochlea, and the facial canal.

The longitudinal sections are unsatisfactory for the study of the external auditory canal and the middle ear.

The longitudinal projection is obtained with the patient supine or prone and the patient's head rotated 45° toward the opposite side being examined. The long axis of the pyramid becomes parallel to the film plane.

Two representative sections in each projection are shown. The complete series of six projections were published previously in Valvassori, G. E. and Buckingham, R. A.: Tomography and Cross Sections of the Ear. Saunders, Philadelphia; Thieme, Stuttgart, 1975.

Horizontal Projection

The horizontal tissue, tomographic and microradiographic sections are at a level approximately 6 mm inferior to the arcuate eminence, Figures 2.1–2.4. Mastoid air cells surround the antrum and extend laterally to the epitympanum.

At this level the epitympanum has a triangular shape with the apex lying posteriorly in the region of the aditus. The lateral epitympanic wall forms a 10° angle, open anteriorly, with a sagittal plane passing through the aditus.

The medial epitympanic wall forms a 20° to 25° angle with the same sagittal plane.

The head of the malleus and body of the incus occupy part of the epitympanic space. The horizontal semicircular canal which opens into the vestibule forms the medial wall of the aditus.

The posterior semicircular canal extends posterolaterally from the crus commune.

The facial and superior vestibular nerves occupy the upper portion of the internal auditory canal.

The petrous portion of the facial nerve extends from the fundus of the internal auditory canal to the geniculate ganglion where it turns sharply posteriorly along the medial wall of the epitympanum.

The cochlea appears in the tomogram anterior to the fundus of the internal auditory canal.

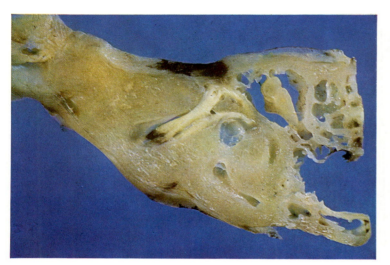

Fig. 2.**1**   Horizontal macrosection (Figs. 2.1–2.48 from Valvassori GE, Buckingham RA: Tomography and Cross-Sections of the Ear. Saunders, Philadelphia; Thieme, Stuttgart 1975)

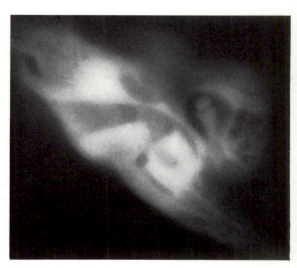

Fig. 2.**2**   Tomograph corresponding to Fig. 2.1

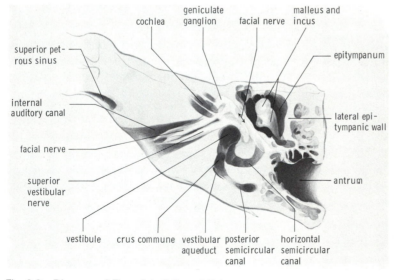

Fig. 2.**3**   Diagram of Figs. 2.1, 2.2, and 2.4

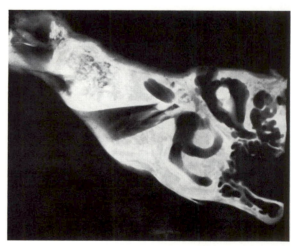

Fig. 2.**4**   Microradiograph of Fig. 2.1

These horizontal sections, Figures 2.5–2.8, lie 4 mm inferior to Figures 2.1–2.4, and cross the oval window and the internal and external auditory canals.

The tympanic cavity lies medial to the external auditory canal and contains the malleus handle and the long process of the incus.

In the tissue section and microradiograph the stapes lies in the oval window which opens into the vestibule. The stapedius tendon passes from the head of the stapes to the pyramidal process.

The vertical portion of the facial nerve lies lateral to the posterior semicircular canal. The cochlear nerve within the inferior portion of the internal auditory canal passes anteriorly into the base of the cochlea. At this level the modiolus is bisected, but is not seen in the tomographs. Three turns of the cochlea are outlined in the tomogram.

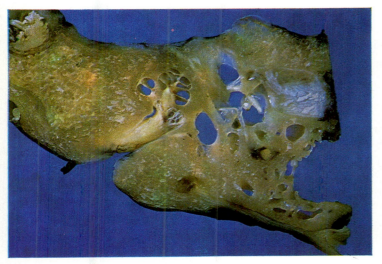

Fig. 2.**5**   Horizontal macrosection

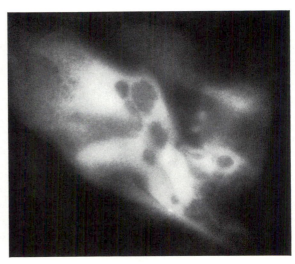

Fig. 2.**6**   Tomograph corresponding to Fig. 2.5

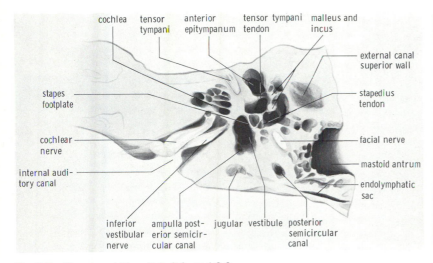

Fig. 2.**7**   Diagram of Figs. 2.5, 2.6, and 2.8

Labels in diagram:
cochlea
tensor tympani
anterior epitympanum
tensor tympani tendon
malleus and incus
external canal superior wall
stapedius tendon
facial nerve
mastoid antrum
endolymphatic sac
stapes footplate
cochlear nerve
internal auditory canal
inferior vestibular nerve
ampulla posterior semicircular canal
jugular
vestibule
posterior semicircular canal

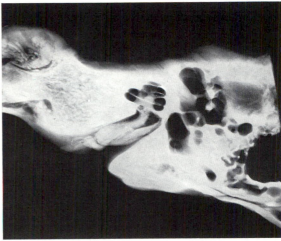

Fig. 2.**8**   Microradiograph of Fig. 2.5

Coronal Projection

These coronal sections, Figures 2.9–2.12, cross the anterior wall of the external auditory canal.

The lateral wall of the epitympanum joins the superior wall of the external auditory canal to form a sharp spur, the scutum, lateral to the neck of the malleus.

The head of the malleus lies in the epitympanum. In the tissue section and microradiograph, the tendon of the tensor tympani stretches across the middle ear from the cochleariform process to the malleus neck.

The cochlea forms the medial wall of the middle ear. In the tomogram only the wall and septa separating the basal and middle coils are recognizable. The rather dense bone of the cochlear capsule sharply outlines the radiolucency of the spiral cochlear canal.

The facial nerve is sectioned just posterior to the geniculate ganglion and both petrous and tympanic segments appear superolateral to the cochlea.

The proximal portion and the external aperture of the carotid canal lie under the cochlea and middle ear.

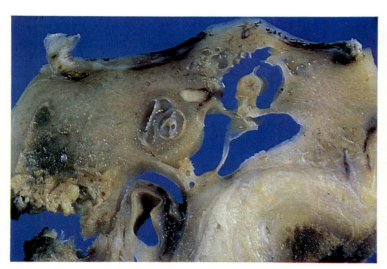

Fig. 2.**9**   Coronal macrosection

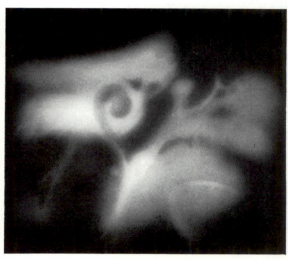

Fig. 2.**10**   Tomograph corresponding to Fig. 2.9

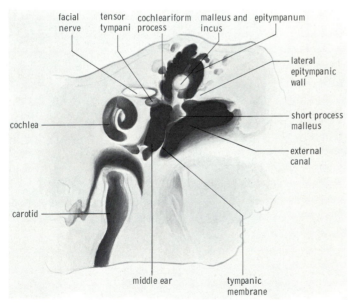

facial nerve — tensor tympani — cochleariform process — malleus and incus — epitympanum — lateral epitympanic wall — cochlea — short process malleus — external canal — carotid — middle ear — tympanic membrane

Fig. 2.**11**   Diagram of Figs. 2.9, 2.10, and 2.12

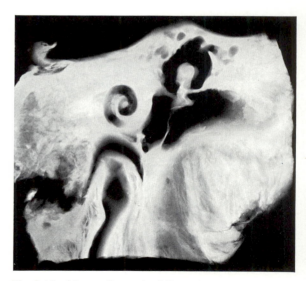

Fig. 2.**12**   Microradiograph of Fig. 2.9

These coronal sections (Figures 2.13–2.16) lie 4 mm posterior to Figures 2.9–2.12, and cross the external and internal auditory canals. The tympanic membrane demarcates the middle and external ears.

The superior wall of the external auditory canal joins the lateral epitympanic wall to form a sharp bony spur, the scutum.

The mastoid antrum extends superiorly and posteriorly from the epitympanum. The posterior portion of the body of the incus lies in the epitympanum medial to the lateral epitympanic wall. The long process of the incus extends toward the stapes. A portion of the footplate appears in the oval window.

The facial canal lies above the oval window and inferior to the horizontal semicircular canal. Both the superior and horizontal semicircular canals open into the vestibule.

The basal turn of the cochlea, which forms the promontory, extends inferiorly from the vestibule. The normal cochlear capsule forms a sharply defined, dense band surrounding the lumen of the basal turn.

The internal auditory canal stretches in its full length medially from the vestibule. Segments of the facial and acoustic nerves lie within the lumen of the internal auditory canal.

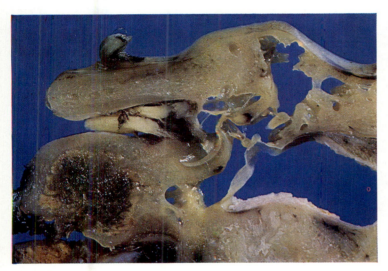

Fig. 2.13 Coronal macrosection

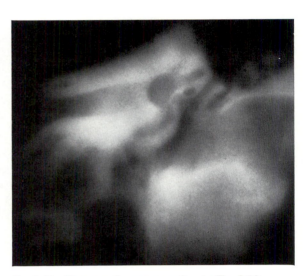

Fig. 2.14 Tomograph corresponding to Fig. 2.13

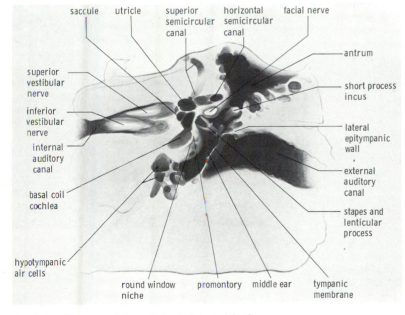

saccule utricle superior semicircular canal horizontal semicircular canal facial nerve

antrum

superior vestibular nerve

short process incus

inferior vestibular nerve

lateral epitympanic wall

internal auditory canal

external auditory canal

basal coil cochlea

stapes and lenticular process

hypotympanic air cells

round window niche promontory middle ear tympanic membrane

Fig. 2.15 Diagram of Figs. 2.13, 2.14, and 2.16

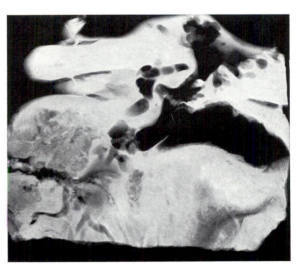

Fig. 2.16 Microradiograph of Fig. 2.13

Semiaxial Projection

The plane of this semiaxial section (Figures 2.17–2.20) lies at the level of the anterior portion of the external and internal auditory canals.

A strip of tympanic membrane divides the external and middle ears. The head of the malleus appears in the epitympanum adjacent to the lateral epitympanic wall. The cochlea forms the medial wall of the tympanic cavity.

The cochlear nerve lies in the internal auditory canal below the facial nerve and enters the base of the modiolus.

These sections cross posterior to the geniculate ganglion and expose both the petrous and tympanic segments of the facial nerve canal. The facial nerve leaves the fundus of the internal auditory canal and passes into the narrow petrous segment toward the geniculate ganglion. The tympanic segment of the facial nerve lies on the medial wall of the middle ear.

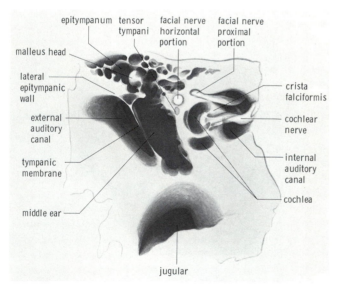

Fig. 2.**17**   Semiaxial macrosection

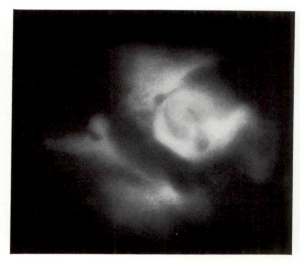

Fig. 2.**18**   Tomograph corresponding to Fig. 2.17

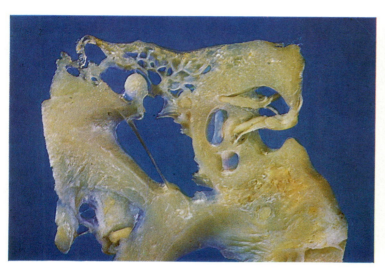

Fig. 2.**19**   Diagram of Figs. 2.17, 2.18, and 2.20

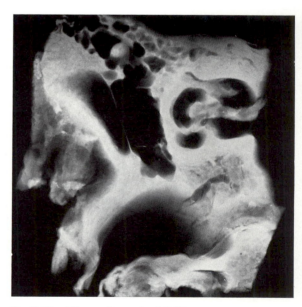

Fig. 2.**20**   Microradiograph of 2.17

These semiaxial sections (Figures 2.21–2.24) lie at the level of the oval window 4 mm posterior to Figures 2.17–2.20. The tympanic membrane separates the middle and external ears. The lateral epitympanic wall projects medially and inferiorly from the tegmen. The body of the incus lies in the epitympanum, and the long process of the incus articulates with the head of the stapes. The anterior crus of the stapes extends from the lenticular process to the footplate which closes the oval window.

The ampullated limbs of the superior and horizontal semicircular canals open into the vestibule. The tympanic segment of the facial nerve lies under the horizontal semicircular canal.

The promontory forms the inferior portion of the labyrinthine wall of the middle ear.

A thin bony plate separates the jugular dome from the hypotympanum.

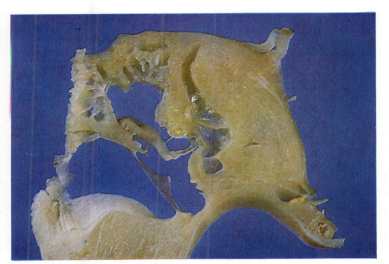

Fig. 2.**21**   Semiaxial macrosection

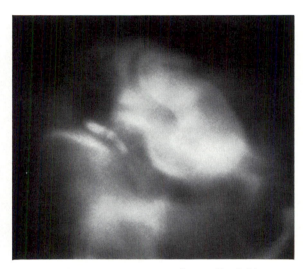

Fig. 2.**22**   Tomograph corresponding to Fig. 2.21

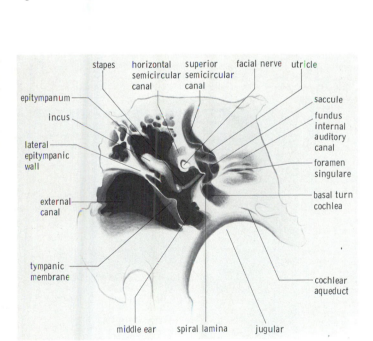

Fig. 2.**23**   Diagram of Figs. 2.21, 2.22, and 2.24

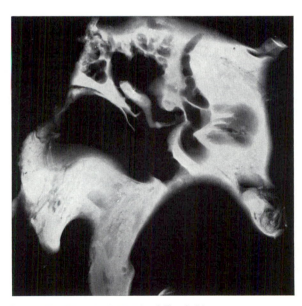

Fig. 2.**24**   Microradiograph of Fig. 2.21

Axial Projection

These axial sections (Figs. 2.25–2.28) cross the middle ear at the malleus handle and stapes.

The tympanic membrane separates external and middle ears. In the tomograph a residual ossicular shadow is present in the epitympanum.

The vestibular aqueduct courses from its outer aperture on the posterior surface of the petrous pyramid toward the crus commune. The entire superior semicircular canal arches through the thickness of the sections from the ampulla to the crus commune.

Both anterior and posterior limbs of the horizontal semicircular canal enter the vestibule. Inferiorly the ampulla of the posterior semicircular canal opens into the vestibule.

The facial nerve canal lies under the horizontal semicircular canal above the oval window niche. The posterior crus and a portion of the footplate of the stapes lie in the oval window and are visible in the tissue section and microradiograph.

The promontory and round window niche are inferior to the oval window.

The jugular fossa lies further inferiorly surrounded by sublabyrinthine air cells.

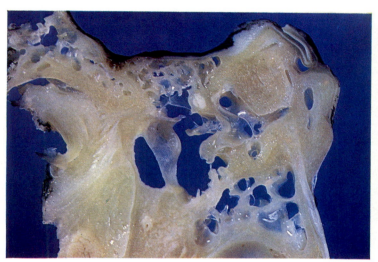

Fig. 2.25   Axial macrosection

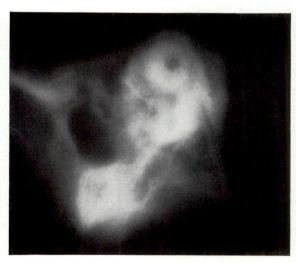

Fig. 2.26   Tomograph corresponding to Fig. 2.25

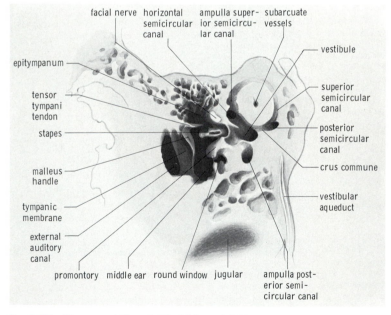

Fig. 2.27   Diagram of Figs. 2.25, 2.26, and 2.28

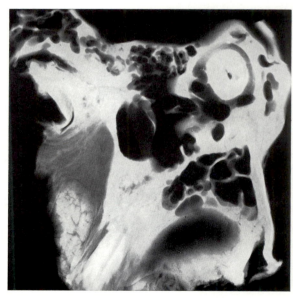

Fig. 2.28   Microradiograph of Fig. 2.25

These axial sections (Figs. 2.29–2.32) lie 7 mm anteromedial to Figures 2.25–2.28. The sections pass through the long axis of the modiolus and expose the three cochlear coils. The septum between the basal and middle coils is visible tomographically, but the modiolus is not sufficiently calcified to be seen. However, the modiolus is clearly seen by the soft x-ray technique of the microradiograph.

The lumen of the cochlear coils is sharply outlined by the surrounding dense cochlear capsule.

The internal carotid artery lies anterior, and the fundus of the internal auditory canal lies posterior to the cochlea. The eustachian portion of the middle ear and the tensor tympani canal lie above the carotid canal.

In the tissue section the cochlear nerve passes from the internal auditory canal into the base of the cochlea. Large air cells appear in the posterior portion of the pyramid. The jugular fossa forms the inferior margin of the pyramid.

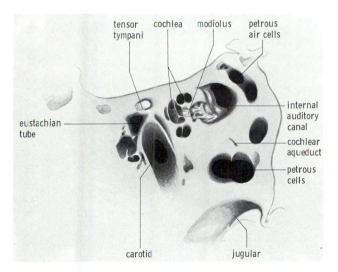

Fig. 2.**29**   Axial macrosection

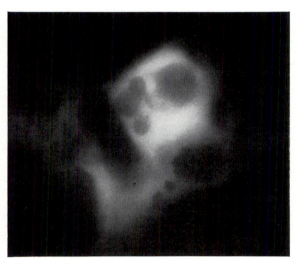

Fig. 2.**30**   Tomograph corresponding to Fig. 2.29

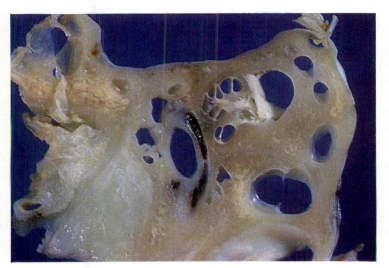

Fig. 2.**31**   Diagram of Figs. 2.29, 2.30, and 2.32

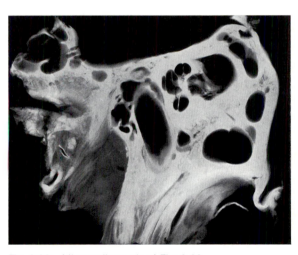

Fig. 2.**32**   Microradiograph of Fig. 2.29

Sagittal Projection

These sagittal sections (Figs. 2.33–2.36) cross the ear at the level of the epitympanum and the ossicles.

A strip of the tympanic membrane attached to the malleus handle separates the external from the middle ears.

A portion of the body of the incus articulates with the malleus head. The long process of the incus extends to the stapes head.

The tegmen of the epitympanum lies over the ossicles.

The anterior mallear ligament passes into the petrotympanic fissure above the anterior tympanic spine.

These sections expose the two limbs of the horizontal semicircular canal and the arch of the posterior semicircular canal. The facial nerve lies under the horizontal semicircular canal and above the stapedius muscle.

Petrous air cells surround the labyrinth. In the tissue section, the endolymphatic sac lies beneath the dura of the posterior surface of the pyramid.

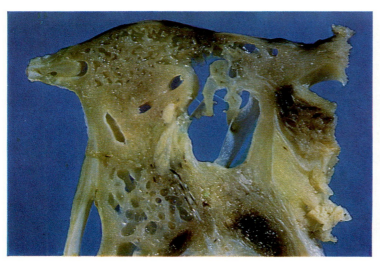

Fig. 2.**33**   Sagittal macrosection

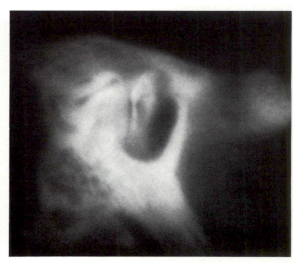

Fig. 2.**34**   Tomograph corresponding to Fig. 2.33

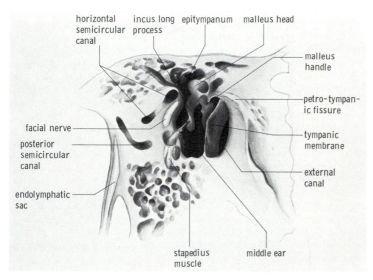

Fig. 2.**35**   Diagram of Figs. 2.33, 2.34, and 2.36

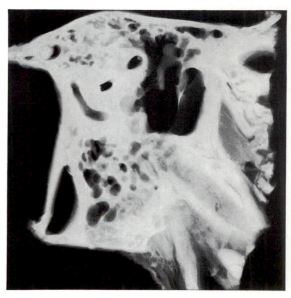

Fig. 2.**36**   Microradiograph of Fig. 2.33

These sagittal sections (Figs. 2.37–2.40) lie 12 mm medial to Figures 2.33–2.36, and cross the internal auditory canal.

The contour of the internal auditory canal is sharply defined except on the posterior aspect because the plane of the section approaches the medial end of the posterior canal wall. It is important to differentiate this normally decreased radiodensity from erosion by acoustic neuromas.

A small portion of the cochlea lies between the carotid and the internal auditory canals. The jugular fossa forms the inferior aspect of the pyramid.

In the tissue section and microradiograph the eustachian tube appears below the tensor tympani canal.

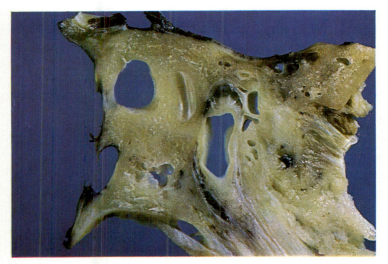

Fig. 2.**37**   Sagittal macrosection

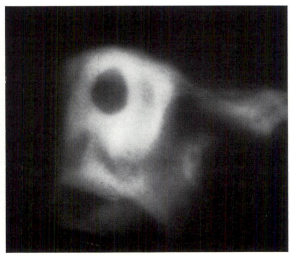

Fig. 2.**38**   Tomograph corresponding to Fig. 2.37

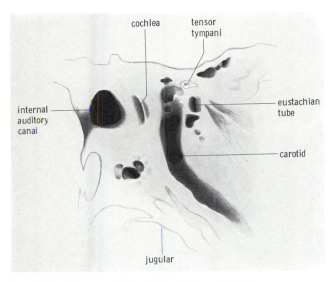

Fig. 2.**39**   Diagram of Figs. 2.37, 2.38, and 2.40

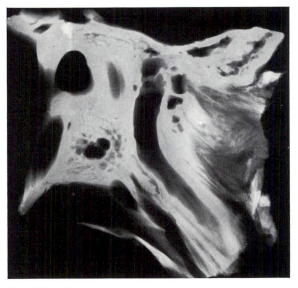

Fig. 2.**40**   Microradiograph of Fig. 2.37

Longitudinal Projection

These longitudinal sections (Figs. 2.41–2.44) cross the modiolus at right angles and expose the basal and middle cochlear coils.

The mastoid air cells and the posterior portion of the middle ear cavity appear laterally. The vertical portion of the facial nerve descends from the posterior genu below the horizontal semicircular canal toward the stylomastoid foramen.

These sections cross the anterior aspect of the vestibule and the ampullated ends of the horizontal and superior semicircular canals. A portion of the stapes footplate lies in the oval window. The round window niche appears in the tomogram below the oval window.

The petrous portion of the facial nerve lies superolateral to the cochlea, and the jugular fossa lies below the cochlea.

The carotid canal arches anteriorly.

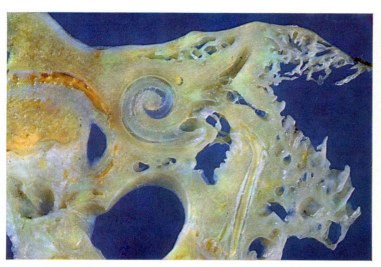

Fig. 2.**41**   Stenvers macrosection

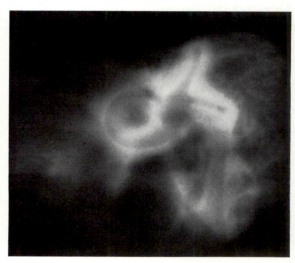

Fig. 2.**42**   Tomograph corresponding to Fig. 2.41

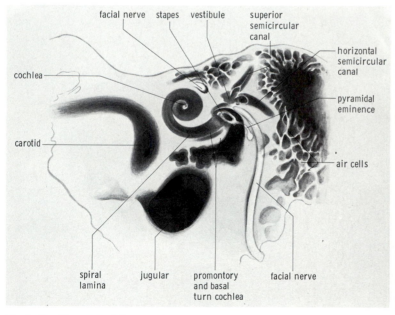

Fig. 2.**43**   Diagram of Figs. 2.41, 2.42, and 2.44

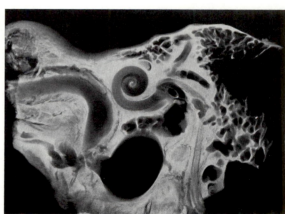

Fig. 2.**44**   Microradiograph of Fig. 2.41

These longitudinal sections (Figs. 2.45–2.48) lie 2 mm posterior to Figures 2.41–2.44. The mastoid air cells are lateral to the horizontal and superior semicircular canals. A thin segment of the basal turn of the cochlea lies below the fundus of the internal auditory meatus. The tympanic sinus lies lateral to the segment of the promontory.

In the tissue section and microradiograph the round window membrane closes the scala tympani in the round window niche.

The membranous utricle and saccule are in the vestibule. The facial and superior vestibular nerves lie above the crista falciformis while the cochlear and inferior vestibular nerves lie below. The jugular bulb forms the inferior margin of the pyramid.

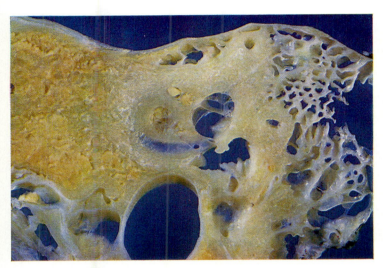

Fig. 2.**45**   Stenvers macrosection

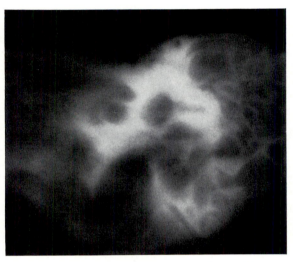

Fig. 2.**46**   Tomograph corresponding to Fig. 2.45

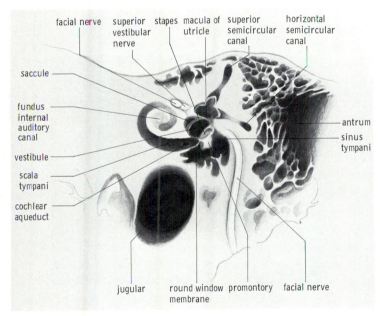

Fig. 2.**47**   Diagram of Figs. 2.45, 2.46, and 2.48

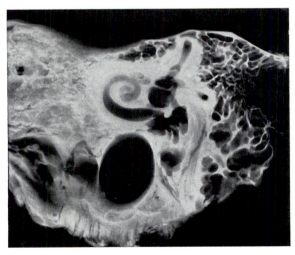

Fig. 2.**48**   Microradiograph of Fig. 2.45

Computerized Tomography of the Normal Temporal Bone

The following CT sections were obtained with a General Electric CT-T 8800 scanner. Sections 1.5 mm thick were obtained in the horizontal and coronal planes from normal ears of living patients. Once obtained the raw data from each image was processed and reconstructed with the new high resolution review program.

Each reconstructed image was matched with a corresponding microradiograph from a set of microradiographs which we obtained from cadaver temporal bone macrosections and used in our previous Atlas.*

* Valvassori, Galdino E., and Buckingham, Richard A.: Tomography and Cross Sections of the Ear. Georg Thieme, Stuttgart, 1975.

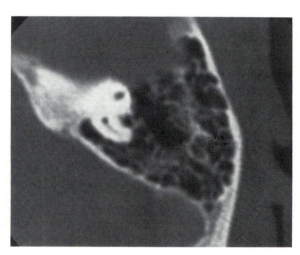

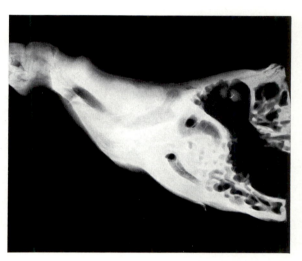

Figs. 2.**49** and 2.**50**   are a horizontal CT section and corresponding microradiograph at a level 4 mm below the arcuate eminence. The sections expose the mastoid and retrolabyrinthine air cells and the mastoid antrum. The section crosses the upper portion of the labyrinth and demonstrates the superior and posterior semicircular canals.

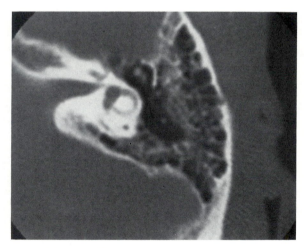

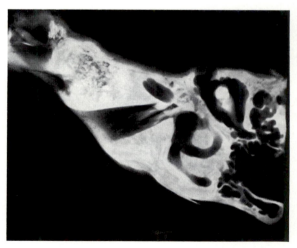

Figs. 2.**51** and 2.**52**   are horizontal CT and microradiograph sections 3 mm inferior to Figures 2.49 and 2.50. The sections show the ossicles in the epitympanum, the aditus and antrum, the vestibule, the horizontal semicircular canal, the posterior semicircular canal and the internal auditory canal. A portion of the basal coil of the cochlea and facial canal at the geniculate ganglion lie anterior to the fundus of the internal canal.

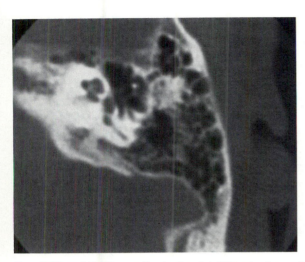

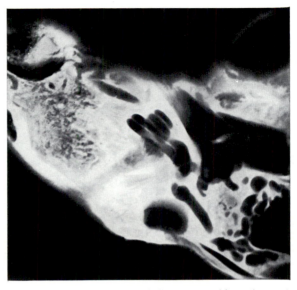

Figs. 2.**53** and 2.**54**   are the horizontal CT and microradiograph sections 5 mm inferior to Figures 2.51 and 2.52. These sections expose the middle ear cavity with the malleus handle, tensor tympani tendon, long process of the incus and incudostapedial joint.

The pyramidal eminence and sinus tympani form the posterior wall of the middle ear. The cochlea, inferior portion of the vestibule and posterior semicircular canal are seen in the labyrinth. The vestibular aqueduct enters the petrous pyramid on the posterior surface.

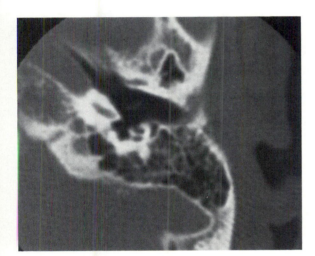

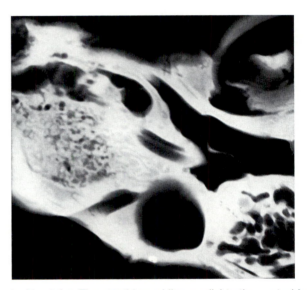

Figs. 2.**55** and 2.**56**   are horizontal CT and microradiograph sections 2 mm inferior to Figures 2.53 and 2.54. The sections show the external auditory canal, the malleus handle and the bony eus-

tachian tube. The carotid canal lies medial to the eustachian tube and anterior to the cochlea. The vertical facial nerve lies adjacent to the posterolateral wall of the middle ear.

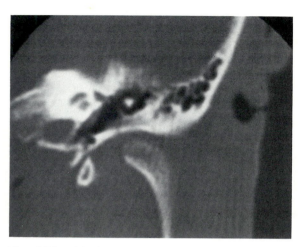

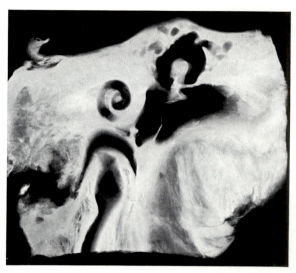

Figs. 2.**57** and 2.**58**   are coronal CT and microradiograph sections at the level of the anterior portion of the cochlea and facial canal at the geniculate ganglion. The malleus head lies in the epitympanum and the carotid canal under the cochlea.

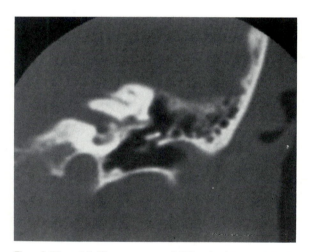

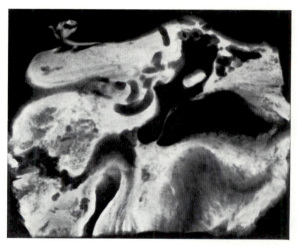

Figs. 2.**59** and 2.**60**   are coronal CT and microradiograph sections 3 mm posterior to Figures 2.57 and 2.58. At this level we see the external canal, the lateral epitympanic wall, and the ossicles. In the labyrinth the section exposes the anterior aspect of the vestibule the horizontal and superior semicircular canals, the basal turn of the cochlea and the internal auditory canal. The jugular fossa lies below the labyrinth.

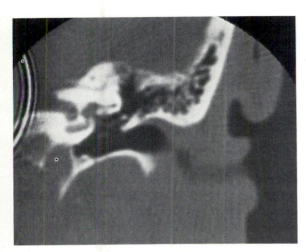

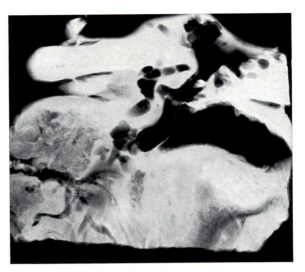

Figs. 2.**61** and 2.**62**   are coronal CT and microradiograph sections 2 mm posterior to Figures 2.59 and 2.60. In these sections the incudostapedial joint and oval window are exposed. The horizontal portion of the facial nerve canal lies under the horizontal semicircular canal.

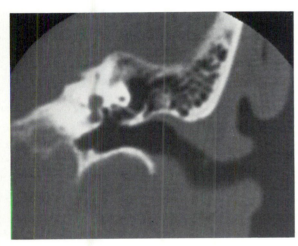

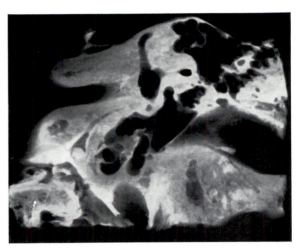

Figs. 2.**63** and 2.**64**   are coronal CT and microradiograph sections 2 mm posterior to Figures 2.61 and 2.62. The round window area and basal turn of the cochlea extend inferior to the vestibule. The facial canal lies under the horizontal semicircular canal. The posterior portion of the lateral epitympanic wall forms the lateral boundry of the aditus ad antrum. The full lenght of the external auditory canal is outlined.

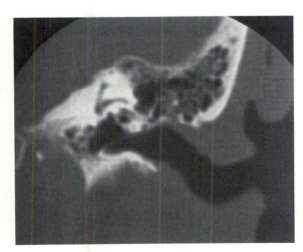

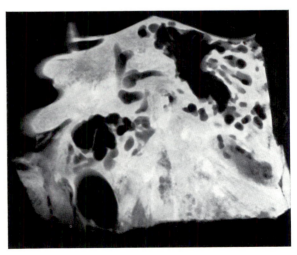

Figs. 2.**65** and 2.**66**   are coronal CT and microradiograph sections 2 mm posterior to Figures 2.63 and 2.64. These sections expose the ampulla of the posterior semicircular canal, the common crus, and the posterior limb of the horizontal semicircular canal. The cochlear aqueduct extends from the under surface of the pyramid to extend laterally in its course to the scala tympani.

Chapter 3   Congenital Abnormalities of the Temporal Bone

Tomography has permitted the accurate evaluation of large numbers of congenital deformities of the temporal bone, since the study can be made in the living patient. Prior to tomography, only a few post mortem specimens of congenital defects were available for study, and surgery was performed without the benefit of knowing the precise type and degree of anomaly present. Congenital malformations are hereditary and transmitted by genetic defects or acquired during fetal life. The severity and degree depend on the causative factor or factors and the age at which the fetus was affected.

Congenital malformations of the temporal bone may be divided into three groups:

1. Defects of the sound conducting apparatus which include the anomalies of the external auditory canal, the middle ear, the ossicles, and the labyrinthine windows.
2. Malformations of the cochleovestibular perceptive apparatus. These include anomalies of one or more structures of the inner ear.
3. Abnormalities of blood vessels and nerves. Included in these lesions are anomalies of the course and position of the carotid artery, the jugular bulb, and the facial nerve.

Radiographic Evaluation

In congenital anomalies of the ear, a radiographic assessment is essential. Otoscopy is of little value in atresia and aplasia of the external auditory canal, and audiometry is unreliable in young children. A proper radiographic study should demonstrate the status of the anatomical structures of the ear. Such information is of value for the otologist in determining the proper treatment for conductive and sensorineural hearing losses.

Conventional radiography is of limited value except for the evaluation of the degree and development of the pneumatization of the mastoid. In agenesis and atresia of the external auditory canal the dense atretic block obscures the middle ear in the Schüller and Owen projections and a tomographic examination should be performed. The tomographic study should include sagittal and coronal projections of both ears. Semiaxial sections are added to evaluate the labryrinthine windows, and horizontal sections are taken in cases of gross spatial distortion of the temporal bone.

In young, restless children sedation is often necessary to immobilize them during tomography.

A good tomographic study will provide the surgeon with the following basic information he needs in his decision about the feasibility of corrective surgery and in determining which type of surgery is indicated.

1. The degree and type of abnormality of the tympanic bone. These abnormalities may range from a relatively minor deformity to a complete agenesis of the external auditory canal.
2. The degree and position of the pneumatization of the mastoid air cells and mastoid antrum.
3. The position of the sigmoid sinus, the jugular bulb, and course of the carotid canal.
4. The development and aeration of the middle ear cavity.
5. The status of the ossicular chain, the size and shape of the ossicles and the presence of fusion or fixation.
6. The patency of the labryrinthine windows.
7. The development and course of the facial nerve.
8. The relationship of the meninges to the mastoid and superior petrous ridge. The middle cranial fossa often forms a deep groove lateral to the labyrinth which results in a low lying dura over the mastoid and epitympanum.
9. The degree of development and the morphology of the inner ear structures. Anomalies of the membranous labyrinth are not visible radiographically, but tomography will detect abnormalities of the bony labyrinthine structures.

We studied more than 400 cases of congenital ear defects. About 60% of these cases had deformities of the external auditory canal, middle ear, or both structures. Inner ear abnormalities accounted for 30% of the congenital defects, and the remaining 10% had mixed defects of the external, middle, and inner ears.

Embryology

A short review of the embryology of the ear should be helpful in understanding the radiographic changes seen in congenital malformations.

The Embryology of the Outer and Middle Ear

In the four-week-old human embryo three branchial arches separated by two branchial grooves appear. While the third arch and second groove disappear the first branchial groove deepens to become the primitive external auditory meatus. Simultaneously the first pharyngeal pouch evaginates, and for a short time comes in contact with the ectoderm of the first branchial groove. Mesenchyme soon grows between and separates these layers of ectoderm and endoderm.

At eight weeks of embryonic life a solid core of epithelial cells grows inward from the primitive external meatus towards the epithelium of the pharyngeal pouch. The thin seam of intervening connective tissue will become the fibrous layer of the definitive tympanic membrane, Figure 3.1.

This core of epithelial tissue from the ectoderm of the first groove remains solid until the seventh month of fetal life when the core of epithelial cells splits, beginning in its deepest portion, where it forms the epithelium of the tympanic membrane. The dissolution of this core of epithelium then proceeds externally to join the lumen of the primitive external meatus. By this time, the other structures of the outer, middle, and inner ear are well formed.

This sequence of embryologic events explains how in some cases of stenosis or atresia of the outer portion of the external canal, the middle ear and tympanic membrane may be well formed.

The first pharyngeal pouch becomes the eustachian tube and middle ear, while the cartilage of the first and second brachial arches form the malleus, incus and part of the stapes. The ossicles grow only during the first half of fetal life after which they ossify having attained full adult size, Figure 3.1.

The air cells of the temporal bone develop as outpouchings from the tympanum, epitympanum, antrum and eustachian tube. These outpouchings may appear in the thirty-four-week old fetus. When air enters the middle ear at birth, pneumatization occurs and cell development continues until early adult life unless arrested by inflammatory processes.

Inner Ear

In the three-week-old human embryo a plate-like ectodermal thickening occurs bilaterally near the hind brain. This is the otic placode which forms in a few days an otic pit. The pit becomes an otocyst by the fourth week. By seven weeks, the otocyst has formed three semicircular canals and by the eleventh week the cochlea, Figure 3.2. The primitive labyrinth enlarges until midterm when it reaches adult form and size. The endolymphatic duct and sac are the earliest appendages of the otic vessicle. They form at four and one half weeks of embryonic life when the otocyst divides into endolymphatic and utriculosaccular portions.

Throughout infancy and childhood the endolymphatic duct and sac continue to change and enlarge to accommodate themselves with the growth of the surrounding temporal bone.

Differentiation of the sensory cells of the semicircular canals, utricle and saccule occur by the eighth week, but development of sensory cells of the cochlea does not begin until the twelfth week and is not complete until after midterm.

By the eighth embryonic week the precartilage surrounding the otic membranous labyrinth changes into an outer zone of true cartilage to form the otic capsule, while the inner zone of precartilage vacuolizes to form the perilymphatic spaces. These spaces appear around the vestibule, the scala tympani and vestibuli and the semicircular canals and coalesce until a continuous perilymphatic space surrounds the entire membranous labyrinth.

Ossification of the otic capsule does not occur until the cartilage has attained maximum growth and maturity at midterm.

The endochondral layer of the bone of the otic capsule is formed from cartilage which is not removed and remodelled into periosteal haversian bone as in other bones of the body.

The first ossification center of the otic capsule appears around the cochlea in the sixteenth week of fetal life when the cochlea has reached adult size. Ossification of the fourteen centers is almost complete by the twenty-third week.

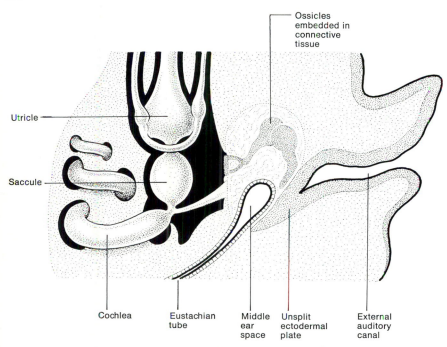

Fig. 3.**1**   Three-month old fetus showing development of middle and external ears. There is a solid core of epithelial cells extending toward the first pharyngeal pouch from the primitive external acoustic meatus. (From Shambaugh GE: *Surgery of the Ear.* 2nd ed. Saunders, Philadelphia and London 1967)

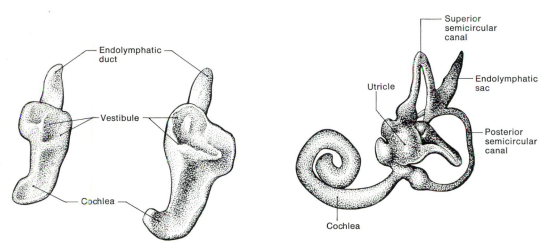

Fig. 3.**2**   Development of the membranous labyrinth during a three-week period a) Five weeks, b) six weeks, c) eight weeks. (From Anson BJ: Morris' Human Anatomy, 12th ed. McGraw-Hill, New York 1966)

Anomalies of the Sound Conducting System

Anomalies of the sound conduction system can affect the external auditory canal, the mastoid, the middle ear cavity, the ossicles, and the labyrinthine windows.

Anomalies of the Tympanic Bone

The degree and type of anomaly of the tympanic bone range from mild stenosis to complete agenesis of the external auditory canal, Figure 3.3–3.19.

Embryologically the definitive external auditory canals begin to form medially at the level of the tympanic membrane. An arrest in this developmental process may leave an atretic plate laterally which causes a complete external canal atresia.

Microtia

Microtia, or varying degrees of deformity of the auricle, is often associated with dysplasia of the external auditory canal. No direct relationship exists between the degree of severity of the auricular and external canal anomalies, though severe microtia is usually associated with severe agenesis of the canal.

In agenesis of the external auditory canal, often a small tissue tag and a small pit are present in place of the normal auricle and external canal.

These pits and tags usually have no topographic relationship to the mastoid and middle ear. To establish the position of the middle ear in relation to the vestigial remnant of the external ear we tape a radiopaque pellet over the pit. The tomogram will show the metallic marker and its relationship to the underlying structures. When the external auditory canal assumes a more verticale course than normal, tomography will reveal this malposition.

The origin of the external auditory canal from the first branchial groove and adjoining branchial arch explains the frequent association of abnormalities of other structures with the same derivation.Mandibular facial dysostoses, the Treacher-Collins and the Franceschetti syndromes frequently are associated with defects of the external canal and auricle.

In many cases of congenital agenesis of the external auditory canal, the temporomandibular joint is displaced posteriorly and lies lateral to the middle ear cavity. In these cases the mandibular condyle is usually hypoplastic and the temporomandibular fossa flat.

Mastoid Pneumatization

Radiography reveals the degree of pneumatization of the mastoid. Pneumatization can be completely absent Figs. 3.7–3.13, limited to a small mastoid antral cell, or be completely normal, Fig. 3.3.

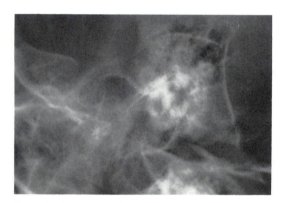

Fig. 3.**3**   Agenesis of external auditory canal, Schüller view, left. The mastoid air cells are well developed and aerated. The middle ear cavity is obscured by the atretic external canal.

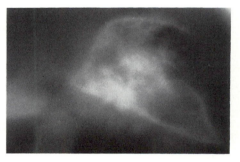

Fig. 3.**4**   Same ear as in Figs. 3.3, 3.5 and 3.6 lateral tomogram. A thick atretic plate closes the middle ear. The fused ossicular mass lies in the aerated epitympanum.

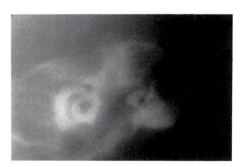

Fig. 3.**5**   Same ear as in Figs. 3.3, 3.4 and 3.6, coronal tomogram. A thick atretic plate closes the slightly hypoplastic, aerated middle ear. The ossicles are fused and fixed to the atretic plate.

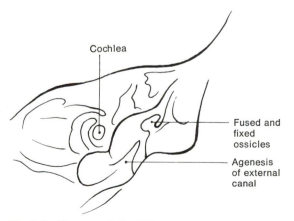

Fig. 3.**6**   Diagram of Fig. 3.5

Conventional Schüller and Owen views and lateral tomographic sections will determine the degree of pneumatization and the position of the sigmoid sinus in relation to the external canal, antrum, and middle ear, Fig. 3.3.

Frontal tomography is necessary to determine the relationship of the tegmental plate to the antrum and middle ear, Figs. 3.7–3.9. A low lying dura is common in congenital atresia as the middle cranial fossa deepens to form a groove lateral to the labyrinth.

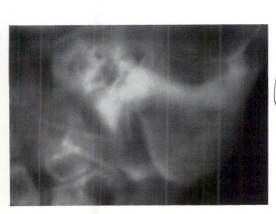

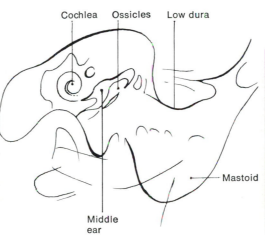

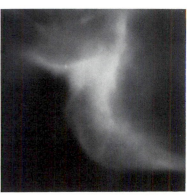

Fig. 3.7   Agenesis of external auditory canal and mastoid, coronal tomogram, left. The middle ear cavity is hypoplastic and the ossicles are fused and fixed. The dura lies well below the level of the epitympanum laterally.

Fig. 3.8   Diagram of Fig. 3.7

Fig. 3.9   Same ear as in Figs. 3.7 and 3.8, sagittal tomogram. The low lying dura forms a deep indentation on the superior surface of the temporal bone.

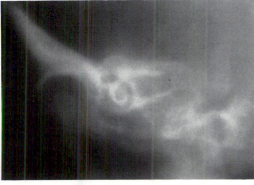

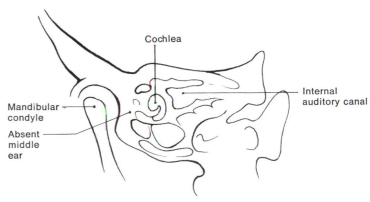

Fig. 3.10   Agenesis of external auditory canal, epitympanum, and mastoid, coronal tomogram, right. The temporomandibular joint lies lateral to the normal cochlea. There are no ossicles.

Fig. 3.11   Diagram of Fig. 3.10

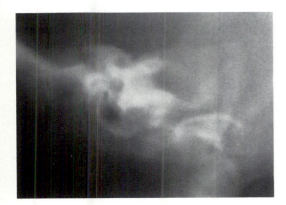

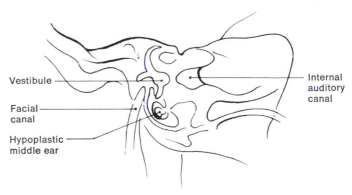

Fig. 3.12   Same ear as in Figs. 3.10, 3.11 and 3.13, coronal tomogram, 6 mm posterior to Fig. 3.10. There is a small inferior middle ear space. The vertical segment of the facial nerve canal is shortened and lies on the lateral surface of the temporal bone.

Fig. 3.13   Diagram of Fig. 3.12

Anomalies of the Middle Ear

The degree of development and aeration of the middle ear is determined by coronal and semiaxial tomographic sections.

The malformations of the middle ear vary from minor hypoplasia, Figs. 3.5–3.6 to almost complete agenesis, Figs. 3.10–3.15. In the majority of cases associated with atresia there is hypoplasia of the hypotympanum while the epitympanic area is well developed. Although hypoplastic, the middle ear is usually well aerated.

Anomalies of the Incus and Malleus

Anomalies of the incus and malleus occur in varying degrees. Coronal and sagittal sections expose these anomalies best. In cases of agenesis of the external auditory canal but relatively normal middle ear development, the malleus and incus are usually well formed. These ossicles are, however, fused together and fixed to the atretic bony plate at the level of the neck of the malleus, Figs. 3.4–3.6.

In these cases the long process of the incus is normal. If the atretic plate lies lateral to the level of the tympanic membrane, the ossicular chain may be entirely normal.

When the middle ear cavity is hypoplastic, the malleus and incus exist as an amalgum of amorphous bone, and the long process of the incus is shortened or absent, Figs. 3.14–3.19.

In severe cases the middle ear may be extremely hypoplastic, and only a rudimentary ossicular mass is present in an ectopic position, Figs. 3.10–3.11.

A congenital anomaly may be confined to the ossicular chain. The external auditory canal, the middle ear, and the ossicles are well formed, but the malleus or incus are fused to the epitympanic wall. The malleus is more commonly fixed than the incus, Figs. 3.20–3.21.

Tomography will demonstrate such an isolated fixation if there is ossified bone between the ossicle and the epitympanic wall or tegmen. In ears with a very low lying tegmental plate, it is difficult to determine the presence of fixation, since the space between the ossicle and the tegmen is very narrow.

Anomalies of the Labyrinthine Windows

Anomalies of the labyrinthine window and the stapes may be the only defect in the middle ear, or such lesions may be associated with other anomalies of the ossicles, the middle ear and the external auditory canal. Stapes and oval window defects are more common than abnormalities of the round window.

In well developed and well aerated middle ear cavities, semiaxial and coronal tomographic sections will detect defects of the stapes superstructure. The most common stapes anomaly diagnosed tomographically is a single, thick monopolar stapes crus.

Congenital fixation of the stapes footplate is a fairly common isolated defect, but tomography can define such a lesion only if the footplate is abnormally thickened and calcified. Tomographically, congenital fixation of the stapes footplate resembles stapedial otosclerosis, Figs. 3.22–3.23.

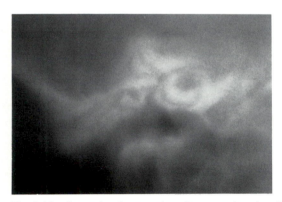

Fig. 3.**14**   Stenosis of external auditory canal and malformation of ossicular chain, coronal tomogram, right. The deformed ossicles lie in the hypoplastic epitympanum. The dysplastic tympanic bone narrows the external canal superiorly. The external canal slopes downward.

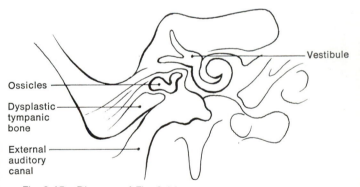

Fig. 3.**15**   Diagram of Fig. 3.14

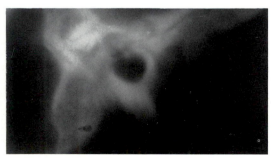

Fig. 3.**16**   Same ear as in Figs. 3.14, 3.15 and 3.17, sagittal tomogram. The grossly deformed ossicles are fixed in the narrow epitympanum.

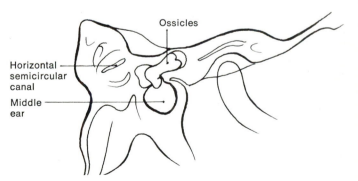

Fig. 3.**17**   Diagram of Fig. 3.16

Anomalies of the Facial Nerve

The course of the facial nerve is affected by the abnormal development of the middle ear, the mastoid, and the external auditory canal. Lateral and anterior displacement of the descending portion of the facial nerve canal is common in atresia of the external auditory canal,

Figs. 3.12–3.13. In cases of atresia and middle ear cavity hypoplasia the tympanic segment of the facial nerve may be shortened and the vertical segment may be grossly ectopic and take an almost horizontal course laterally. Further discussion of facial nerve anomalies are included in Chapter 12.

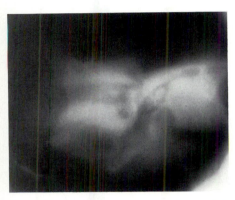

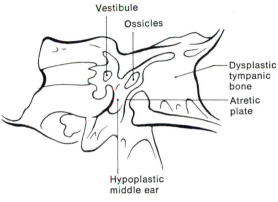

Fig. 3.18   Atresia of external auditory canal and hypoplasia of middle ear cavity, semiaxial tomogram, left. The narrow, deformed external auditory canal is closed medially by a bony atretic plate. The tympanic cavity is hypoplastic, and the deformed ossicles lie in the narrow epitympanum.

Fig. 3.19   Diagram of Fig. 3.18

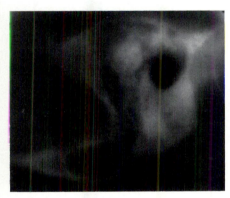

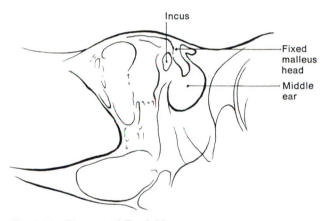

Fig. 3.20   Fixation of malleus, sagittal tomogram, right. The head of the malleus is fixed to the tegmen by a thick bony bar.

Fig. 3.21   Diagram of Fig. 3.20

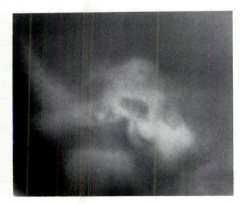

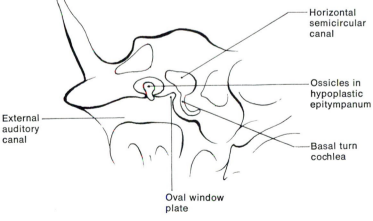

Fig. 3.22   Closure of oval window, semiaxial tomogram, right. A thick bony plate closes the oval window. Stapes superstructure and long process of incus are absent. The epitympanum is hypoplastic, and the horizontal semicircular canal short and dilated.

Fig. 3.23   Diagram of Fig. 3.22

Anomalies of the Inner Ear

Most cases of congenital sensorineural deafness are caused by abnormal development of the membranous labyrinth. These lesions are not detectible by radiography.

Defects in the otic capsule are visible radiographically. Anomalies of the otic capsule may involve a single structure or the entire capsule.

With recent advances in surgical procedures for profound sensorineural deafness, tomography of the labyrinth is indicated for: 1. diagnosis of the status of the otic capsule; 2. detection of cases possibly suitable for surgery of the endolymphatic sac or other inner ear structures and; 3. selection of possible candidates for cochlear implants.

The most severe anomaly of the otic capsule is the Michel type of deformity which is characterized by a hypoplastic petrous pyramid and an almost complete lack of development of the inner ear structures. There is often a single labyrinthine cavity of varying size which occupies the space normally taken by the vestible, cochlea and semicircular canals, Figs. 3.24–3.29. When facial nerve function is normal, the internal auditory canal is present but the lumen of the canal is narrowed to the size of the facial nerve. The external auditory canal and middle ear cavity are usually normal, but appear abnormally large in comparison with the small labyrinthine vestiges. The Michel deformity is usually bilateral. We have found this deformity associated with the Klippel-Feil anomaly in several cases.

A less severe deformity of the labyrinthine capsule is the Mondini type which is characterized by an abnormal development of the cochlea and often is associated with an abnormality of the vestibular aqueduct, the vestibule and the semicircular canals. The cochlea may be hypoplastic or of normal size, but the bony partition between the cochlear coils is hypoplastic or absent, which gives the tomographic appearance of an "empty cochlea", Figs. 3.30–3.31. The vestibular aqueduct is often shortened and dilated, Figs. 3.34–3.35. The vestibule appears larger and the contour more globular than normal. There is often dilatation of the ampullated ends of the horizontal and superior semicircular canals, Figs. 3.32–3.33. The Modini deformity may be unilateral or bilateral.

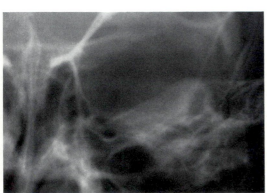

Fig. 3.**24** Michel anomaly, transorbital view, left. A single labyrinthine cavity lies in a hypoplastic petrous pyramid.

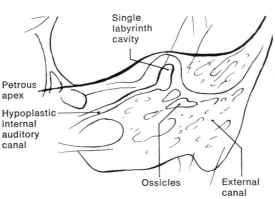

Fig. 3.**25** Diagram of Figs. 3.24 and 3.26

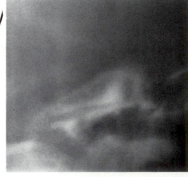

Fig. 3.**26** Same ear as in Figs. 3.24 and 3.25, coronal tomogram. The hypoplastic internal auditory canal passes inferior to the anomalous labyrinthine cavity. Middle ear and external canal are normal.

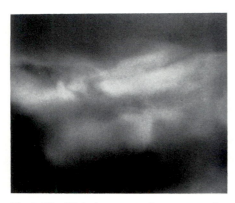

Fig. 3.**27** Michel anomaly, coronal tomogram, right. There is no cochlea. External canal and middle ear are normal.

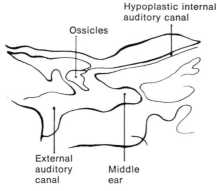

Fig. 3.**28** Diagram of Figs. 3.27 and 3.29

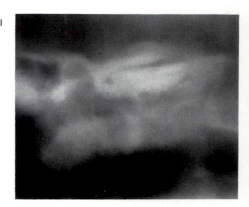

Fig. 3.**29** Same ear as in Figs. 3.27 and 3.28, 4 mm posterior, coronal tomogram. A minute cavity represents the remnant of the labyrinth. The internal auditory canal is hypoplastic.

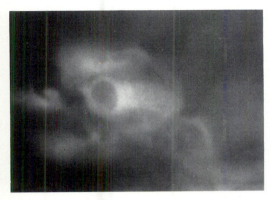

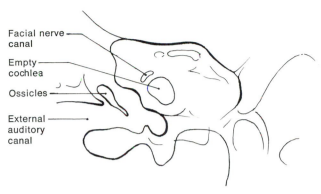

Fig. 3.**30**   Mondini anomaly, coronal tomogram, right. There is an "empty cochlea" due to absence of the bony partition between the cochlear coils.

Fig. 3.**31**   Diagram of Fig. 3.30

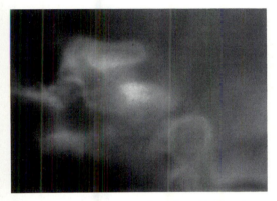

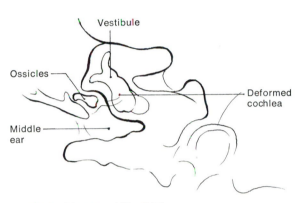

Fig. 3.**32**   Same ear as in Figs. 3.30, 3.31 and 3.33, 4 mm posterior, coronal tomogram, right. The deformed cochlea lies below the dilated vestibule. The superior and horizontal semicircular canals are enlarged.

Fig. 3.**33**   Diagram of Fig. 3.32

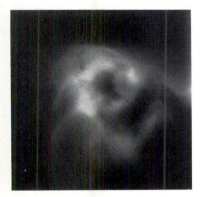

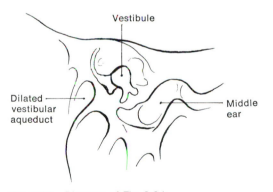

Fig. 3.**34**   Mondini anomaly, sagittal tomogram, right. The vestibular aqueduct is grossly dilated.

Fig. 3.**35**   Diagram of Fig. 3.34

Vestibular Aqueduct and Semicircular Canals

A dilated and shortened vestibular aqueduct, similar in tomographic appearance to that of the Mondini deformity, is occasionally present without other radiographically visualized abnormalities, Figs. 3.34–3.35. To diagnose dilatation of the vestibular aqueduct we measure the aqueduct at its midpoint between the outer aperture and the common crus. An aqueduct is abnormally dilated when the anteroposterior diameter at the midpoint of the postisthmic segment measures more than 1.5 mm.

The horizontal semicircular canal is often congenitally deformed. This anomaly may be isolated or associated with other malformations of the bony labyrinth. The horizontal canal may be shortened and dilated or, in more severe defects, exist merely as a lateral outpouching of the vestibule. In these cases there is absence of the bony core around which the canal normally loops. An isolated anomaly of the horizontal canal may occur with normal cochlear and vestibular function.

Hypoplasia or aplasia of the vestibule and semicircular canals can be present with or without other inner ear anomalies. This condition often occurs in association with the Waardenburg syndrome, Figs. 3.36–3.39.

Anomalies of the Internal Auditory Canal

The most common anomaly of the internal auditory canal is an hypoplasia of the canal. The hypoplasia can be isolated or be associated with other anomalies, Figs. 3.29, 3.38, 3.39.

Rarely the canal is abnormally dilated and shortened. A dilated and shortened internal canal at times is associated with chronic hydrocephalus. In these cases the dilatation is secondary to increased intracranial pressure and is not a congenital defect.

Anomalies of the Cochlear Aqueduct

In about 20% of the ears with congenital anomalies of the otic capsule, the cochlear aqueduct is abnormally dilated. A dilated cochlear aqueduct occurs occasionally as an isolated defect, Figs. 3.40–3.41.

Isolated dilation of the aqueduct can cause a "labyrinth gusher" of cerebrospinal fluid which sometimes occurs during stapedectomy for otosclerosis or congenital footplate fixation.

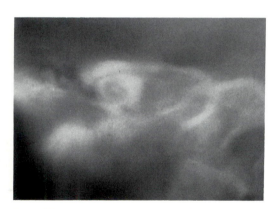

Fig. 3.**36** Multiple anomalies of labyrinth, Waardenburg syndrome, coronal tomogram, right. The cochlea is hypoplastic and the bony partition between the coils is incomplete.

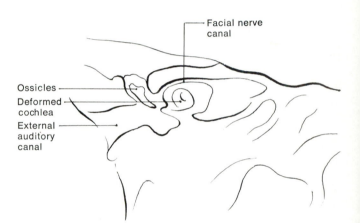

Fig. 3.**37** Diagram of Fig. 3.36

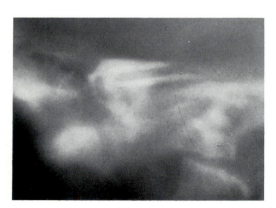

Fig. 3.**38** Same ear as in Figs. 3.36, 3.37 and 3.39, 4 mm posterior, coronal tomogram. The vestibule is rudimentary and the semicircular canals are absent. The internal auditory canal is hypoplastic.

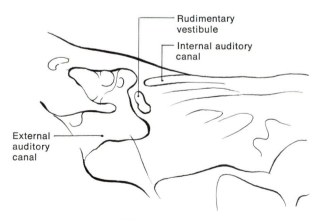

Fig. 3.**39** Diagram of Fig. 3.38

Congenital Obliterative Labyrinthitis

A lesion acquired late in fetal life may cause bony obliteration of the lumen of one or more of the inner ear structures which are already well formed, Figs. 3.42–3.45. This type of obliteration cannot be differentiated radiographically from obliterative labyrinthitis secondary to postnatal infections.

Congenital Cerebrospinal Fluid Otorrhea

Congenital cerebrospinal fluid otorrhea occurs rarely and often causes repeated bouts of meningitis. The etiology is varied. In some instances, a defect in the tegmen and dura result in cerebrospinal fluid leaks. More rarely the otorrhea is the result of defects at the fundus of the internal auditory canal and in the stapes footplate with

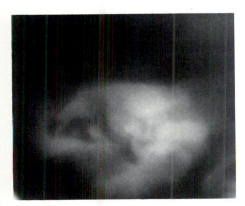

Fig. 3.40   Dilated cochlear aqueduct, semiaxial tomogram, right. The cochlear aqueduct is abnormally dilated throughout the course.

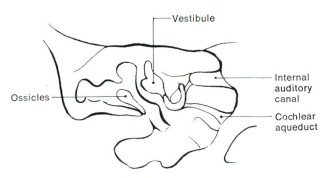

Fig. 3.41   Diagram of Fig. 3.40

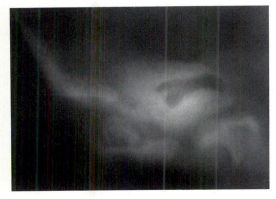

Fig. 3.42   Obliterative labyrinthitis, coronal tomogram, right. The lumen of the labyrinth is obliterated. There is a bony mass in the middle ear, and another bony mass obstructs the external auditory canal.

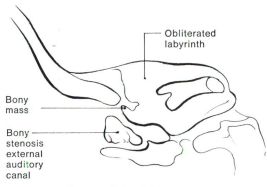

Fig. 3.43   Diagram of Fig. 3.42

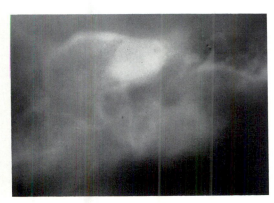

Fig. 3.44   Obliterative labyrinthitis, coronal tomogram, left. The lumen of the cochlea is completely obliterated, the external canal and middle ear are normal.

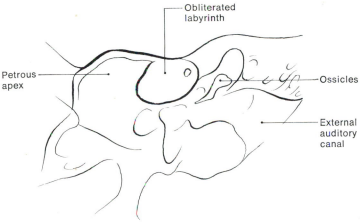

Fig. 3.45   Diagram of Fig. 3.44

consequent communication between the subarachnoid space and the middle ear via the internal auditory canal and the vestibule. These patients are profoundly deaf.

Congenital Vascular Anomalies

Various radiographic techniques visualize anomalies of the jugular vein and the carotid artery as these structures course through the temporal bone.

Jugular Vein

There is a tremendous variation in the size of the jugular vein and bulb. These variations occur not only from patient to patient but from one side to the other in the same patient. The size of the jugular fossa is not a criterion of a pathologic process.

A normal jugular fossa may produce only a slight indentation on the undersurface of the petrous bone or extend upwards as high as the superior petrous ridge posterior to the labyrinth and the internal auditory canal, Figs. 3.46–3.49. In these instances the jugular bulb projects so high that the vein blocks access to the internal auditory canal by the translabyrinthine route.

The jugular bulb at times projects into the hypo- or mesotympanum. There may be a bony cover over the jugular bulb, Figs. 3.50–3.51, or the vein may lie exposed in the middle ear in contact with the medial surface of the tympanic membrane. In these cases such a high jugular bulb can be misdiagnosed as a glomus tumor.

There are three variations of high jugular bulbs projecting into the mesotympanum, which the radiologist should differentiate from pathological conditions.

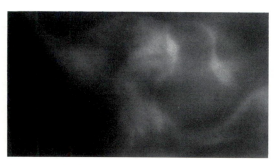

Fig. 3.**46**   High jugular fossa, coronal tomogram, right. The jugular bulb extends to the superior petrous ridge posterior to the internal auditory canal.

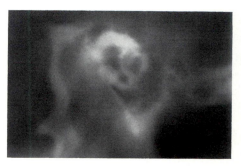

Fig. 3.**47**   High jugular fossa, sagittal tomogram, right. The jugular bulb reaches the superior petrous ridge posterior to the labyrinth.

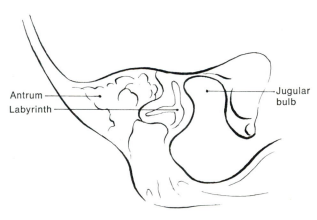

Fig. 3.**48**   Diagram of Fig. 3.46

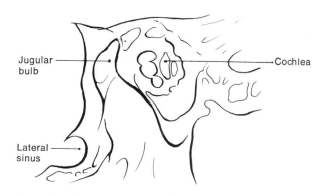

Fig. 3.**49**   Diagram of Fig. 3.47

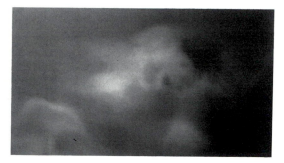

Fig. 3.**50**   High jugular bulb, coronal tomogram, left. The jugular bulb covered by a thin bony shell projects into the mesotympanum.

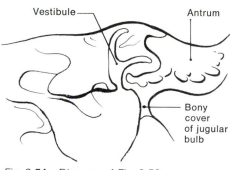

Fig. 3.**51**   Diagram of Fig. 3.50

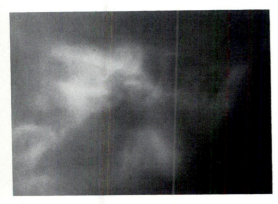

Fig. 3.**52** High jugular bulb, coronal tomogram, left. There is a large defect in the hypotympanic floor through which the jugular bulb herniates into the middle ear.

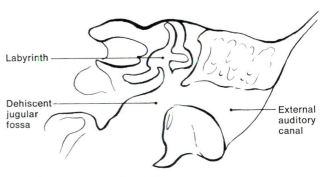

Fig. 3.**53**   Diagram of Fig. 3.52

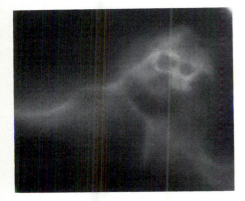

Fig. 3.**54** High jugular bulb, sagittal tomogram, left. Same ear as in Figs. 3.52 and 3.53. The jugular bulb protrudes into the posteroinferior quadrant of the middle ear.

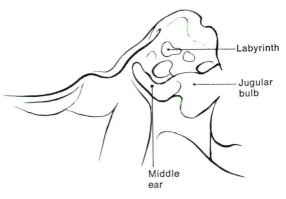

Fig. 3.**55**   Diagram of Fig. 3.54

1. The jugular fossa and bulb are high and a soft tissue mass protrudes into the middle ear but is covered by a thin bony shell, Figs. 3.50–3.51.
2. The jugular fossa and bulb are high, but there is an incomplete bony shell surrounding the soft tissue mass which protrudes into the middle ear, Figs. 3.52–3.55.
3. The jugular fossa is not high but there is a large defect in the dome of the fossa. The jugular bulb herniates into the middle ear where it appears as a soft tissue mass. This variation may be confused with a glomus tumor but for the fact that the contour of the jugular fossa is normal except for the defect. In the few cases where the diagnosis is in doubt, retrograde jugular venography will resolve the question. Jugular venography will show a normal jugular vein projecting into the middle ear to the level of the soft tissue mass appearing in the tomographs, Fig. 3.56.

Ectopic Carotid Artery

Minor variations in the intratemporal course of the internal carotid artery are not uncommon but are of no clinical significance.
The carotid artery may take an ectopic course through the middle ear. This anomaly is rare but is of clinical importance. If surgery is contemplated the otologic surgeon should be aware of the abnormal position of the

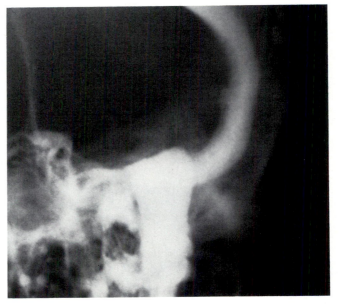

Fig. 3.**56** Retrograde jugular venogram, left. The jugular bulb protrudes into the middle ear to the level of the vestibule.

artery in his surgical field. This lesion also may be misdiagnosed as a glomus or other type of middle ear tumor. We have recognized eight cases of this rare vascular anomaly. All were confirmed by angiographic studies.

Microscopic otoscopy shows a pinkish or white-blue mass lying in the inferior mesotympanum in contact with the medial surface of the tympanic membrane. The mass may or may not pulsate.

The tomographic findings of an ectopic intratemporal carotid artery are:

1. There is a soft tissue mass extending throughout the entire length of the inferior portion of the middle ear cavity, Figs. 3.57, 3.61, 3.63.
2. There may be a thin bony wall partially surrounding the artery.
3. Contact of the mass with the tympanic membrane causes lateral bulging of the membrane. Medially the mass may cause indentation of the promontory, Figs. 3.61–3.63.
4. The arterial tissue mass may encroach on the incudostapedial joint and cause conductive deafness.
5. The normal proximal portion of the carotid canal is absent. The normal canal is always clearly visible below the cochlea in coronal and semiaxial sections, Figs. 3.57–3.58.
6. The anomalous carotid artery enters the temporal bone through a canal or dehiscent area in the floor of the posterior portion of the hypotympanum between the jugular fossa medially and the vertical portion of the facial canal laterally, Figs. 3.59–3.60.

Only arteriography can confirm the tomographic findings. The arteriographic findings are, Figs. 3.64–3.67:

1. There is narrowing or tapering of the internal carotid artery at the site where the artery enters the base of the skull;
2. The proximal ectopic arterial segment lies at least 1 cm more laterally and posteriorly than normal. In the coronal plane this arterial segment lies lateral rather than medial to the vertical plane which passes through the vestibule;
3. The proximal anomalous carotid artery segment follows a straight vertical course while the proximal segment of a normal internal carotid artery curves gently medially and anteriorly;
4. The anomalous carotid artery makes a sharp 90° turn into the middle ear cavity. The artery then runs anteriorly throughout the middle ear and exits inferior to the cochlear apex where it usually regains the normal course in the petrous pyramid.

In these cases of ectopic internal carotid artery the jugular venogram is normal.

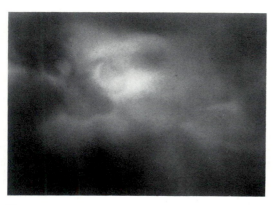

Fig. 3.**57** Ectopic carotid artery, coronal tomogram, right. The proximal portion of the carotid canal normally seen under the cochlea is absent. The ectopic artery causes a soft tissue density in the lower middle ear.

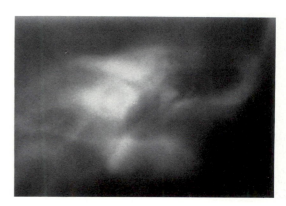

Fig. 3.**58** Corresponding tomogram of normal left ear of Fig. 3.57 for comparison

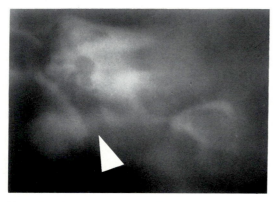

Fig. 3.**59** Same ear as in Fig. 3.57, 4 mm posterior, coronal tomogram. The ectopic artery enters the middle ear through a canal in the floor of the posterior hypotympanum.

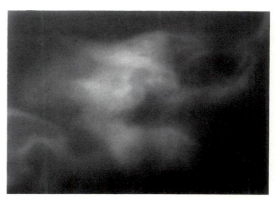

Fig. 3.**60** Corresponding tomogram of normal left ear of Fig. 3.59 for comparison

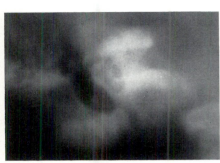

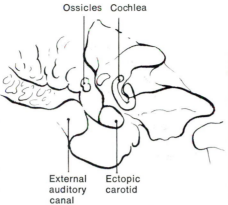

Ossicles Cochlea

External   Ectopic
auditory   carotid
canal

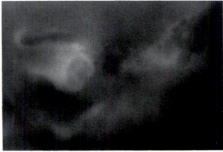

Fig. 3.**61** Ectopic carotid artery, semiaxial tomogram, right. The ectopic artery appears as a soft tissue mass in the lower middle ear and causes a concavity on the promontory.

Fig. 3.**62** Diagram of Fig. 3.61

Fig. 3.**63** Ectopic carotid artery, semiaxial tomogram, left. The findings are similar to those in Fig. 3.61 and 3.62.

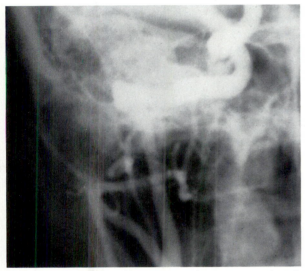

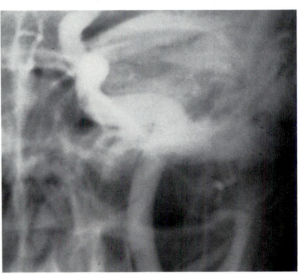

Fig. 3.**64** Ectopic carotid artery, arteriogram, coronal projection, right, same ear as in Figs. 3.57, 3.59, 3.61, 3.62 and 3.66. The narrow proximal internal carotid artery enters the middle ear and courses lateral to the vestibular plane.

Fig. 3.**65** Corresponding arteriogram of normal left carotid for comparison

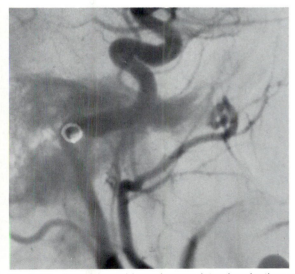

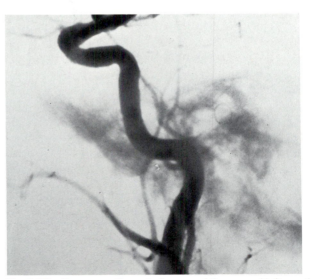

Fig. 3.**66** Ectopic carotid arteriogram, lateral projection, with subtraction. Same ear as in Figs. 3.57, 3.59, 3.61, 3.62 and 3.64. The ectopic carotid enters the posterior middle ear and makes a 90° turn anteriorly. The marker corresponds to the region of the vestibule.

Fig. 3.**67** Corresponding arteriogram of the normal left carotid for comparison

Chapter 4   Temporal Bone Trauma

Radiographic studies of the temporal bone following head trauma are indicated when there is cerebrospinal fluid otorrhea or rhinorrhea, hearing loss, or facial nerve paralysis.

Demonstration of temporal bone fractures is important for therapeutic and medicolegal reasons.

In fractures of the base of the skull, the temporal bone is usually involved. The temporal bone can also be affected by fractures of the calvarium which extend into the skull base.

Temporal bone fractures are difficult to visualize radiographically. Conventional radiography is helpful in demonstrating fractures of the temporal squama and mastoid. When fractures involve the middle ear and petrous pyramid, tomography is indispensible in demonstrating the extent of the lesion.

In acute head trauma with unconsciousness or neurologic findings a CT should be performed as the first radiologic examination to rule out the possibility of intracranial hemorrhage. This examination, if performed with the later generation of scanners, will also demonstrate any temporal bone fractures.

Classification

Temporal bone fractures are divided into longitudinal and transverse lesions depending on the direction of the fracture line. Longitudinal fractures occur more frequently than transverse fractures in a ratio of 5:1. Classification of temporal bone fractures into longitudinal and transverse types is somewhat arbitrary, since most fractures follow a serpiginous tract into the temporal bone.

Localized fractures of the mastoid and external canal are the result of direct trauma. An isolated fracture of the anterior wall of the external canal may result from indirect trauma from a blow to the mandible.

The typical longitudinal fracture involves the temporal squama and extends into the mastoid. The fracture usually reaches the external auditory canal and passes medially into the epitympanum. Medial extension into the petrosa from the epitympanum may occur, and the fracture line pursue an intra-or extralabyrinthine course.

An intralabyrinthine course of the fracture is rare since the labyrinthine bone is relatively resistant to trauma. Extralabyrinthine extension of a longitudinal fracture occurs either anterior or posterior to the labyrinth, though anterior extension is more common.

A transverse fracture of the temporal bone typically crosses the petrous pyramid at right angles to the longitudinal axis of the pyramid. The fracture line usually follows the line of least resistance and runs from the dome of the jugular fossa through the labyrinth to the superior petrous ridge.

Clinical Findings

Clinical findings depend on the type of fracture. Hemotympanum and bleeding from the ear occur when the external auditory canal or tympanic membrane are involved.

When the tegmen is involved and the tegmental dura is torn, cerebrospinal fluid otorrhea occurs if the tympanic membrane is also ruptured. If the tympanic membrane is intact, the cerebrospinal fluid will flow into the eustachian tube and a cerebrospinal rhinorrhea will result.

When the fracture line crosses the epitympanum, there usually is disruption of the ossicular chain with a conductive deafness. Conductive deafness also occurs following displaced fractures of the anterior external canal wall and consequent canal stenosis. When the fracture line extends into the labyrinth a total sensorineural deafness and vestibular paralysis occur. When the fracture runs into the petrous pyramid adjacent to but not involving the labyrinth, partial sensorineural deafness or vestibular paresis often result from labyrinthine concussion. In a longitudinal fracture with extralabyrinthine extension into the petrous pyramid mixed hearing loss can result from simultaneous ossicular disruption and labyrinthine concussion.

Facial paralysis occurs immediately or after a period of a few hours or days following trauma.

Immediate onset of facial paralysis is the result of bisection of the nerve by the fracture. Delayed facial paralysis is due to fracture of the facial canal and post-traumatic edema of the nerve.

Radiographic Technique

Fractures with wide separation and displacement of the fragments are easily visualized radiographically. Microfractures and fractures with minimal separation and displacement can only be recognized if the radiographic plane passes at right angles to the plane of the fracture. For this reason, the radiographic projections vary for longitudinal and transverse fractures, and multiple conventional and tomographic projections are needed to demonstrate the contour of a serpiginous fracture.

The radiographic evaluation of a temporal bone fracture should begin with conventional views including the Schüller, Towne-Chamberlain, Stenvers, and basal views. When a fracture line is detected in the temporal squama on the Schüller view and extends into the pyramid the fracture will be of the longitudinal type, Fig. 4.1. If a fracture line is seen in the occipital bone in the Towne-Chamberlain or Stenvers projection, pyramidal extension of the fracture will be of the transverse type, Fig. 4.18.

Tomography

Tomography permits precise evaluation of the course of fractures into the middle ear and petrous bone. This technique will show displacement and disruption of the ossicular chain, the site of facial nerve lesions and tegmental injuries.

In longitudinal fractures, the most revealing projections are the lateral and axial views of the petrous pyramid, since the plane of the fracture will lie at right angles to the tomographic sections, Fig. 4.2–4.3.

Coronal and Stenvers projections are required for demonstrating transverse fractures.

Horizontal sections are useful in both longitudinal and transverse fractures.

A fracture line may disappear at a certain level only to reappear a few millimeters distant. This apparent gap is not due to interruption of the fracture but rather to the fact that the plane of the fracture line changes course and becomes invisible in some of the tomographic sections.

In those cases where conventional radiography fails to show a fracture but clinical findings indicate a disruption of middle or inner function, multiple tomographic projections are required to demonstrate the lesion. Four tomographic projections, approximately 45° apart are used to screen the petrous pyramid. These projections are coronal, axial, sagittal, and Stenvers. A horizontal series may be indicated if the four vertical projections fail to demonstrate a lesion.

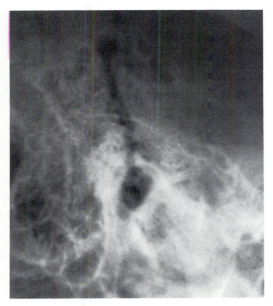

Fig. 4.1   Longitudinal fracture, Schüller view, right. A wide fracture line extends from the temporal squama through the mastoid to the posterosuperior wall of the external auditory canal.

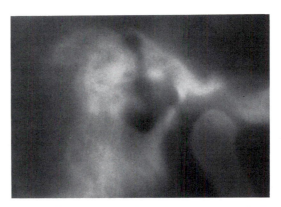

Fig. 4.2   Same ear as in Figs. 4.1 and 4.3, sagittal tomogram. The fracture extends from the tegmen to the anterosuperior portion of the external canal and passes anterior to the horizontal semicircular canal.

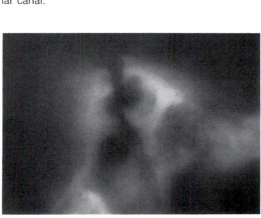

Fig. 4.3   Same ear as in Figs. 4.1 and 4.2, sagittal tomogram. The fracture follows an intralabyrinthine course and splits the internal auditory canal. ▶

Radiographic Findings in Longitudinal Fractures

Longitudinal fractures of the temporal bone involve the mastoid and extend from the floor of the middle cranial fossa and tegmen downward and often forward to the posterosuperior wall of the external auditory canal, Fig. 4.8. There often is an extension of the fracture to the anterior wall of the external auditory canal and temporomandibular fossa, Figs. 4.2, 4.4, 4.5, 4.11.

A fracture of the posterior wall of the external auditory canal may extend medially to the facial nerve canal at or distal to the pyramidal turn of the nerve with a resultant facial paralysis, Figs. 4.9, 4.10, 4.12, 4.13.

Medial extension of a longitudinal fracture into the epitympanum results in a disruption of the ossicular chain, a tegmental fracture, and often a cerebrospinal otorrhea, Figs. 4.4–4.13.

We have observed luxation of the incus where the short process was propelled into the facial canal and paralyzed the facial nerve distal to the pyramidal turn.

A longitudinal fracture may extend into the petrous pyramid through the labyrinth, Figs. 4.2–4.3, but more commonly anterior to the labyrinth. Anterior petrous extension occasionally causes a lesion of the facial nerve and canal at the superficial geniculate ganglion area. Our data show that in longitudinal fractures the facial nerve is most commonly injured at the geniculate ganglion area, Figs. 12.5–12.8.

Anterior extension of the longitudinal fracture may reach the carotid canal, injure the internal carotid, and lead to a post-traumatic aneurysm.

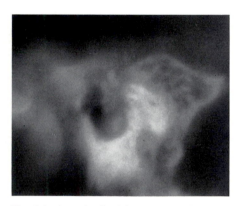

Fig. 4.4   Longitudinal fracture, sagittal tomogram, left. The fracture extends from the tegmen through the epitympanum to the anterior canal wall and disrupts the ossicles.

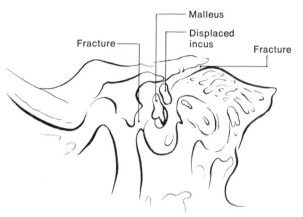

Fig. 4.5   Diagram of Fig. 4.4

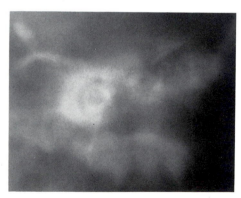

Fig. 4.6   Same ear as in Fig. 4.4, coronal tomogram. The tegmen is fractured and the incus dislocated from the malleus.

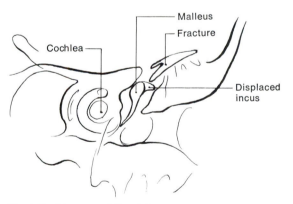

Fig. 4.7   Diagram of Fig. 4.6

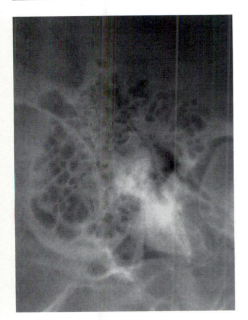

Fig. 4.**8** Longitudinal fracture, Schüller view, right. A thin fracture crosses the mastoid and passes through the posterior and anterior walls of the external auditory canal.

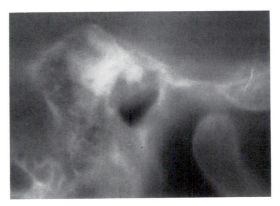

Fig. 4.**9** Same ear as in Fig. 4.8, sagittal tomogram. The tomogram demonstrates a fracture which passes inferior to the horizontal semicircular canal and involves the facial canal just distal to the pyramidal turn. The ossicles are disrupted.

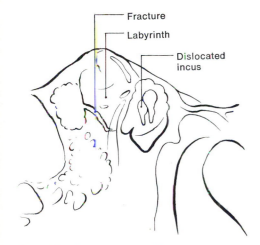

Fig. 4.**10** Diagram of Fig. 4.9

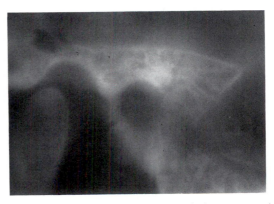

Fig. 4.**11** Longitudinal fracture, sagittal tomogram, left. The fracture line runs from the tegmen to the posterosuperior and anteroinferior walls of the external auditory canal.

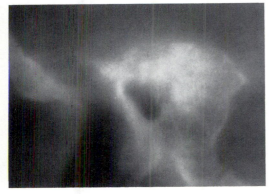

Fig. 4.**12** Same ear as in Fig. 4.11, sagittal tomogram, 10 mm medial. The fracture involves the facial canal at the second turn. The incus is dislocated.

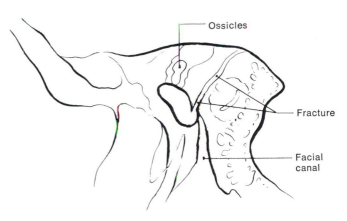

Fig. 4.**13** Diagram of Fig. 4.12

Radiographic Findings in Transverse Fractures

Most transverse fractures of the temporal bone lie medial to the middle ear cavity and therefore usually involve the inner ear structures. The fracture may extend anteriorly into the floor of the middle cranial fossa and posteriorly into the occipital bone.

Most commonly transverse fractures reach from the dome of the jugular fossa to the superior petrous ridge either medial or lateral to the arcuate eminence. Laterally placed fractures involve the promontory, the vestibule, the horizontal and posterior semicircular canals, and occasionally the tympanic segment of the facial nerve. Medially situated fractures involve the vestibule, the cochlea, the fundus of the internal auditory canal, and the crus commune, Figs. 4.14–4.25.

A more unusual type of transverse fracture occurs medial to the vestibule and bisects the internal auditory canal.

Direct Mastoid Fractures

Direct mastoid trauma produces a comminuted fracture of the mastoid cortex and trabeculae and diffuse clouding of the air cells from accompanying hemorrhage. Occasionally the fractures extend to the external canal and to the vertical segment of the facial canal and cause facial nerve paralysis.

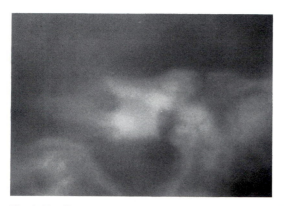

Fig. 4.**14**   Transverse fracture, coronal tomogram, left. The fracture extends from the superior petrous ridge lateral to the arcuate eminence to the jugular fossa and splits the vestibule.

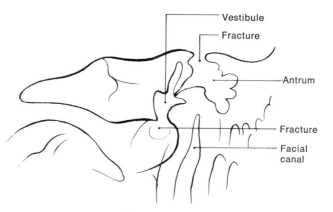

Fig. 4.**15**   Diagram of Fig. 4.14

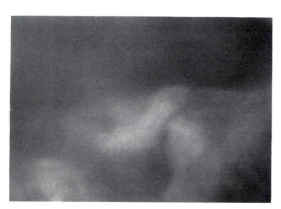

Fig. 4.**16**   Same ear as in Fig. 4.14, coronal tomogram, 4 mm posterior. The wide fracture crosses the posterior aspect of the labyrinth.

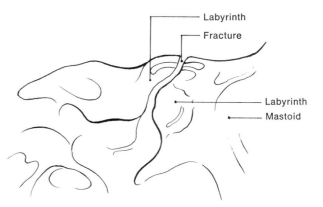

Fig. 4.**17**   Diagram of Fig. 4.16

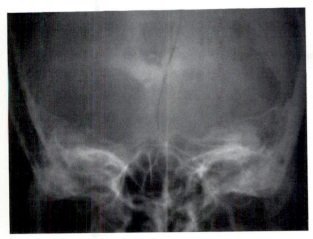

Fig. 4.18 Transverse fractures, both temporal bones, Towne view. There are fractures of both petrous pyramids and a linear fracture of the occipital bone extending to the foramen magnum.

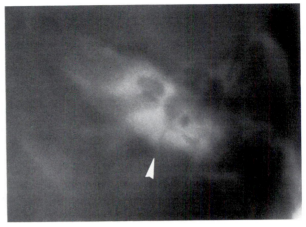

Fig. 4.19 Left ear of Fig. 4.18, horizontal tomogram. The fracture extends through the vestibule to the posterior surface of the petrous pyramid.

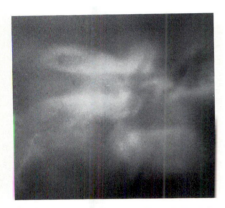

Fig. 4.20 Same ear as in Figs. 4.19, 4.21 and 4.22, coronal tomograms 4 mm apart. The fracture crosses the promontory of the cochlea.

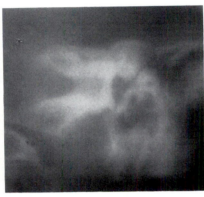

Fig. 4.21 The fracture extends from the horizontal semicircular canal across the vestibule and involves the ampulla of the posterior semicircular canal.

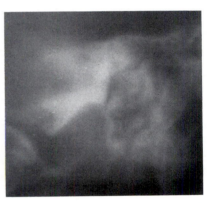

Fig. 4.22 The fracture extends from the superior petrous ridge, crosses the labyrinth and reaches the jugular fossa.

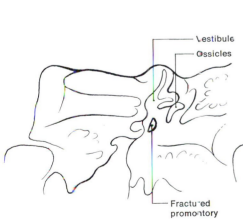

Vestibule
Ossicles

Fractured promontory

Fig. 4.23 Diagram of Fig. 4.20

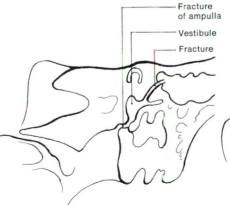

Fracture of ampulla
Vestibule
Fracture

Fig. 4.24 Diagram of Fig. 4.21

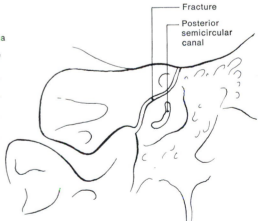

Fracture
Posterior semicircular canal

Fig. 4.25 Diagram of Fig. 4.22

Ossicular Dislocation

Following a temporal bone fracture, some patients develop a persistant conductive deafness which is usually secondary to disruption of the ossicular chain. The disruption is associated with radiographic evidence of a fracture, usually of the longitudinal type. In some cases radiographic evidence of a fracture is absent, but disruption of the ossicles is evident in the tomograms.

Ossicular disruption can also occur following direct trauma to the ear by foreign bodies perforating the tympanic membrane, from previous mastoid surgery, or by projectile missiles.

Dislocation of the malleus is rare because of the firm attachment of the malleus to the tympanic membrane and the strong anterior mallear ligament.

The incus is most commonly dislocated since its attachments to the malleus and stapes are easily torn, Figs. 4.26–4.29.

When the incudomallear joint is disrupted, the body of the incus is usually rotated and displaced superiorly, posteriorly, and laterally. More rarely the incus body is displaced inferolaterally to abut against the superior portion of the tympanic membrane. Otoscopically the dislocated incus appears as a bony mass in the upper portion of the middle ear.

The most common site of ossicular chain disruption is the incudostapedial joint area. The disruption exists as a fracture of the lenticular process of the incus, a dislocation of the incudostapedial joint, or a fracture through the stapes superstructure.

Radiographic detection of disruption of the incudostapedial joint area is rarely made by visualization of the separation of the incus long process from the stapes head, but by recognition of lateral rotation of the long process of the incus away from the stapes.

Isolated fractures of the stapes footplate, crural fractures, or dislocation of the stapes footplate are not visible radiographically.

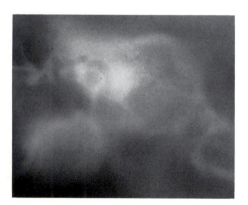

Fig. 4.**26** Ossicular dislocation, coronal tomogram, right. The body of the incus is displaced inferolaterally and protrudes into the external auditory canal.

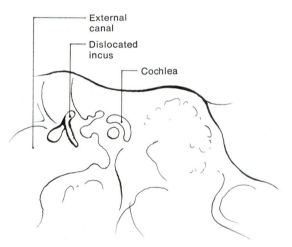

Fig. 4.**27** Diagram of Fig. 4.26

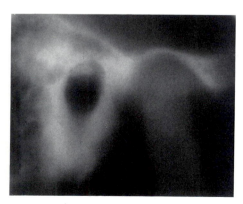

Fig. 4.**28** Same ear as in Fig. 4.26, sagittal tomogram

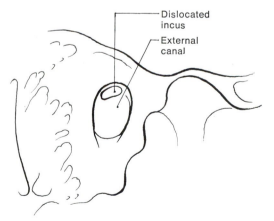

Fig. 4.**29** Diagram of Fig. 4.28

Projectile Missiles

Missiles such as bullets or metallic fragments from industrial accidents penetrate into the temporal bone and cause severe injury. The injury depends on the trajectory of the bullet and the site where the bullet fragments come to rest. Following industrial accidents, we usually find radio-opaque fragments lodged in the external auditory canal or middle ear, Figs. 4.30–4.31. Bullet wounds cause comminution of the temporal bone. There are mul-

tiple metallic bullet fragments, since bullets usually shatter on impact with the hard bone of the petrosa, Figs. 4.32–4.36.

Some bullet wounds cause mastoid and middle ear trauma with cerebrospinal fluid leaks, conductive deafness, and facial paralysis. When lesions involve the inner ear structures there will be total sensorineural deafness and loss of vestibular function.

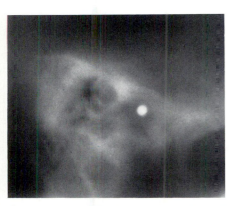

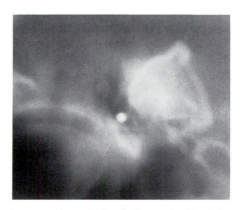

Fig. 4.30 and 4.31   Foreign body, Fig. 4.30 sagittal tomogram, Fig. 4.31 semiaxial tomogram, right. A metallic foreign body, a large weld spark, lies in the eustachian tube portion of the middle ear.

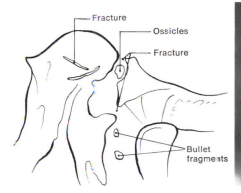

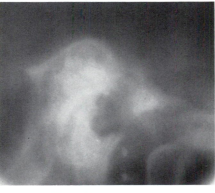

Fig. 4.32 and 4.33   Bullet wound, Fig. 4.32 diagram and Fig. 4.33 sagittal tomogram, right. There is a comminuted fracture involving the external canal, middle ear and petrous pyramid. Bullet fragments are present in the temporomandibular joint space.

4.34

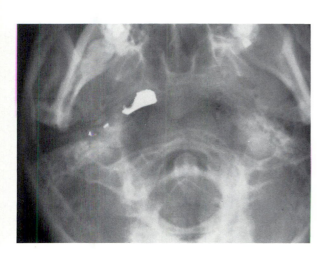

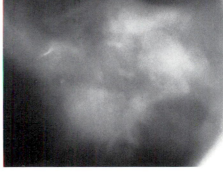

4.35

Fig. 4.34 and 4.35   Same ear as in Figs. 4.33 and 4.36, semiaxial tomogram. The bullet has splintered the cochlea.

◀ Fig. 4.36   Same ear as in Figs. 4.33 and 4.35, basal view. The main portion of the bullet is lodged in the petrous apex. Metallic fragments outline the trajectory.

Chapter 5   Acute Otitis Media and Mastoiditis

Acute mastoiditis occurs as a complication or extension of an acute otitis media. Acute otitis media is an infection which begins in the upper respiratory tract and nasopharynx, ascends the eustachian tube, and affects the middle ear. Probably even in the early stages of acute otitis media, the inflammatory process extends to some extent into the epitympanum and mastoid antrum. Depending on the virulence of the infecting organism, the resistance of the host, and the type of treatment, the infection may or may not extend to involve the mastoid air cells and the air cells of the petrous pyramid.

Further progress of the infectious process, uncontrolled by proper therapy, leads to suppuration and destruction of air cell septa in the mastoid and petrous pyramid. This results in areas of coalescence and abscess formation.

In the preantibiotic era, acute suppurative mastoiditis often extended beyond the borders of the temporal bone. Erosion of the posterior wall of the mastoid over the sigmoid sinus resulted in extradural abscess formation and septic thrombophlebitis of the sigmoid sinus. Similar erosions of the cortex of the mastoid resulted in subperiosteal abscesses over the mastoid process and under the superior attachment of the sternocleidomastoid muscle. Extension of the infection from the mastoid or from deep infected cells in the petrous pyramid often caused serious intracranial complications.

Otoscopically the tympanic membrane in acute otitis media is inflamed, reddened, and most often bulges externally due to seropurulent fluid under increased pressure in the middle ear. The mucosa of the middle ear becomes thickened and inflamed due to the infection. In those cases which develop mastoiditis the mucosal thickening extends from the middle ear into the epitympanum, antrum, and air cells.

Radiographic Technique

Conventional x-rays are sufficient to study acute inflammatory disorders of the mastoid air cells. We use Schüller, Owen and Towne views. The Chausse III projection exposes the middle ear space.

These views are usually sufficient to determine the degree of clouding of the air cells, cell wall destruction and sinus plate erosion.

Coronal and sagittal tomographic sections are indicated when further information is required to determine the presence of erosion of the tegmen or petrositis.

Computerized tomography is indicated when there is a suspicion of petrositis or extratemporal spread of the infection.

Radiographic Findings

The radiographic findings of acute mastoiditis depend on the stage of the inflammatory process and the extent of pneumatization of the temporal bone. Acute mastoiditis does not occur in acellular mastoids.

The earliest findings of an acute mastoiditis are a haziness of the middle ear cavity and the mastoid air cells. As the infective process worsens diffuse clouding of the middle ear cavity and mastoid air cells occur. In the initial stage of the disease, the trabecular pattern of the mastoid air cells is intact, Figs. 5.1–5.2. However, mucosal edema and seropurulent fluid cause the trabecular pattern to be less well defined due to lack of the normal air bone interface between cells and trabeculae. A similar involvement usually occurs in the petrous air cells of well pneumatized petrous bones.

With progression of the disease, the trabecular pattern first becomes ill defined due to demineralization. This phase is followed by destruction of the trabeculae with formation of coalescent areas of suppuration, Figs. 5.3–5.5.

When a severe coalescent mastoiditis extends posteriorly, the sinus plate becomes poorly defined and partially eroded. These findings indicate possible septic thrombophlebitis of the lateral sinus. Dissolution of the bony tegmen is difficult to demonstrate in conventional radiographic views, but the defect is usually demonstrated in tomographic sections.

When intracranial complications due to spread of infection from the mastoid to the posterior or middle cranial fossae are suspected, CT becomes the method of choice. CT will show bony defects and intracranial extensions of the infection.

Differential Diagnosis

On conventional radiography the early findings of acute mastoiditis may be identical to the features of serous otitis media. In serous otitis media, sterile serous fluid fills the middle ear and at times the entire mastoid air cell system. Since the clinical features of serous otitis and acute otitis media are quite different, it is imperative that the radiologist have sufficient clinical information to avoid misdiagnosis.

Reticuloendotheliosis in the form of eosinophilic granuloma may cause a breakdown of the trabecular pattern similar to that of acute coalescent mastoiditis or petrositis. Clinical history and otoscopic findings will enable the radiologist to diagnose this lesion correctly.

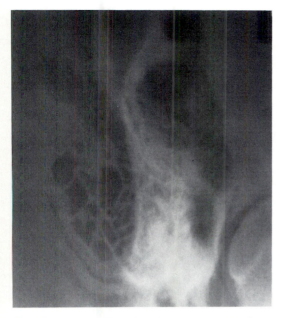

Fig. 5.1   Acute mastoiditis, Owen view, right. There is a diffuse homogeneous clouding of the mastoid air cells with intact trabeculae.

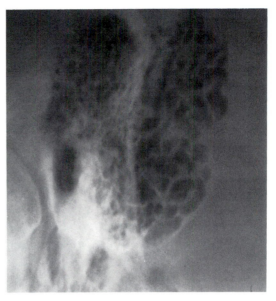

Fig. 5.2   Same patient as in Fig. 5.1, normal mastoid, Owen view, left, for comparison.

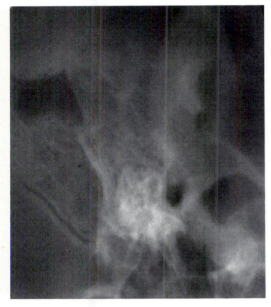

Fig. 5.3   Acute mastoiditis, Schüller view, right. There is diffuse clouding of the mastoid air cells, and there is a large coalescent area of trabecular destruction superiorly.

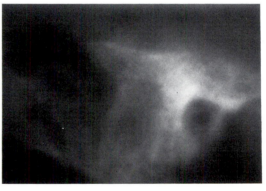

Fig. 5.4   Same ear as in Figs. 5.3 and 5.4, sagittal tomogram. There is diffuse clouding of the air cells with loss of definition and partial destruction of the trabeculae. There is a coalescent area of trabecular destruction posterior to the external canal.

Malignant External Otitis

Malignant external otitis is an acute osteomyelitis of the temporal bone which occurs in aged diabetic patients and is caused by the pseudomonas bacterium. The infection begins as an external otitis but spreads rapidly to involve the surrounding walls of the external canal. The process often extends into the middle ear and mastoid. The infection usually breaks through the floor of the

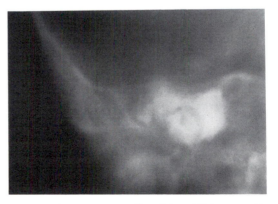

Fig. 5.5   Same ear as in Figs. 5.3 and 5.4, coronal tomogram. The middle ear is diffusely clouded, but the contour of the middle ear and ossicles is intact.

external canal at the bony and cartilagenous junction, and spreads along the under surface of the temporal bone to involve the facial nerve at the stylomastoid foramen. Further medial extension involves the jugular fossa and cranial nerves IX, X, XI, and XII. Anterior spread of the infection affects the temporomandibular joint.

Radiographic Findings

Tomography is essential when studying malignant otitis. Coronal, sagittal, and semiaxial projections are indicated. Computerized tomography is indicated when the infection spreads outside the temporal bone.

The radiographic findings of malignant external otitis resemble those of carcinoma of the external auditory canal. The bony external canal appears eroded and partially destroyed. The floor of the canal is usually the first area to be involved, Fig. 5.6.

When facial nerve paralysis occurs, the facial canal in the early stage is normal, since the nerve is first affected at the stylomastoid foramen. Tomography a few days after the onset of the paralysis usually shows erosion of the contour of the stylomastoid foramen and of the adjacent mastoid segment of the facial canal, Figs. 5.9–5.10. The lateral wall of the jugular fossa becomes eroded as the infection passes medially, Fig. 5.7.

If the anterior wall of the external canal is destroyed and the infection involves the mandibular fossa, the mandibular condyle is displaced anteriorly, Fig. 5.8.

The mastoid air cells may become involved by direct posterior extension or via the middle ear. The lateral attic wall and floor of the middle ear often are destroyed. In severe, advanced cases the entire petrous pyramid may be involved in a severe demineralizing, osteomyelitic process which may spread to the adjacent occipital bone and cervical spine.

Healing Stages

If surgical and antibiotic therapy is successful in arresting the spread of and eliminating the infection, follow-up tomographic studies show remineralization of the petrous pyramid, mastoid, occipital bone and other involved structures.

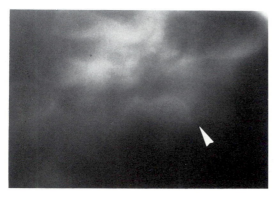

Fig. 5.6   Malignant external otitis, coronal tomogram, left. There is erosion of the lateral portion of the floor of the external auditory canal, arrow, and soft tissue swelling in the lumen of the canal.

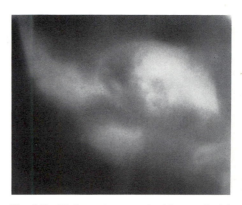

Fig. 5.7   Malignant external otitis, semiaxial tomogram, right. The middle ear cavity is cloudy and the floor destroyed by extension of the disease process into the jugular fossa.

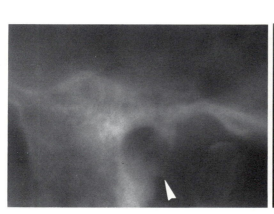

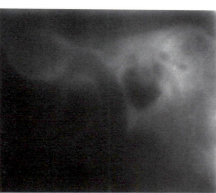

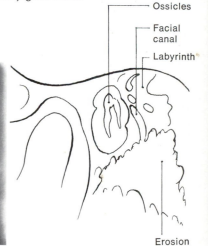

Fig. 5.8   Malignant external otitis, sagittal tomogram, right. There is a soft tissue density within the lumen of the external auditory canal. The anterior bony canal wall is partially destroyed, arrow, with extension of the infection into the temporomandibular joint. The mandibular condyle is displaced anteriorly.

Fig. 5.9   Malignant external otitis, sagittal tomogram, left. The undersurface of the mastoid, the stylomastoid foramen and the distal segment of the facial canal are eroded.

Fig. 5.10   Diagram of Fig. 5.9

Chapter 6 Chronic Otitis Media and Mastoiditis

Chronic otitis media and mastoiditis are the result of an infection by an organism of low virulence or of an acute infection with incomplete resolution. In the United States today due to improved general health, antibiotics and vaccines, acute otitis rarely progresses to chronic otitis media. In the preantibiotic era a single, severe infection by a virulent organism associated with decreased host resistance often resulted in severe destruction of the middle ear and scarring which led to chronic suppuration. Another type of chronic otitis media is the result of faulty middle ear aeration and eustachian malfunction. This is chronic adhesive otitis media and is relatively more common today in the United States.

Clinical Findings

The clinical findings in chronic otitis media and mastoiditis are perforation of the tympanic membrane, chronic suppurative discharge and poor hearing in the affected ear. The mucosa of the middle ear is involved in a chronic inflammatory process which also affects the epitympanum, mastoid antrum and mastoid air cells. Chronic suppurative otitis media and mastoiditis must be differentiated from chronic adhesive otitis media in which there are varying degrees of middle ear atelectasis with suppuration. In adhesive otitis the causative factor is chronic eustachian tube malfunction.

Otoscopic Findings

In chronic otitis media and mastoiditis, there is a central type of tympanic membrane perforation and a suppurative discharge from the middle ear. The tympanic membrane remnant is thickened and reddened and the mucosa of the middle ear is edematous, and hyperemic. There often is a granulomatous polyp of varying size which arises from the margin of the tympanic membrane perforation or from the mucosa of the medial wall of the middle ear.

In chronic adhesive otitis media there usually is a deep atelectatic, retracted pocket in a portion of the tympanic membrane which appears as a perforation. Careful microscopic otoscopy, however, will show that the atelectatic pocket is an area of retracted, ectatic atrophic tympanic membrane and not a perforation. Chronic adhesive otitis media may evolve into a cholesteatoma, another form of chronic mastoiditis which we shall discuss separately.

Radiographic Findings

Conventional radiography is usually sufficient to evaluate the degree of development of the mastoid, the trabecular pattern, and the degree of involvement of the air cells. The Schüller, Owen, and Towne projections are

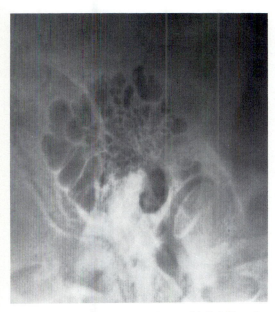

Fig. 6.1　Normal pneumatized mastoid, Schüller view, right. Large clear air cells occupy the entire mastoid.

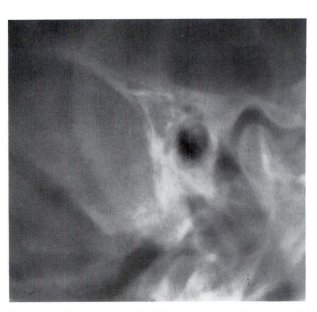

Fig. 6.2　Diploic mastoid, Schüller view, right. The pneumatization is limited to a large mastoid antrum and a few periantral cells. The overlying dense bone obscures the radiolucency of the antrum. There is diploic bone in the mastoid process.

used to study the mastoids. The Chaussee III adds details of the status of the middle ear cavity, but for more precise evaluation of the middle ear, tomography is necessary.

Coronal, semiaxial and sagittal tomographic sections are obtained to study the middle ear cavity and mastoid air cells. For unilateral disease we take tomographs in the three projections of the involved side but only coronal tomographs of the uninvolved side for comparison.

Variations of Mastoid Pneumatization

The radiographic findings of chronic otitis media and mastoiditis depend on the size and the degree of pneumatization of the mastoid. Mastoid pneumatization varies from extensive cellularity which may extend beyond the limits of the temporal bone to a single antral cell in a markedly constricted mastoid, Figs. 6.1–6.2.

There are two types of constricted mastoids, the diploic and the compact. In the diploic type the mastoid process contains a spongy diploe which is far less dense than the surrounding cortex. In the compact type the mastoid process is densely ossified and has the same density as the cortex.

A poorly pneumatized but noninfected mastoid must be differentiated from chronic mastoiditis and cholesteatoma. In conventional lateral radiographs of poorly pneumatized mastoids the overlying dense bone obscures the mastoid antrum. In conventional coronal radiographs such as the Towne, the mastoid antrum in a poorly pneumatized mastoid will appear as a single, smooth cavity. This single smooth cavity is often mis-

diagnosed as a cholesteatoma while in reality the ear is free of disease. In these cases tomography is essential for making a correct diagnosis. Tomographs will demonstrate a large clear antral cavity with either a smooth or slightly scalloped margin. The bone surrounding the antrum will be diploic or compact. The most important finding in the differential from cholesteatoma will be the presence of a normal middle ear and ossicular chain.

The radiographic findings of chronic mastoiditis consist of a nonhomogeneous clouding of the mastoid antrum and air cells with varying degrees of change of the mastoid trabeculae.

Mastoid inflammation produces thickening of some trabeculae secondary to reactive new bone formation and at the same time demineralization of other trabeculae. At this stage of the process, the air cells appear cloudy and fewer than normal, and the residual trabeculae thickened, Fig. 6.3.

As the chronic inflammatory process continues, the air cells become constricted as reactive new bone thickens the remaining trabeculae. In the final stage of the process, the air cells are obliterated and the mastoid appears completely sclerotic, Fig. 6.4.

The lumen of the mastoid antrum and residual air cells is usually filled with granulation tissue and appears cloudy. An acquired sclerotic mastoid caused by chronic inflammation should be differentiated from a compact mastoid. In a sclerotic mastoid the overall size is normal while in the underdeveloped compact mastoid the overall size is small. In addition, the mastoid antrum and periantral cells are clear in the compact mastoid, but cloudy in the chronic mastoiditis.

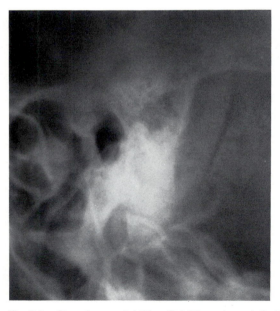

Fig. 6.3 Chronic mastoiditis, Schüller view, left. There is a nonhomogeneous clouding of the mastoid air cells with thickening of the trabeculae. Some air cells appear constricted by reactive new bone formation.

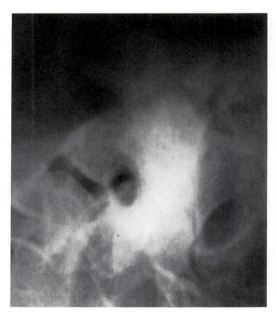

Fig. 6.4 Chronic mastoiditis, acquired sclerotic type, Schüller view, left. The air cells are completely obliterated by reactive new bone formation.

The Middle Ear

For proper evaluation of the middle ear in chronic otitis media, we utilize tomography. The radiographic appearance of the middle ear depends on the degree of inflammatory changes in the mucosa and the aeration of the middle ear.

In chronic suppurative otitis media and mastoiditis the residual portion of the tympanic membrane is usually thickened and visible tomographically. The middle ear is partially or completely cloudy during active suppuration. If there is no active infection the middle ear is aerated.

In chronic adhesive otitis media, tomographic sections demonstrate thickened portions of the tympanic membrane retracted to the promontory and a contracted middle ear space, Figs. 6.5–6.6.

Erosion of the long process of the incus commonly occurs in chronic otitis media and mastoiditis, and the malleus handle is often foreshortened. Erosion of the malleus head and incus body in the epitympanum is rare unless cholesteatoma is present.

Cholesterol Granuloma

Cholesterol granuloma is a nonspecific chronic inflammation of the middle ear and mastoid. Histologically a cholesterol granuloma consists of a mass of chronic inflammatory tissue containing clefts of cholesterol crystals surrounded by giant cells.

When a cholesterol granuloma occurs in the middle ear behind an intact tympanic membrane otoscopically it resembles a glomus tumor. Tomographically the granuloma appears as a well defined soft tissue mass when the middle ear is aerated. Unfortunately the middle ear mucosa is usually inflamed and the granuloma cannot be discerned. The bony contour of the middle ear is intact, but the ossicles are often eroded by the granulomatous process, Figs. 6.7, 6.8.

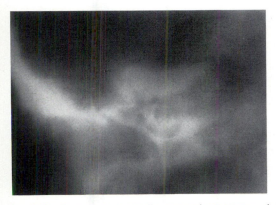

Fig. 6.5   Chronic otitis media, coronal tomogram, right. The tympanic membrane is retracted onto the promontory and the middle ear space contracted. The lateral epitympanic wall is intact, but the malleus handle lies almost horizontally.

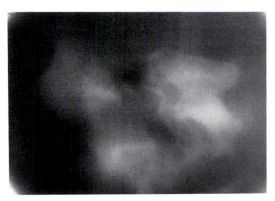

Fig. 6.7   Cholesteral granuloma, semiaxial tomogram, right. A soft tissue mass is present in the posterosuperior quadrant of the tympanic cavity surrounding the intact long process of the incus.

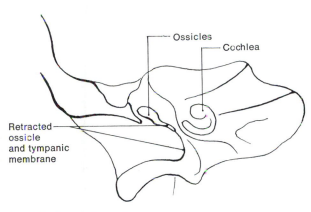

Fig. 6.6   Diagram of Fig. 6.5

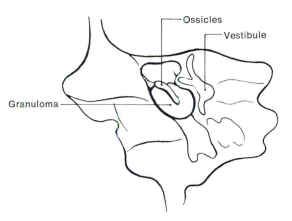

Fig. 6.8   Diagram of Fig. 6.7

Tympanosclerosis

Tympanosclerosis consists of deposits of hyalinized and often calcified fibrotic granulation tissue in the middle ear, epitympanum, and tympanic membrane.

Tympanosclerosis occurs most commonly as deposits of thickened hyalinized tissue within the layers of the tympanic membrane, on the promontory, and in the epitympanum surrounding and fixing the ossicles.

Tympanosclerotic deposits, if large enough and calcified, are demonstrated tomographically. The deposits appear as punctate or linear densities within the tympanic membrane or applied to the contour of the promontory, Fig. 6.9.

Large deposits of tympanosclerosis in the epitympanum appear as ill defined calcified masses which surround the ossicles. The normal ossicular contour is lost.

An isolated plaque of tympanosclerosis in the anterior or superior epitympanum may ankylose the malleus head. Thes findings can be seen on semiaxial and sagittal tomographic sections, Figs. 6.10–6.11.

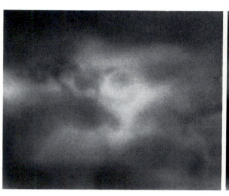
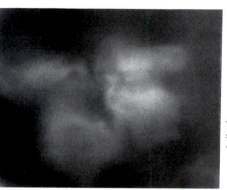
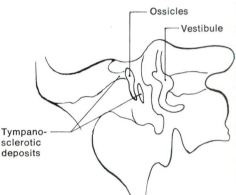

Fig. 6.**9** Tympanosclerosis, middle ear, coronal tomogram, right. A calcified deposit of tympanosclerosis lies in the upper portion of the middle ear adjacent to the promontory.

Fig. 6.**10** Tympanosclerosis, middle ear, semiaxial tomogram, right. An isolated plaque of tympanosclerosis fixes the malleus head to the lateral epitympanic wall. There is another deposit medial to the ossicle.

Fig. 6.**11**   Diagram of Fig. 6.10

Chronic Granulomatous Disorders

Tuberculosis

Tuberculosis of the ear is rarely seen in the United States today. In the few cases we have studied radiographically, the findings were similar to chronic otitis media and mastoiditis. The diagnosis of tuberculosis is made by biopsy and bacteriologic studies, Figs. 6.12, 6.13.

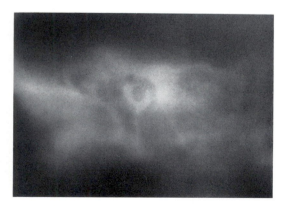
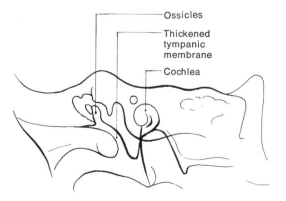

Fig. 6.**12**   Tuberculosis, middle ear and mastoid, coronal tomogram, right. The middle ear cavity is partially cloudy, and the tympanic membrane markedly thickened. There is no bony erosion.

Fig. 6.**13**   Diagram of Fig. 6.12

Chapter 7   Cholesteatoma of the Middle Ear and Mastoid

A cholesteatoma is an epidermoid cyst which histologically consists of an inner layer of desquamating stratified squamous epithelium apposed on an outer layer of subepithelial connective tissue. The lumen of the cyst is filled with desquamated epithelial debris. The subepithelial connective tissue layer is usually involved by a chronic inflammatory process characterized by deposition of cholesterol crystals, and infiltration of giant cell and round cells.

The epithelial cyst enlarges progressively because of accumulation of epithelial debris within its lumen. As the cyst enlarges and comes in contact with contiguous bony structures of the middle ear, mastoid, and petrous pyramid, erosion of these structures occurs due to pressure necrosis and enzymatic lysis of bone.

Cholesteatomas may be congenital or acquired. Congenital cholesteatomas arise from epithelial rests within or adjacent to the temporal bone. Acquired cholesteatomas originate in the middle ear and extend into the mastoid and occasionally into the petrous pyramid. There is another distinct form of cholesteatoma which arises in the external auditory canal and often follows previous irradiation of the head.

Acquired Cholesteatoma of the Middle Ear and Mastoid

The etiology of acquired cholesteatoma is not known, and there are four main theories which attempt to explain the pathogenesis. Each theory describes a different origin of cholesteatoma. Regardless of their etiology, acquired cholesteatomas slowly expand to erode middle ear and mastoid structures.

The pathogenesis of acquired cholesteatoma may occur in one of the four following manners:

1. *Negative pressure theory.* Poor aeration of the middle ear, probably related to malfunction of the eustachian tube, results in a relative negative pressure in the middle ear. This negative pressure causes medialward retraction of the pars flaccida or of atrophic areas of the pars tensa of the tympanic membrane. The retracted areas deepen to form pits and epithelial debris collects within the lumen of the retracted pockets. When egress of the debris is impaired, encystment and cholesteatoma formation ensues. Many authors call this type of lesion occuring in the pars flaccida a primary acquired cholesteatoma.

2. *Migration theory.* This theory postulates that a previous necrotic otitis media destroys the marginal portion of the pars tensa of the tympanic membrane. Epithelium from the external auditory canal grows into the middle ear at the margin of the perforation, encysts and forms a cholesteatoma. Most authors refer to this type of cholesteatoma as a secondary acquired cholesteatoma.

Epithelium from the surface of the tympanic membrane may also migrate into the middle ear from the rim of a central perforation of the pars tensa to form a cholesteatoma.

3. *Metaplasia theory.* Following middle ear infection, the middle ear mucosa undergoes a metaplasia to desquamating stratified squamous epithelium. Encystment follows, and a cholesteatoma is formed.

4. *Papillary ingrowth theory.* This theory has been advanced by Rüedi. An inflammatory stimulus causes invasive hyperplasia of the basal layer of the stratified squamous epithelium of the pars flaccida. The hyperplastic basal cells infiltrate into the subepithelial connective tissues of the pars flaccida, extend into the epitympanum, desquamate, encyst, and form a cholesteatoma.

Clinical and Otoscopic Findings

Most cholesteatomas originate from the stratified squamous epithelium of the tympanic membrane or external auditory canal and develop in the middle ear or epitympanum. As they enlarge, they destroy the ossicles and adjacent bony structures and extend into the mastoid.

Acquired cholesteatomas are characterized by a tympanic membrane perforation of the pars flaccida, the pars tensa or a combined perforation of both pars flaccida and pars tensa. There is usually an associated chronic infection, a history of chronic aural discharge, and a conductive or mixed deafness.

Most perforations are of the marginal type since part of their circumference lies in contact with the bony margin of the tympanic sulcus or notch of Rivinus. Some cholesteatomas occur with central perforations of the pars tensa.

The characteristic of cholesteatoma is that the lumen of the tympanic membrane perforation contains varying amounts of epithelial debris. In chronically infected cholesteatomas, granulomatous tissue and polyps accompany the epithelial debris.

The otologist can diagnose most cholesteatomas otoscopically. However, he cannot determine otoscopically the size and extent of the lesion in the epitympanum and mastoid. The otologist can make a qualitative diagnosis of cholesteatoma, but the quantitative evaluation of the lesion requires tomographic study of the middle ear and mastoid.

Once the otologist has diagnosed a cholesteatoma he must determine the size and extent of the lesion in the mastoid and the status of the ossicular chain by tomographs. A small epitympanic perforation filled with epithelial debris may be the only otoscopic evidence of a large cholesteatoma that will be visualized by tomography. On the contrary a large tympanic membrane perforation filled with debris may on tomography be found to be associated with a relatively small lesion.

Without a tomographic evaluation the otologist has no insight into the size of the lesion, the status of the ossicles, the presence of fistulae of the labyrinth, or an anomalous course of the facial nerve.

Radiographic Techniques

Radiographic evaluation of the middle ear and mastoid for cholesteatoma can be done with conventional or tomographic techniques. Tomography is the method of choice since tomography reveals the presence of soft tissue masses and erosion of the bony structures such as ossicles and labyrinth far better than conventional radiographs. Conventional radiography should only be used when multidirectional tomography is not available.

Computerized tomography is useful to demonstrate extension of the cholesteatoma into the petrous apex and erosion of the tegmen and sinus plates. In cases of acute exacerbations CT will show intracranial complications such as extradural and cerebral abscesses.

Conventional Radiography

The most useful projections for the study of cholesteatomas are the Schüller, Owen, and Chausse III, Fig. 7.21.

The Schüller and Owen projection show extension of the cholesteatoma into the mastoid. The Owen will occasionally show erosion of the ossicles and of the posterosuperior wall of the bony external canal.

The Chausse III is useful for the study of cholesteatomas of the pars flaccida because this projection demonstrates erosion of the anterior portion of the lateral epitympanic wall.

Limitations of Conventional Radiography

The most serious limitation of conventional radiography in the study of cholesteatoma is the superimposition of many complex and minute structures on a single plane. Ossicles, antrum, mastoid, and other skull structures are superimposed and difficult to differentiate. In cholesteatoma details recognizable in special conventional views such as the Owen and Chausse III when the middle ear is normally aerated are obscured. Epithelial debris, fluid and inflammatory tissue in the middle ear obliterate the air bone interfaces and prevent delineation of the ossicles and the middle ear spaces.

Tomography

The projections required for a tomographic study depend on whether the lesion is unilateral or bilateral.

In unilateral lesions, coronal, semiaxial, and sagittal sections of the middle ear and mastoid of the affected side are taken. Coronal sections of the opposite normal ear are obtained for comparison. A Schüller view of both mastoids is taken for evaluation of the pneumatization. In bilateral cases the three projections of both sides as well as the Schüller views are utilized.

At times modified sagittal views are needed to improve visualization of the ossicles. To free the incus from superimposition of the overlying posterosuperior canal wall the head is rotated 20° toward the axial projection. To demonstrate the entire long process of the incus the vertex of the skull can be inclined 10°–15° toward the table top.

When CT is employed, high definition horizontal and coronal sections, 1.5 mm thick should be obtained. Computer reconstructed sagittal sections are useful in definition of the tegmen.

Classifications and Radiographic Findings

Tomography allows the radiologist to diagnose the presence of cholesteatoma and to establish the extent of the lesion. The diagnosis of acquired cholesteatoma is based on detection of soft tissue lesions in the middle ear and erosion of bony structures. The evaluation of the extent of the lesion depends on the recognition of changes in the aditus, antrum, and mastoid.

Diagnosis of Cholesteatoma – Erosion of Bony Structures

The evaluation of fine bony structures is essential in the diagnosis of cholesteatoma.

These structures are: 1. the lateral epitympanic wall; 2. the anterior tympanic spine; 3. the posterosuperior wall of the bony external canal; 4. the malleus head; and 5. the body of the incus.

Erosion of one or more of these structures is found in the great majority of cholesteatomas.

Erosion of the long process of the incus occurs commonly in chronic otitis media as well as in cholesteatoma and is not a specific finding for cholesteatoma.

The superstructure of the stapes may be eroded in cholesteatomas. The radiographic detection of stapes erosion is difficult because of the small size of this structure and because cholesteatoma and inflammatory tissue in the middle ear obscure the stapes.

Soft Tissue Lesions

With cholesteatoma there is a soft tissue mass in the meso or epitympanum. If the middle ear cavity is aerated, the soft tissue mass is visible tomographically and can be diagnosed. When fluid or inflammatory tissue fill the middle ear cavity the cholesteatoma mass is obscured, since the radiographic density is the same for cholesteatoma and the inflammatory tissue and fluid.

Patterns of Radiographic Findings

We have observed different patterns of radiographic findings in the study of cholesteatomas. When we analyzed these patterns and compared them with the site of the perforation of the tympanic membrane we found patterns which correspond to the site of the perforation. Cholesteatomas of the pars flaccida, known as primary acquired cholesteatomas, have a characteristic radiographic pattern.

Cholesteatomas arising from the pars tensa, usually the posterosuperior portion, known as secondary acquired cholesteatomas, have a radiographic pattern distinct from pars flaccida lesions.

At times a cholesteatoma may involve both the pars flaccida and pars tensa. These lesions produce a radiographic pattern that is a combination of the two types. In extensive, far advanced cholesteatomas of either the pars flaccida or pars tensa there is destruction of most of the structures in the meso- and epitympanum and no distinct pattern remains.

Pars Flaccida Cholesteatoma

Cholesteatomas arising from the pars flaccida are the easiest lesions to diagnose radiographically because the lateral epitympanic wall is eroded.

The typical radiographic pattern of a pars flaccida cholesteatoma consists in one or more of the following findings, Figs. 7.1–7.4, 7.7–7.10.

1. There is erosion of the anterior portion of the lateral epitympanic wall in the coronal and semiaxial projections;
2. There is erosion of the anterior tympanic spine in the sagittal sections;
3. A soft tissue mass lies in the epitympanum lateral to the ossicles. The mass is visible in the coronal and semiaxial projections;
4. There is an increased distance between the lateral epitympanic wall and the ossicles. This increase is due to medial displacement of the ossicles and to erosion of the lateral epitympanic wall;

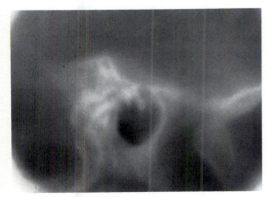

Fig. 7.1   Cholesteatoma, pars flaccida, coronal tomogram, right. The inferior margin of the lateral epitympanic wall is eroded, and there is a small soft tissue mass between the lateral epitympanic wall and the lateral surface of the malleus head. The tympanic membrane is thickened.

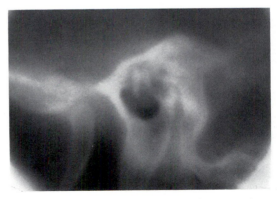

Fig. 7.2   Same patient as in Fig. 7.1, corresponding coronal tomogram of normal left ear for comparison

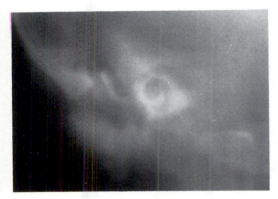

Fig. 7.3   Same ear as in Fig. 7.1, sagittal tomogram. A small soft tissue mass occupies the anterior epitympanic space. The anterior tympanic spine and the anterior aspect of the malleus head are eroded.

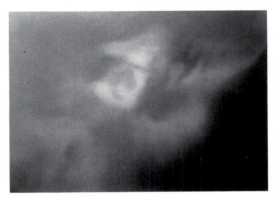

Fig. 7.4   Same patient as in Figs. 7.1 and 7.3, corresponding sagittal tomogram of normal left ear for comparison

5. In more advanced lesions the malleus head and incus body are eroded;

6. When the cholesteatoma fills the epitympanum and extends to the tegmen, the epitympanum acquires a smooth shell-like outline.

When the cholesteatoma is limited to the anterior portion of the epitympanum, only the adjacent aspect of the malleus head is eroded and will have a concave rather than convex outline.

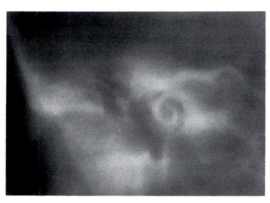

Fig. 7.5 Epitympanic retraction pocket, coronal tomogram, right. The inferior margin of the lateral epitympanic wall is eroded, but there is no soft tissue mass in the epitympanum lateral to the malleus head.

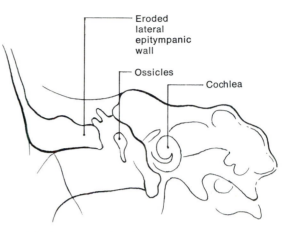

Fig. 7.6 Diagram of Fig. 7.5

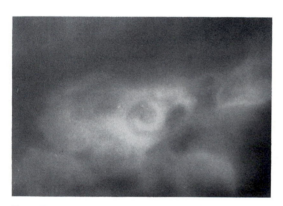

Fig. 7.7 Cholesteatoma, pars flaccida, coronal tomogram, left. There is a pronounced erosion of the lateral epitympanic wall and soft tissue mass in the epitympanum. The ossicles are eroded slightly and displaced medially. See Fig. 7.2 for comparison with a normal ear.

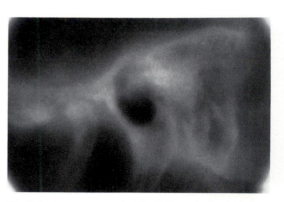

Fig. 7.8 Same ear as in Fig. 7.7, sagittal tomogram. The cholesteatomatous soft tissue mass erodes the anterior tympanic spine and the adjacent aspect of the malleus head. The lesion extends superiorly and posteriorly along the tegmen. See Fig. 7.4 for comparison with a normal ear.

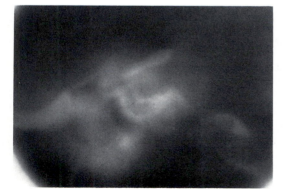

Fig. 7.9 Cholesteatoma, pars flaccida, semiaxial tomogram, right. The cholesteatomatous mass partially fills the epitympanic cavity and erodes the lateral epitympanic wall and ossicles. In this ear the dura is low lateral to the epitympanum.

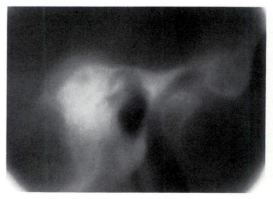

Fig. 7.10 Same ear as in Fig. 7.9, sagittal tomogram. The anterior tympanic spine and the malleus head are completely eroded by a mass which fills the anterior epitympanic space. See Fig. 7.4 for comparison with a normal ear.

If the cholesteatoma extends into the posterior epitympanum, the body of the incus will be eroded.

The long process of the incus is usually spared in pars flaccida cholesteatomas unless the cholesteatoma sac is large and extends into the posterior middle ear.

In pars flaccida cholesteatomas the tympanic cavity is usually contracted and narrowed by retraction of the pars tensa of the tympanic membrane. Since the pars tensa is usually thickened, the retracted membrane becomes visible.

Epitympanic Retraction Pockets

An epitympanic retraction pocket is an invagination of the pars flaccida of the tympanic membrane without accumulation of epithelial debris. Since these lesions can be precursor of a cholesteatoma they must be followed carefully by the otologist.

Blunting of the lateral epitympanic wall is observed in simple retraction pockets of the pars flaccida. If the pars flaccida is thickened, the membrane is clearly visible. There is no soft tissue mass, since there is no encystment of accumulated debris within the lumen of the pocket, Figs. 7.5–7.6.

Pars Tensa Cholesteatomas

Cholesteatomas of the pars tensa are more difficult to diagnose than pars flaccida lesions because the lateral epitympanic wall may be intact. In early cases bony erosion is limited to the long process of the incus and this is not a specific finding for cholesteatomas.

The radiographic pattern for cholesteatoma of the pars tensa consists in findings common to all pars tensa cholesteatomas and of findings which depend on the site of origin of the lesion in the pars tensa.

Findings common to all pars tensa cholesteatomas are, Figs. 7.11–7.18:

1. There is a soft tissue mass in the middle ear;
2. The long process of the incus is eroded;
3. The soft tissue mass of the middle ear extends into the epitympanum medial to the ossicles;
4. The malleus head and incus body are displaced laterally by the soft tissue mass of the cholesteatoma sac. The malleus head is usually displaced but intact while the displaced incus body is often eroded.

The most frequently occurring type of pars tensa cholesteatoma arises from the posterosuperior margin of the membrane. In these cases there is often blunting of the

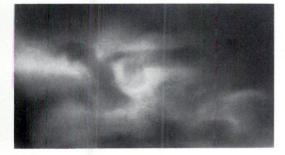

Fig. 7.11   Cholesteatoma, pars tensa, coronal tomogram, right. A cholesteatomatous soft tissue mass fills the mesotympanum and extends into the epitympanum medial to the ossicles. The ossicles are eroded partially and displaced laterally.

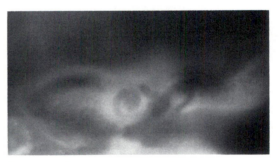

Fig. 7.12   Same patient as in Fig. 7.11, corresponding coronal tomogram of normal left ear for comparison.

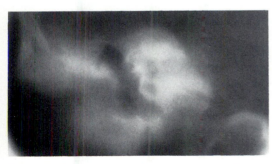

Fig. 7.13   Same ear as in Fig. 7.11, semiaxial tomogram. A soft tissue mass fills the posterosuperior quadrant of the tympanic cavity, extends into the epitympanum and displaces the incus laterally.

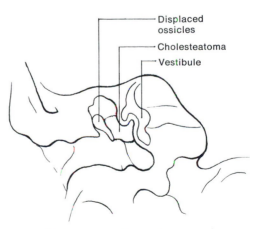

Displaced ossicles
Cholesteatoma
Vestibule

Fig. 7.14   Diagram of Fig. 7.13

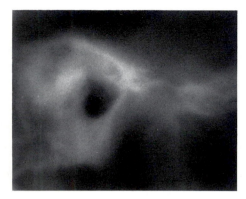

Fig. 7.**15**   Same ear as in Figs. 7.11 and 7.13, sagittal tomogram. A soft tissue fills the posterior two-thirds of the epitympanum and extends into the antrum. The ossicles are partially eroded and the long process of the incus is shortened. The anterior tympanic spine is intact.

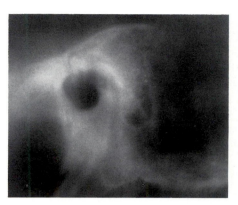

Fig. 7.**16**   Same patient as in Figs. 7.11–7.15, corresponding sagittal tomogram of normal left ear for comparison

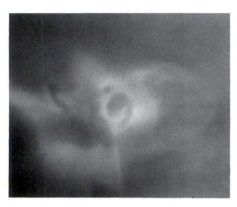

Fig. 7.**17**   Cholesteatoma, pars tensa, coronal tomogram, right. The soft tissue mass of cholesteatoma fills the upper portion of the tympanic cavity and extends medial to the ossicles into the epitympanum. The epitympanic space lateral to the ossicles is clear. See Fig. 7.12 for comparison with a normal ear.

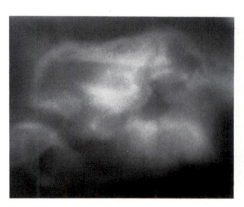

Fig. 7.**18**   Cholesteatoma, pars tensa, coronal tomogram, left. A soft tissue mass of cholesteatoma fills the posterosuperior quadrant of the middle ear and erodes the long process of the incus. The mass extends into the epitympanum medial to the ossicles which are displaced laterally.

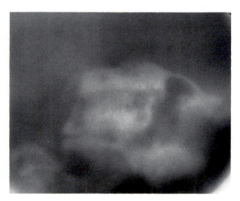

Fig. 7.**19**   Cholesteatoma, combined pars tensa and pars flaccida, semiaxial tomogram, left. In this projection the features of a pars tensa cholesteatoma are prominent. The eroded ossicles are displaced laterally by a soft tissue mass extending into the epitympanum medial to the ossicles.

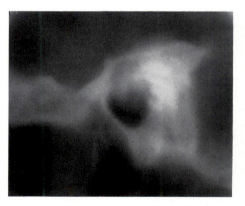

Fig. 7.**20**   Same ear as in Fig. 7.19, sagittal tomogram. In the sagittal projection the findings of a pars flaccida cholesteatoma prevail: the anterior tympanic spine and the ossicles are eroded, and there is a soft tissue mass in the epitympanum.

posterior portion of the lateral epitympanic wall and erosion of the posterosuperior bony canal wall.

Cholesteatomas may arise from central and from anterosuperior perforations of the pars tensa. In these cases the posterosuperior bony wall of the external auditory canal is intact, but the other findings of pars tensa cholesteatoma are present.

Combined Pars Flaccida and Pars Tensa Cholesteatomas

In cholesteatomas which arise from combined perforations of the pars tensa and pars flaccida the radiographic findings are a combination of the two patterns, Figs. 7.19–7.20.

The predominance of the findings depends on which portion of the tympanic membrane is more extensively involved. In combined cholesteatomas with a large pars flaccida perforation, the radiographic pattern of a pars flaccida cholesteatoma will predominate. Greater pars tensa involvement results in a chiefly pars tensa pattern.

Total Perforation

At times the entire pars flaccida and pars tensa are perforated. The pattern of bony erosion in these cases is similar to that of combined perforations. The mesotympanum appears aerated because of total atelectasis of the tympanic membrane which is in contact with the medial wall of the middle ear.

Evaluation of the Extent of Cholesteatoma

The radiographic detection of the extent of a cholesteatoma beyond the limits of the meso- and epitympanum depends on the recognition of certain bony changes in the aditus, the antrum, and the mastoid.

Aditus

Enlargement of the aditus is best seen in semiaxial tomographs and indicates extension of the cholesteatoma posterosuperiorly. The short process of the incus which lies in the adjacent fossa is usually eroded, Fig. 7.23.

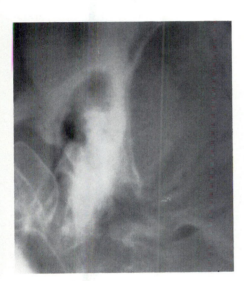

Fig. 7.**21** Cholesteatoma, Owen view, left. The cholesteatoma erodes the posterosuperior wall of the external auditory canal and creates a smooth walled cavity in the upper portion of the mastoid. The remaining portion of the mastoid is sclerotic and acellular.

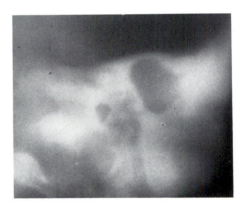

Fig. 7.**22** Same ear as in Figs. 7.21, 7.23 and 7.24, coronal tomogram. The mastoid antrum is cloudy, enlarged and the contour is smooth. The Körner's septum is absent.

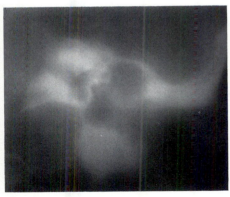

Fig. 7.**23** Same ear as in Figs. 7.21, 7.22 and 7.24, semiaxial tomogram. The aditus is markedly enlarged, and the posterior portion of the lateral epitympanic wall is grossly eroded. There is a large soft tissue mass filling the aditus and extending inferiorly.

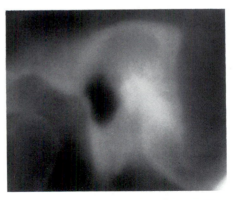

Fig. 7.**24** Same ear as in Figs. 7.21–7.23, sagittal tomogram. The cholesteatoma erodes the posterosuperior canal wall and produces a smooth cavity in the upper portion of the sclerotic mastoid.

Antrum

When the cholesteatoma extends into the mastoid antrum, the lumen of the antrum becomes cloudy. As the cholesteatoma erodes the air cells which line the walls of the antrum, the contour becomes smooth. Further extension of the cholesteatoma results in enlargement of the antral cavity, Figs. 7.21–7.24.

Superior extension of the cholesteatoma causes progressive erosion of the Körner's septum. The Körner's septum is a rather constant landmark in pneumatized mastoids and appears as a thick bony septum extending from the tegmen medially and inferiorly into the antrum and aditus. Erosion of the septum is best seen in coronal tomographs. Complete amputation of the septum indicates extension of the cholesteatoma to the tegmen of the antrum. In unilateral cholesteatoma comparison of the involved and normal side confirms the presence of erosion of the Körner's septum.

Mastoid

Further extension of the cholesteatoma into the mastoid causes progressive destruction of the trabecular pattern and formation of a large, smooth-walled cloudy cavity, Figs. 7.21–7.24.

Occasionally, the cholesteatoma may insinuate itself into the mastoid air cells without eroding the bony trabeculae. This type of involvement, usually seen in children, causes a cloudiness of the mastoid air cells which cannot be distinguished radiographically from simple mastoiditis.

Occasionally, an extensive mastoid cholesteatoma will erode the posterior portion of the lateral epitympanic wall and the posterosuperior wall of the bony external auditory canal. The cholesteatoma exteriorizes itself, discharges into the external auditory canal and forms a "natural radical" mastoid cavity. Tomographically in these cases there is a defect of varying size in the mastoid and adjacent posterosuperior external canal wall.

Complications

Complications of cholesteatomas occur when the lesion erodes the anatomical boundaries of the middle ear, antrum and mastoid or involves the facial nerve.

The most common complications are:

1. Erosion of the tegmen or sinus plate;
2. Erosion of the labyrinthine wall with fistula formation;

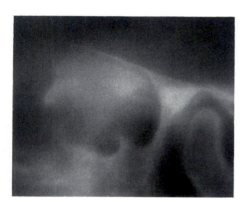

Fig. 7.**25** Cholesteatoma, sinus plate erosion, sagittal tomogram, right. A large cholesteatoma fills the entire mastoid and erodes the sinus plate posteriorly.

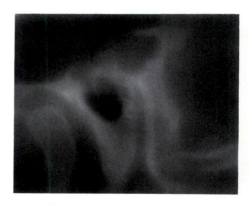

Fig. 7.**26** Cholesteatoma, tegmen erosion, sagittal tomogram, left. The cholesteatoma fills the attic and extends into the upper portion of the constricted mastoid. The tegmen is eroded superiorly.

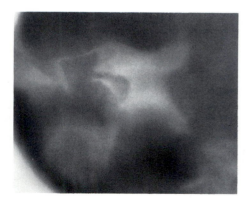

Fig. 7.**27** Cholesteatoma, labyrinthine fistula, semiaxial tomogram, right. The cholesteatoma enlarges the aditus and antrum and erodes the lateral aspect of the bony capsule of the horizontal semicircular canal.

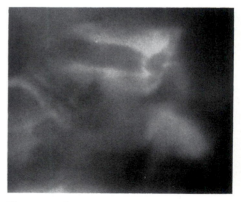

Fig. 7.**28** Cholesteatoma, tegmen erosion and labyrinthine fistula, coronal tomogram, left. A huge cholesteatoma erodes the tegmen and the bony wall of the horizontal semicircular canal.

3. Extension of the cholesteatoma into the petrous pyramid; and
4. Erosion of the facial nerve canal.

Tegmen and Sinus Plate Erosion

Erosion of the tegmen usually occurs in large cholesteatomas. In the sagittal tomographic sections there is a defect of varying size in the tegmen of the epitympanum or mastoid, Figs. 7.25–7.26. In coronal sections, the tegmen slopes downward anteriorly and is not well visualized in this projection.

Meningeal and intracranial complications may occur in association with tegmental erosions, but computerized tomography is needed to show such lesions as otogenic abscesses.

Erosion of the posterior wall of the mastoid and of the sinus plate occurs in extensive cholesteatomas and may lead to septic thrombophlebitis of the lateral sinus or to cerebellar abscess formation.

Fistulae

Labyrinthine fistulae occur most commonly in the lateral portion of the horizontal semicircular canal which bulges into the antrum. Radiographically a fistula of the horizontal simicircular canal is characterized by flattening of the normal convex contour of the canal and by a dehiscence in the labyrinthine capsule over the lumen of the canal.

Fistulae at the lateral prominence of the horizontal semicircular canal are best seen in coronal and semiaxial tomographs, Figs. 7.27–7.28. Fistulae of either the anterior or posterior aspects of the horizontal canal are exposed best in the sagittal projection, 7.32.

Fistulae in other areas of the labyrinth are rare and usually occur in large cholesteatomas which erode into the pyramid.

Horizontal semicircular canal fistulae are rare in pars flaccida cholesteatomas because the ossicles are interposed between the sac and the bony horizontal. In far

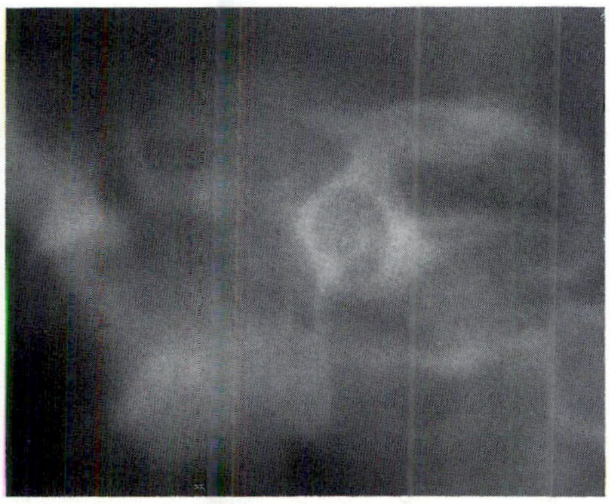

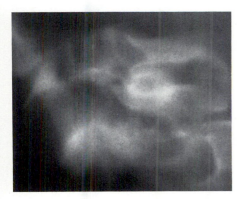

Fig. 7.29   Cholesteatoma, petrous extension and facial canal erosion, coronal tomogram, right. The cholesteatoma erodes into the petrous pyramid above the cochlea and involves the facial canal at the geniculate ganglion area.

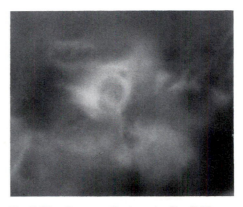

Fig. 7.30   Same patient as in Fig. 7.29, corresponding coronal tomogram of the normal left ear for comparison

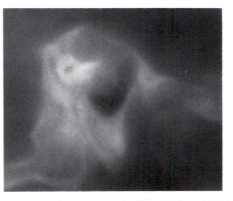

Fig. 7.31   Same ear as in Figs. 7.29 and 7.32, coronal tomogram, 4 mm posterior to Fig. 7.29. The cholesteatoma extends into the petrous pyramid to the level of the fundus of the internal auditory canal. The vestibule, horizontal and superior semicircular canals are severely eroded.

Fig. 7.32   Same ear as in Figs. 7.29 and 7.31, sagittal tomogram, right. The petrous extension of the cholesteatoma has destroyed the ampullated limbs of the horizontal and superior semicircular canals.

advanced cases a fistula may occur in association with dissolution of the ossicles.

Fistulae of the horizontal semicirucular canal are not uncommon in pars tensa cholesteatoma, because extension of the cholesteatoma from the middle ear is medial to the ossicles and in contact with the bony horizontal semicircular canal.

Petrous Extension of Cholesteatoma

Extension of acquired cholesteatomas into the petrous pyramid is rare. This extension occurs in large cholesteatomas which arise in well pneumatized petrous bones. In the medialward extension, the cholesteatoma follows the course of least resistance and erodes the thin walls of the petrous air cells, Figs. 7.29–7.32.

The paths most commonly followed by petrous extensions are:

1. Anterosuperiorly, above the cochlea, involving the geniculate ganglion and extending to the suprameatal area of the petrous bone;
2. Posterosuperiorly, between the limbs of the superior semicircular canal to reach the fundus of the internal auditory canal. These lesions may broach the wall of the internal auditory canal;
3. Infralabyrinthine, inferior to the cochlea and internal auditory canal. Such lesions may break into the jugular fossa.

The cholesteatoma may extend to reach the petrous apex by any of these routes.

Facial Nerve

Facial nerve paralysis is rare except in extensive cholesteatomas. The cholesteatomas may erode the facial nerve canal, and expose the nerve. Facial paralysis occurs when the exposed nerve is compressed by the cholesteatoma or affected by an inflammatory process.

The demonstration of erosion of the facial nerve canal is important to the otologic surgeon, since he should be aware of the erosion preoperatively to avoid damage to the exposed nerve.

The most common site of facial nerve canal erosion is the area extending from the oval window to the pyramidal eminence and the proximal portion of the vertical segment. Erosion of the anterior portion of the tympanic

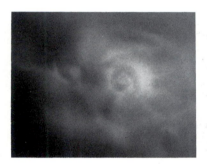

Fig. 7.**33** Cholesteatoma, congenital, coronal tomogram, right. A well defined soft tissue mass lies in the mesotympanum in contact with the tympanic membrane and promontory. There is no bony erosion.

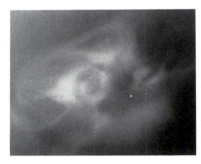

Fig. 7.**34** Normal coronal tomogram, left, for comparison with Figs. 7.33 and 7.35

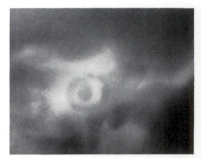

Fig. 7.**35** Cholesteatoma, congenital, coronal tomogram, left. A large soft tissue mass of cholesteatoma fills the upper portion of the tympanic cavity and extends into the epitympanum medial to the ossicles. The lateral epitympanic wall is intact.

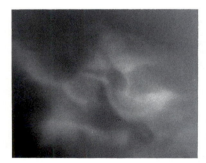

Fig. 7.**36** Cholesteatoma, congenital, coronal tomogram, right. There is a cholesteatomatous soft tissue mass in the epitympanum which erodes the medial aspect of the lateral epitympanic wall. The incus is eroded and the mastoid antrum enlarged.

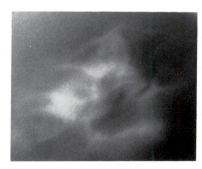

Fig. 7.**37** Normal coronal tomogram, left, for comparison with Figs. 7.36 and 7.38

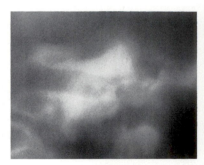

Fig. 7.**38** Cholesteatoma, congenital, coronal tomogram, left. A cholesteatomatous soft tissue mass fills the upper portion of the tympanic cavity and erodes the long process of the incus. The lateral epitympanic wall is intact, but the lesion causes the intact tympanic membrane to bulge laterally.

segment and geniculate ganglion may occur in large anterior epitympanic lesions, Fig. 7.29. Erosion of the mastoid segment of the nerve occurs in lesions which involve the entire mastoid.

Involvement of the tympanic segment of the nerve is best seen in semiaxial sections, and mastoid segment erosion best in sagittal sections.

In 50% of cases the bony canal of the horizontal portion of the facial nerve may be congenitally dehiscent. Therefore tomographic evidence of defects of the bony canal of this segment of the nerve does not indicate erosion by cholesteatoma. But erosions of the bony canal in the vertical portion or the geniculate ganglion area are significant, since they usually indicate erosion by cholesteatoma.

Congenital Cholesteatoma

Congenital cholesteatomas histologically are epidermoid tumors originating from embryonic epidermoid rests located anywhere in the temporal bone or adjacent epidural and meningeal spaces.

The clinical symptomatology of congenital cholesteatoma depends on the site and size of the lesion.

Middle Ear Cholesteatoma

Otoscopically congenital middle ear cholesteatomas appear as whitish globular masses lying medial to an intact tympanic membrane. There is usually no history of antecedent inflammatory ear disease. Occasionally there is an associated serous otitis media.

Tomographic study shows a well defined soft tissue mass within the middle ear, Figs. 7.33–7.38. If the cholesteatoma involves the entire middle ear space or if there is an accompanying serous otitis media, the entire tympanic cavity appears cloudy.

The cholesteatoma mass may erode portions of the ossicular chain. In congenital cholesteatoma the tympanic membrane often bulges laterally, Fig. 7.38. This lateral bulging seen on coronal and semiaxial tomographs enables the radiologist to differentiate the mass of the congenital cholesteatoma from serous otitis media. In both instances the middle ear will appear cloudy, but in serous otitis media the tympanic membrane is retracted medially.

The inferior margin of the lateral epitympanic wall which is typically eroded in acquired cholesteatoma is intact in congenital lesions. The medial aspect of the lateral epitympanic wall is often eroded from within when the congenital lesion extends into the epitympanum, Fig. 7.36.

Congenital cholesteatomas arising in the mastoid are very rare and appear as areas of destruction of the trabecular pattern produced by the cystic mass in the mastoid. In such cases the middle ear cavity is normal in contradistinction to acquired cholesteatoma where the middle ear is always involved.

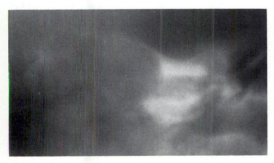

Fig. 7.**39** Cholesteatoma, congenital, petrous pyramid, coronal tomogram, left. A large expansile cholesteatoma arising from within the petrosa involves the entire petrous apex and erodes the medial portion of the internal auditory canal.

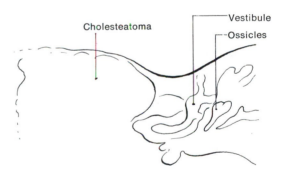

Fig. 7.**40** Diagram of Fig. 7.39

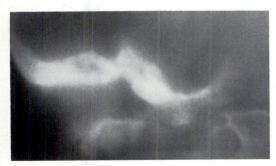

Fig. 7.**41** Cholesteatoma, congenital, petrous pyramid, coronal tomogram, right. A large cholesteatoma arising from the epidural space erodes the superior aspect of the petrous pyramid, the labyrinth and internal auditory canal are markedly eroded.

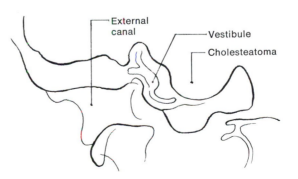

Fig. 7.**42** Diagram of Fig. 7.41

Petrous Pyramid Cholesteatoma

Clinically the first sign of a congenital cholestatoma of the petrous pyramid is a facial paralysis of slow onset followed by sensorineural hearing loss caused by erosion of the labyrinth. In the early stages the middle ear may be normal.

Radiographic findings depend on whether the cholesteatoma arises from within the petrous apex or from the adjacent epidural or meningeal spaces.

When the cholesteatoma arises from within the petrous apex, multidirectional or computerized tomography will show an expansile, cystic lesion in the apex. The involved

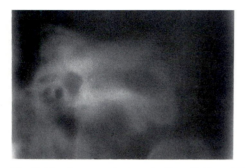

Fig. 7.**43** Same patient as in Figs. 7.44 and 7.45, corresponding coronal tomogram of normal right ear for comparison

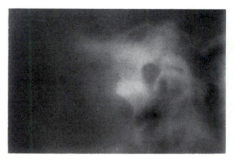

Fig. 7.**44** Cholesteatoma, congenital, jugular fossa, coronal tomogram, left. The jugular fossa and the posteroinferior aspect of the petrous pyramid are eroded by a large cholesteatoma. The hypotympanic floor is intact.

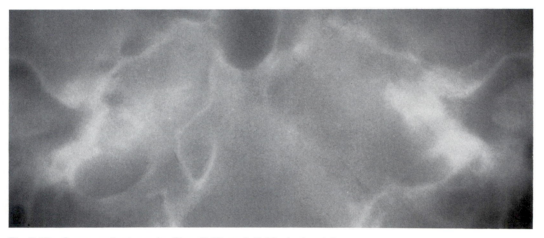

Fig. 7.**45** Same patient as in Figs. 7.43 and 7.44, horizontal tomogram. The left jugular fossa is expanded. The clivus and hypoglossal canal on the left are eroded.

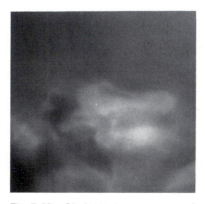

Fig. 7.**46** Cholesteatoma, congenital, cerebellopontile angle, coronal tomogram, right. The medial portion of the internal auditory canal measures 1.5 mm wider than the corresponding segment of the left internal canal, Fig. 7.47.

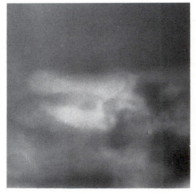

Fig. 7.**47** Same patient as in Fig. 7.46, corresponding coronal tomogram of normal left ear for comparison

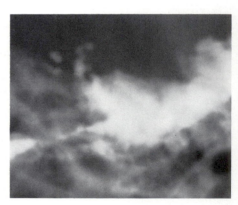

Fig. 7.**48** Same patient as in Figs. 7.46 and 7.47, cerebellopontile cisternogram, right. A lobulated mass of the cholesteatoma is outlined in the cerebellopontile cistern. There is no filling of the internal auditory canal.

area of the pyramid is expanded, and the superior pet-rous ridge is usually elevated and thinned out. As the lesion expands the internal auditory canal and the laby-rinth become eroded, Figs. 7.39–7.40.

Cholesteatomas arising from the epidural or meningeal spaces on the superior aspect of the pyramid cause a scooped out defect of the superior aspect of the pyramid. The defect is caused by erosion of the pyramid from without, and there is no bony rim as in lesions arising from within the pyramid, Fig. 7.41–7.42.

Cholesteatoma of the epidural or meningeal spaces originating in the jugular fossa area can mimic glomus jugulare tumors clinically and radiographically, Figs. 7.44–7.45. Similar to glomus jugular tumors, these pri-mary cholesteatomas expand the jugular fossa and erode the posteroinferior aspect of the petrous pyramid and adjacent occipital bone. The differentiation between cholesteatoma and glomus tumor can often be made tomographically, since congenital cholesteatomas of the jugular area usually do not erode the floor of the hypotympanum and extend into the middle ear as glomus jugulare do. In doubtful cases angiography is indicated.

Congenital cholesteatomas of the cerebellopontine angle produce signs and symptoms similar to an acoustic neuroma.

In cholesteatoma of the angle the lumen of the internal auditory canal usually is not expanded, but here is ero-sion and shortening of the posterior wall of the internal canal, Figs. 7.46–7.47.

Cerebellopontine cisternography in congenital choles-teatoma reveals a mass which usually blocks the aperture of the internal auditory canal. The mass has a charac-teristic lobulated appearance quite different from the smooth contour of acoustic neuroma, Fig. 7.48.

Computerized Tomography

Computerized tomography is especially useful in the study of epidural cholesteatomas. Preinfusion sections usually show an area of decreased absorption in the affected area, Fig. 7.49.

Post infusion sections in epidural cholesteatomas reveal a ring-like area of enhancement which corresponds to the capsule of the cholesteatoma, Figs. 7.50–7.51.

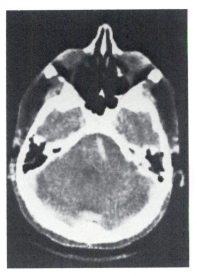

Fig. 7.**50**   Same ear as Figs. 7.49 and 7.51, Horizontal CT sec-tion, post-infusion. A band-like area of enhancement is demons-trated in the capsule of the cholesteatoma. The fourth ventricle is slightly displaced to the right.

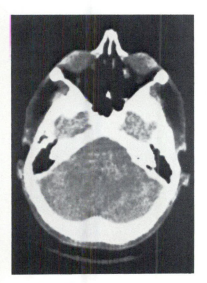

Fig. 7.**49**   Cholesteatoma, congenital, cerebellopontile angle, computerized tomography, axial section, pre-infusion, left. There is an area of slightly decreased absorption in the region of the left cerebellopontile angle.

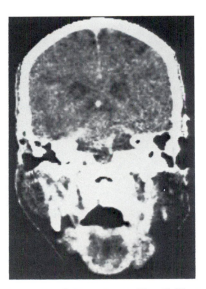

Fig. 7.**51**   Same ear as Figs. 7.49 and 7.50, coronal sections, post-infusion. A ring-like area of enhancement outlines the cholesteatoma.

Cholesteatoma of the External Auditory Canal

There are two types of cholesteatoma of the external auditory canal. The first type, keratosis obliterans, is caused by osteomas, stenosis of the canal or hard masses of cerumen. Blockage of the external canal for a long period permits epithelial debris to accumulate in the canal and enlarge the bony contour of the external canal. Tomographically there is concentric enlargement of the bony external auditory canal by a soft tissue mass medial to the site of the canal stenosis or obstruction, Figs. 7.52–7.53.

The other type of cholesteatoma of the external canal is called invasive keratitis and is characterized by localized accumulations of desquamated debris which occur on the floor of the bony canal, Figs. 7.54–7.56.

Removal of the debris reveals deep localized erosions of the bony canal wall and areas of exposed, necrotic bone. Occasionally the lesions extend and involve almost the entire circumference of the external canal. There is a history of antecedent radiotherapy to the area of the ear in approximately 50% of these cases. In invasive kerotitis, tomography shows erosion of the cortex of the involved portion of the canal. In larger lesions there are scooped out defects of the bony canal wall. When the lesion is diffuse, there is expansion of the involved canal segment without obstruction of the canal lumen.

When the external canal cholesteatoma is large and reaches the anulus, the lesion erodes into the middle ear and attic. Erosion of the lateral attic wall is often seen in the tomograms, Figs. 7.52–7.53.

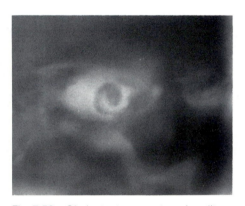

Fig. 7.**52**   Cholesteatoma, external auditory canal, coronal tomogram, left. The external canal is grossly expanded, and the contour of the floor is markedly excavated. There is a soft tissue mass in the lumen of the canal. The cholesteatoma extends into the epitympanum through an erosion of the lateral epitympanic wall.

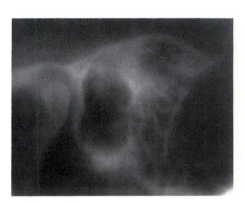

Fig. 7.**53**   Same patient as in Fig. 7.52, sagittal tomogram, left. There is a deep excavation of the canal floor and extension of the lesion into the epitympanum.

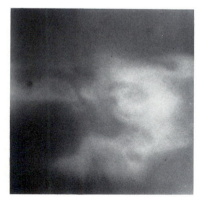

Fig. 7.**54**   Cholesteatoma, external auditory canal, invasive keratitis, coronal tomogram, right. There is a smooth erosion of the lateral portion of the floor of the bony external canal. The medial portion of the bony canal is intact.

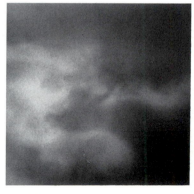

Fig. 7.**55**   Same patient as in Figs. 7.54 and 7.56, normal left coronal tomogram for comparison.

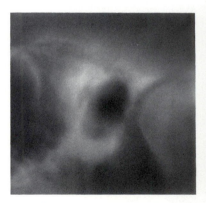

Fig. 7.**56**   Same ear as in Fig. 7.54, sagittal tomogram. The floor of the lateral portion of the external canal is excavated causing a double contour inferiorly.

Chapter 8   Postoperative Radiology of the Mastoid

Postoperative radiographs of the ear are difficult to interpret. The bony landmarks are usually missing, and there is often clouding of the mastoid cavity because of recurrent pathologic changes or because tissue grafts or flaps were used to fill the mastoidectomy cavity. In addition, with passage of time new bone formation may partially fill in the surgical defects.

To understand and interpret the postoperative radiographic findings of the ear the radiologist should be acquainted with the basic techniques of middle ear and mastoid surgery.

Simple and Radical Mastoidectomy

Mastoid surgery may be divided into simple and radical procedures.

Simple Mastoidectomy

A simple mastoidectomy consists in drilling away the external mastoid cortex and exenterating the mastoid air cells.

Air cell exenteration extends to the mastoid antrum. When indicated by the pathology the dissection will extend anterosuperiorly to the epitympanum. The surgeon drills between the dural plate and the superior wall of the external auditory canal and leaves the inferior margin of the lateral epitympanic wall intact.

At times the surgeon may only explore the antrum and epitympanum. In these cases he removes only enough mastoid cortex and mastoid air cells to expose these areas.

Radical and Modified Radical Mastoidectomies

The essential feature which differentiates a simple mastoidectomy from one of the various types of radical mastoidectomies is that in the radical procedure the mastoid bridge is removed. During the surgical dissection of the mastoid, the lateral portion of the posterosuperior bony canal wall and upper portion of the lateral epitympanic wall are first drilled away. This leaves a bony arch called the mastoid bridge which is made up of the medial portion of the posterosuperior bony canal wall and the inferior margin of the epitympanic wall.

This bridge is removed during one of the last stages of the operation and converts a simple mastoidectomy into a radical mastoidectomy. Removal of the bridge transforms the mastoid cavity and the external canal into a common cavity.

The modified radical mastoidectomy is the most commonly performed type of radical mastoidectomy. In the modified radical mastoidectomy remnants of the tympanic membrane and ossicles are retained to preserve hearing.

In the true radical mastoidectomy, which is rarely performed, all middle ear structures and tympanic membrane remnants are removed.

Tympanoplasty

Tympanoplasties are surgical procedures of the middle ear and mastoid designed to improve hearing. There are five classical types of tympanoplasties. In Type I and II a graft is used to cover defects of the tympanic membrane. In Type III and IV usually some form of mastoidectomy and ossicular reconstruction are performed. Type V is rarely performed and consists of a fenestration of the horizontal semicircular canal and preservation of a reduced middle ear space.

Radiographic Findings

Postoperative radiography of the ear is difficult and tomography is essential to evaluate pathology correctly.

The postoperative radiographic evaluation of the ear requires a knowledge of: 1. the pathology for which the surgery was performed; 2. the type of surgery performed; and 3. the clinical and otoscopic findings that make further x-ray studies necessary.

In postoperative radiography of the ear an almost infinite spectrum of findings may occur depending on variables of the preoperative pathology, the surgical procedure, and recurrent or residual disease.

Ideally whenever the surgeon feels that, at the end of the surgery, there is residual disease he should secure a postoperative tomographic study which can serve as a base line for subsequent evaluations.

A disease-free surgical cavity appears as a well defined and sharply outlined defect in the mastoid, epitympanum and external canal depending on the type of surgery performed. Small defects in the tegmen produced during surgery are of no significance.

The mastoid cavity is usually clear unless some form of fibromuscular flap was used to fill the mastoid. The radiologist must be informed about the use of such flaps. The middle ear cavity may be normal in size or contracted. The ossicles may be normal, completely absent, or transposed.

The facial nerve canal is intact or exposed depending on the type of surgery and preoperative disease.

Postoperative Pathology

Postoperative pathologic changes in the ear involve bony and soft tissue structures.

Bony changes in the mastoid depend on whether infection, cholesteatoma or both are present.

If there is persistent or recurrent infection in the mastoid, the outline of the cavity becomes poorly defined and irregular due to osteitis of the walls. The trabeculae of residual air cells become demineralized and in longstanding infection sclerotic.

If recurrent cholesteatoma is filling the mastoidectomy cavity there is expansion of the cavity and thinning of the walls which leads to erosions in the tegmen and sinus plates, Figs. 8.6–8.7.

Fistulae of the labyrinth may be present. However, without a description of the pre- and intraoperative findings, the radiologist will be unable to tell if such fistuale existed prior to surgery.

Ossicles

Radiographic appearance of the ossicular chain will depend on whether the ossicles have been removed at surgery, left in place, or transposed.

The body of the incus is the ossicle most often transposed. When properly transposed the body of the incus can be easily seen lying in the posterosuperior quadrant of the middle ear between the tympanic membrane or malleus handle and the oval window region.

With recurrent infection the incus may be resorbed. Placement of the incus between the tympanic membrane or malleus handle and the stapes may fail, and the incus migrate inferiorly where it is visualized tomographically. Recurrent cholesteatoma can displace a transposed incus inferiorly, Figs. 8.1–8.3.

Soft Tissue Changes

Following radical mastoidectomy the mastoid and external ear common cavity must be cleaned periodically to prevent accumulation of necrotic epithelial debris and cerumen. Usually the cavity is not completely filled with debris so that the tomographs show only partial cloudiness. If debris has been allowed to accumulate over a period of years the cavity will appear completely cloudy.

Infection and recurrent cholesteatomas will also fill and opacify the mastoid cavity, Figs. 8.6–8.7.

The middle ear is often decreased in size but aerated following a successful mastoid surgery. Clouding of the constricted middle ear cavity is evidence of recurrent infection or cholesteatoma.

At times, following tympanoplasty, the graft used to reconstruct the tympanic membrane becomes displaced in an abnormally lateral position. Thickened and scarred lateralized grafts can be seen in coronal and semiaxial tomographs, Figs. 8.4–8.5.

Meningocele and Meningoencephalocele

A soft tissue mass contiguous to a defect in the tegmen of the mastoid suggests the possibility of a meningocele or meningoencephalocele. If the brain and meninges herniate into the relatively small space of the antrum or epitympanum, the constant pulsation of the cerebrospinal fluid is transmitted through the walls of the meningocele to cause a gradual resorption of the surrounding bony walls. This results in a typical rounded bony defect seen in the tomographs, Figs. 8.8–8.11.

Computerized tomography is useful in differentiating the soft tissue mass of a meningocele or meningoencephalocele from a recurrent cholesteatoma, since recurrent cholesteatoma will also produce a smooth bony defect. The density of a meningocele will be the same as cerebrospinal fluid, the density of an encephalocele that of brain tissue, but the density of a cholesteatoma will be greater than that of the two former conditions.

Stenosis of the External Auditory Canal

At times following myringoplasty and tympanoplasty where the external canal is preserved, the canal becomes filled with a fibrous scar. The tympanic membrane graft may also heal in a position far lateral to the bony sulcus.

Tomographically when scar tissued fills the canal the air column of the external canal ends in a blind sac lateral to the bony sulcus.

When there is lateralization of the graft the external canal is air-filled, and the lateralized graft, if thick, will be visible on the tomographs.

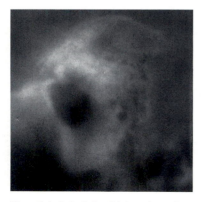 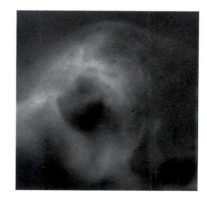 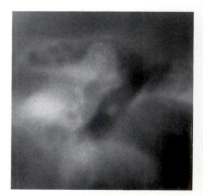

Figs. 8.**1**, 8.**2**, 8.**3**   Dislocation of transposed incus, left: 8.1 only malleus present in epitympanum. 8.2 and 8.3 incus displaced inferiorly, below level of oval window.

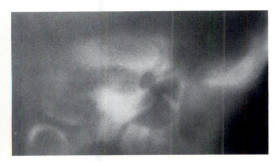

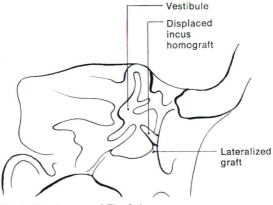

Fig. 8.4 Lateralization of tympanic membrane graft with lateral displacement of transposed incus, coronal tomogram, left

Fig. 8.5 Diagram of Fig. 8.4

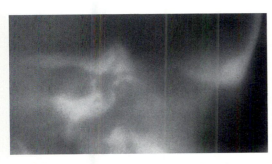

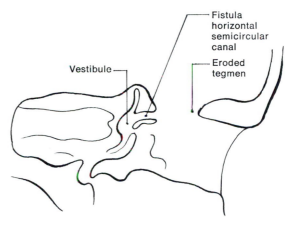

Fig. 8.6 Recurrent cholesteatoma, coronal tomogram, left. The tegmen of the mastoidectomy cavity is eroded and there is a fistula of the horizontal semicircular canal. A soft tissue mass fills the entire mastoid cavity and middle ear.

Fig. 8.7 Diagram of Fig. 8.6

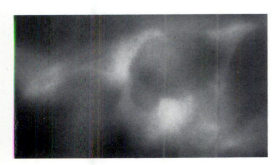

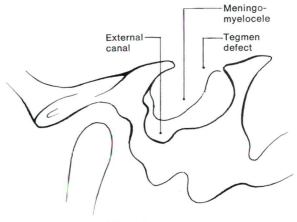

Fig. 8.8 Postmastoidectomy meningocele, sagittal tomogram, left. A soft tissue mass herniates into the mastoid cavity through a large tegmental defect. The cavity contour is rounded and the margins of the tegmental defect are sharp.

Fig. 8.9 Diagram of Fig. 8.8

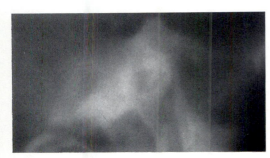

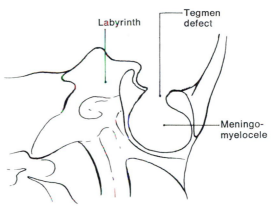

Fig. 8.10 Same patient as in Fig. 8.8, coronal tomogram. A well defined soft tissue mass lies within the smooth-walled mastoidectomy cavity.

Fig. 8.11 Diagram of Fig. 8.10

Chapter 9   Benign Tumors

Benign tumors of the temporal bone originate in the squama, the mastoid and the petrous pyramid or from adjacent structures such as the meninges, the jugular vein and cranial nerves.

Acoustic neuromas and glomus jugulare tumors will be discussed in more detail separately.

Exostoses

Exostoses are the most common tumor of the external auditory canal. Exostoses represent local or diffuse areas of hyperostosis often caused by frequent swimming. They are usually multiple, large or small, and often are bilateral. Small lesions cause no symptoms, while large lesions obstruct the canal.

Tomographically exostoses have a variable appearance. Small lesions appear as dense nodules, protruding into the lumen of the external auditory canal. More diffuse lesions appear as dense bony ridges which stretch along the canal walls. Occasionally the entire circumference of the canal is thickened and the lumen is constricted, Fig. 9.1.

Osteoma

Osteomas are benign bony tumors which are usually single and may occur anywhere in the temporal bone. There are two types, the cancellous and the compact. Radiographically the compact lesion appears as a well defined, occasionally lobulated dense bony mass. Cancellous osteomas appear as partially ossified masses.

A common site is the external auditory canal where the osteoma appears as a single bony mass occluding the lumen. This lesion may cause retention of epithelial debris and cerumen which results in cholesteatoma of the external auditory canal, Fig. 9.2.

Osteomas may also occur as a solitary lesion in the squama, mastoid, middle ear and petrous pyramid.

In the squama, an osteoma produces a hard bony mass on the surface of the bone usually above and posterior to the auricle. When they occur in the mastoid, osteomas are usually asymptomatic unless they encroach upon the facial nerve.

Osteomas may lie in the middle ear and cause conductive hearing loss by impinging upon the ossicular chain, Fig. 9.3.

In the petrous pyramid, osteomas usually are situated in the region of the porus of the internal auditory canal. Rarely they may encroach on the neurovascular structures of the internal auditory canal and cause hearing and vestibular disturbances.

Adenoma

Adenomas usually occur in the fibrocartilagenous portion of the external auditory canal. As with other benign tumors of the external canal, radiography is not indicated unless the lesion obstructs the canal and obscures the view of the tympanic membrane and middle ear.

Middle ear adenomas are rare. The lesion has a tendency to recur after surgery and may degenerate into a adenocarcinoma.

Tomographically an adenoma appears as a diffuse or localized nonspecific soft tissue mass in the tympanic cavity. There is no bony erosion unless malignant degeneration of the adenoma into an adenocarcinoma has occurred, Figs. 9.4, 9.5.

Hemangioma

Hemangiomas are rare tumors of the temporal bone. The clinical and radiographic features depend on the anatomical location.

They may occur in the temporal squama where they produce an area of radiolucency with typical spoke-like trabeculation.

A hemangioma of the external canal can fill and enlarge the bony canal. A radiographic diagnosis can be made if there are phleboliths within the lesion.

A hemangioma of the middle ear results in a poorly defined soft tissue mass which may be associated with ossicular erosion, Figs. 9.6, 9.7. A hemangioma can be differentiated from a glomus jugulare tumor because hemangiomas do not erode the hypotympanic floor.

Hemangiomas of the petrous pyramid produce a diffuse mottled demineralization with multiple honeycombed radiolucencies.

A hemangioma may lie in the internal auditory canal and cerebellopontine angle and mimic an acoustic neuroma. Differentiation can be made by computerized tomography or subtraction arteriography.

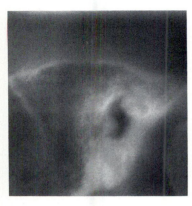

Fig. 9.**1**   Exostosis, external auditory canal, sagittal tomogram, right. The lumen of the canal is stenosed by exostoses arising from the anterior and posterior walls of the canal.

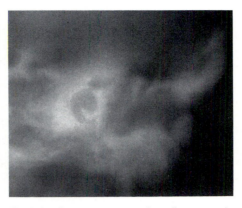

Fig. 9.**2**   Osteoma, external auditory canal, coronal tomogram, left. A well defined bony mass narrows the lumen of the canal laterally.

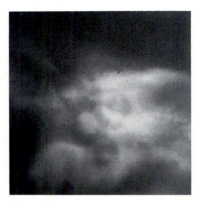

Fig. 9.**3**   Osteoma, middle ear, coronal tomogram, right. A well defined bony mass arises from the promontory and lies in contact with the tympanic membrane.

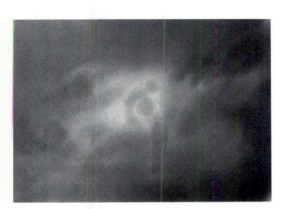

Fig. 9.**4**   Adenoma, middle ear, coronal tomogram, left. A soft tissue mass fills the tympanic cavity to the level of the malleus head.

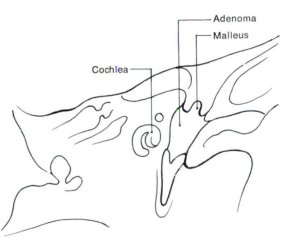

Fig. 9.**5**   Diagram of Fig. 9.4

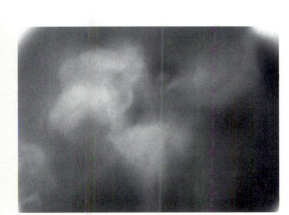

Fig. 9.**6**   Hemangioma, middle ear, semiaxial tomogram, left. A soft tissue mass fills the posterosuperior portion of the tympanic cavity and erodes the long process of the incus.

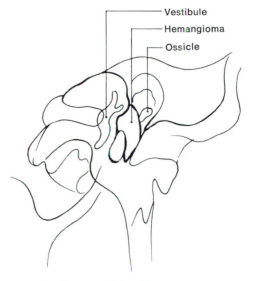

Fig. 9.**7**   Diagram of Fig. 9.6

Meningioma

Meningiomas arise from the meningeal covering of the temporal bone and from meningeal extension within the internal auditory canal.

The most common type of meningioma arises from the dura covering the petrous ridge. Radiographically the findings vary from hyperostosis to moth-eaten erosion which can progress to frank destruction of the petrous bone. Often there is a combination of these findings, Figs. 9.12–9.15.

One form of hyperostotic meningioma is the en plaque lesion. A characteristic manifestation of this lesion is the presence of a calcified layer separated from the surface of the temporal bone by a radiolucent band, Figs. 9.8–9.11. Some meningiomas erode the tegmen and break into the middle ear cavity. Occasionally a meningioma can involve the middle ear cavity without apparent erosion of the tegmen, Fig. 9.8. The facial nerve is often involved in the region of the geniculate ganglion. Erosion of the labyrinth is rare.

Computerized tomography is indicated in cases where a meningioma is suspected, since this technique will demonstrate the involvement of the base of the skull and the presence of any intracranial component of the tumor, Figs. 9.18–9.21.

Meningiomas arising within the internal auditory canal and cerebellopontine angle cistern mimic acoustic neuromas clinically and radiographically. Differential diagnosis can be made if there is hyperostosis of the walls of the internal auditory canal and of the crista falciformis or if there are calcifications scattered within the mass, Figs. 9.16, 9.17.

Cerebellopontine cisternography will outline the size of the mass but will not differentiate the type of lesion.

Computerized tomography and arteriography are required to differentiate meningioma from acoustic neuroma and other cerebellopontine angle masses, Figs. 9.20, 9.21.

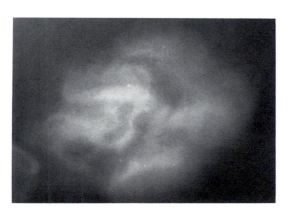

Fig. 9.**8** Meningioma, temporal bone, semiaxial tomogram, left. There is a marked hyperostotic meningioma of the superior aspect of the petrous pyramid. The lesion extends into the middle ear cavity which is cloudy.

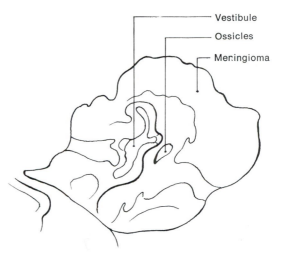

Fig. 9.**9** Diagram of Fig. 9.8

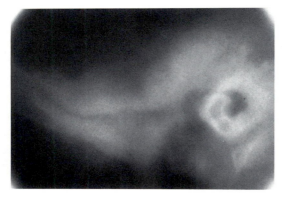

Fig. 9.**10** Same ear as in Fig. 9.8, sagittal tomogram. The hyperostotic process extends from the petrous pyramid along the floor of the middle cranial fossa. A radiolucent band separates the lesion from the underlying surface of the base of the skull.

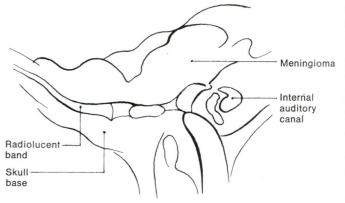

Fig. 9.**11** Diagram of Fig. 9.10

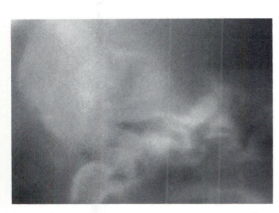

Fig. 9.**12** Meningioma, petrous pyramid, coronal tomogram, left. A large, poorly calcified mass involves the petrous pyramid. There is a combination of hyperostotic and destructive changes.

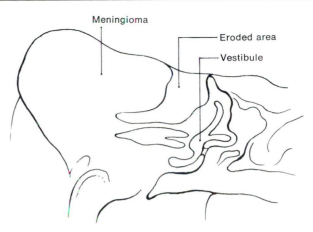

Fig. 9.**13** Diagram of Fig. 9.12

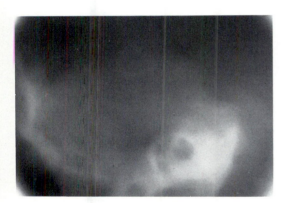

Fig. 9.**14** Same ear as in Fig. 9.12, sagittal tomogram. There is a severe erosion of the anterior portion of the petrous pyramid and adjacent floor of the middle cranial fossa by a large, poorly calcified meningioma.

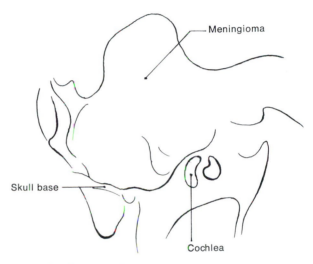

Fig. 9.**15** Diagram of Fig. 9.14

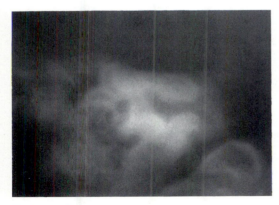

Fig. 9.**16** Meningioma, petrous pyramid and internal auditory canal, coronal tomogram, right. There is hyperostosis of the petrous bone forming the walls of the internal auditory canal. The porus is narrow, and the posterior canal wall shortened.

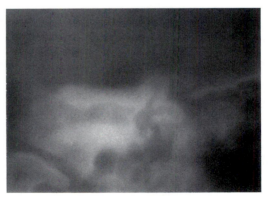

Fig. 9.**17** Same patient as in Fig. 9.16, corresponding coronal tomogram of normal left ear for comparison

Neuromas of the Cranial Nerves V, IX, X, XII

Neuromas of the cranial nerves V, VII, VIII, IX, X, XI, XII may involve the petrous pyramid. Neuromas of the VIIth and VIIIth cranial nerves are discussed in Chapters 10 and 12.

These tumors which are usually neuromas or neurofibromas arise within the temporal bone or in adjacent spaces such as the jugular fossa, cerebellopontine cistern, and the Meckel's cave, Figs. 9.22–9.24.

Vth Nerve Neuromas

Neuromas of the Vth nerve arising from the gasserian ganglion tend to enlarge superiorly into the middle cranial fossa. Occasionally these tumors cause indentation and erosion of the superior petrous ridge medial to the internal auditory canal.

Coronal, sagittal, and Stenvers tomographic projections will demonstrate the site and degree of bony involvement.

Arteriography with and without subtraction will show displacement of vessels in the region of the middle cranial fossa. There will be a blush if the lesion is vascular.

Postinfusion computerized tomography is also useful to demonstrate the tumor mass.

IXth, Xth, XIth, XIIth Nerve Neuromas

Neuromas of the IXth, Xth, XIth, XIIth nerves arise in the jugular fossa or in the hypoglossal canal. They produce paralytic lesions of varying types. As the tumor

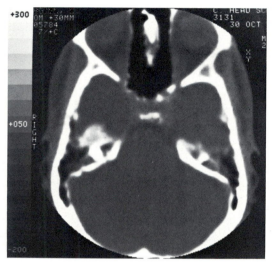

Fig. 9.18   Meningioma, petrous pyramid, computerized tomography, horizontal section. The meningioma produces thickening and hyperostosis of the anterior aspect of the right petrous pyramid.

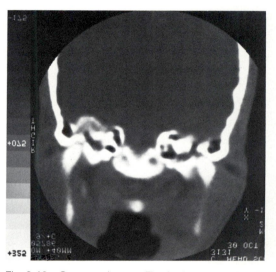

Fig. 9.19   Same patient as Fig. 9.18, coronal CT. The coronal CT shows the hyperostosis of the superior aspect of the right petrous pyramid at the level of the tegmen tympani.

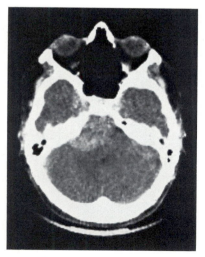

Fig. 9.20   Meningioma, cerebellopontine angle, CT, horizontal section. Following infusion of contrast material there is enhancement of a large soft tissue mass of the right cerebellopontine and prepontine cisterns.

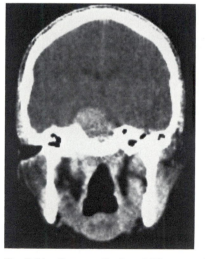

Fig. 9.21   Same patient as 9.20, coronal CT. The enhanced mass extends through the tentorial notch into the middle cranial fossa.

enlarges it produces a progressive expansion of the jugular fossa and hypoglossal canal similar to the lesion of a glomus jugulare tumor, Figs. 9.22–9.24. Neuromas can also extend intracranially into the posterior cranial fossa and the foramen magnum.

Neuromas of the IXth, Xth, XIth, XIIth nerves are differentiated from glomus tumors by the following tomographic features:

1. In neuromas the contour of the bone surrounding the lesion is smooth and sharply demarcated. In glomus tumors the contour of the eroded jugular fossa is poorly defined.
2. Neuromas do not erode the floor of the middle ear while glomus tumors erode the middle ear.
3. Expansion rather than erosion of the hypoglossal canal is pathognomonic of a neuroma of the XIIth nerve. As the lesion enlarges the hypoglossal canal becomes completely destroyed. Glomus tumors erode the jugular end of the hypoglossal canal.

Conventional radiography and tomography are necessary to demonstrate the site and extent of the involvement of the base of the skull. Tomography demonstrates the erosion much better than conventional radiographs. Coronal, sagittal, horizontal and Stenvers tomographic projections expose the involved areas.

If the tumor is large, arteriography will demonstrate displacement of the vessels of the posterior cranial fossa. Since neuromas are poorly vascularized, the tumor mass cannot be outlined by arteriography.

Posterior fossa myelography is useful to demonstrate defects or blockage of the subarachnoid space at the foramen magnum or posterior cranial fossa cisterns.

Computerized tomography will demonstrate bony erosions caused by the tumors. If the density of the mass is enhanced after infusion, computerized tomography will outline the lesion.

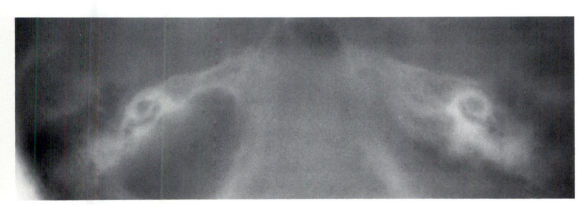

Fig. 9.22 Neuroma, XIIth nerve, horizontal tomogram, right. A neuroma of the XIIth nerve causes a large, smooth-walled lesion in the region of the jugular fossa. The posterior surface of the petrosa is eroded.

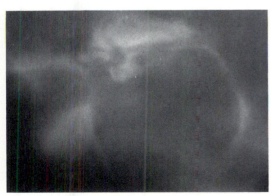

Fig. 9.23 Same patient as in ig. 9.22, coronal tomogram. The large neuroma erodes the inferior aspect of the petrous bone and hypoglossal canal. The bony floor of the middle ear is elevated, but preserved.

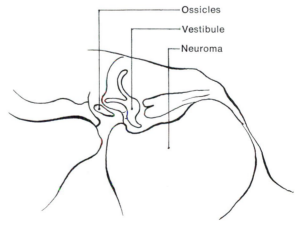

Fig. 9.24 Diagram of Fig. 9.23

Eosinophilic Granuloma

Eosinophilic granuloma is a benign chronic granuloma related to other diseases of the reticuloendothelial system such as Letterer-Siwe, Hand-Schüller-Christian, and histiocystosis X. The etiology is unknown, but eosinophilic granuloma is commonly classified as a benign tumor.

Eosinophilic granuloma of the temporal bone usually involves the mastoid. Radiographically the findings are similar to an acute mastoiditis with areas of coalescence. The involved mastoid air cells appear cloudy, and the trabecular pattern is destroyed with formation of a cav-

ity. The mastoid cortex may be thinned, destroyed, or expanded, Figs. 9.25–9.28.

The differential diagnosis from acute mastoditis is made by clinical history. In acute mastoiditis, there are fever, tenderness, and draining from the ear. In eosinophilic granuloma there are no systemic symptoms and the swollen mastoid is not tender. There may be discharge from the ear and granulation in the middle ear and external canal.

When the disorder affects the squama, eosinophilic granuloma causes lytic areas of variable size. There is no reactive new bone at the margins of the lesion.

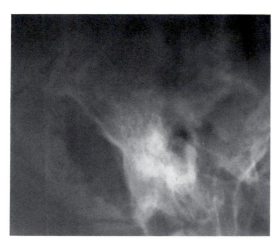

Fig. 9.**25**   Eosinophilic granuloma, Schüller view, right. There is a large coalescent lesion in the posterior aspect of the mastoid. The eroded cavity and mastoid cells are cloudy.

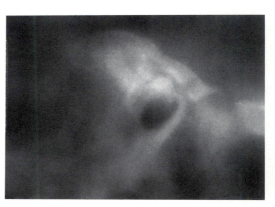

Fig. 9.**26**   Same ear as in Figs. 9.25 and 9.27, sagittal tomogram. A large destructive lesion is present in the mastoid. The sinus plate is partially eroded.

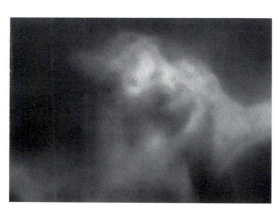

Fig. 9.**27**   Same ear as in Figs. 9.25 and 9.26, sagittal tomogram, 6 mm medial to Fig. 9.26. Multiple areas of destruction are present in the petrous pyramid.

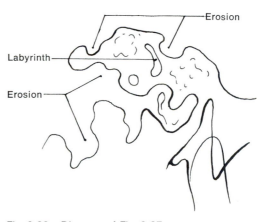

Fig. 9.**28**   Diagram of Fig. 9.27

Glomus Tumors

Glomus tumors, also called chemodectomas and non-chromaffin paragangliomas, are benign tumors arising in the middle ear or jugular fossa from minute glomus bodies which are found chiefly in the jugular fossa and on the promontory of the middle ear.

The symptomatology depends on the site and size of the lesion. Lesions arising in the jugular fossa, called glomus jugulare tumors, encroach upon the adjacent cranial nerves and may cause paralysis of these nerves. The tumor usually involves the middle ear where it may cause conductive deafness by encroaching upon the ossicular chain. As the lesion enlarges it extends into the mastoid and external auditory canal. Involvement of the labyrinth causes tinnitus, sensorineural deafness and vertigo. Glomus tympanicum is a lesion which arises from glomus bodies along the Jacobson's nerve on the promontory. Early these lesions are small and confined to the middle ear, where they may encroach upon the ossicles. If the lesion enlarges inferiorly and destroys the hypotympanic floor they become indistinguishable from glomus jugulare tumurs.

Otoscopic Findings

The characteristic finding of a glomus tumor is the presence of a reddish purple mass in the middle ear. In the early stages the mass lies medial to the intact tympanic membrane. Contact of the tumor with the tympanic membrane often causes a curvilinear air-tumor interface. Since both glomus jugulare and glomus tympanicum tumors arise in the inferior portion of the middle ear, otoscopic differentiation between the two types is impossible.

As the lesions enlarge, the tympanic membrane is sloughed, and reddish purple polypoid masses appear in the external auditory canal. These polypoid lesions bleed easily and profusely when manipulated, while inflammatory polyps of chronic otitis media bleed only slightly. The diagnosis should be confirmed by biopsy. This procedure should be performed after radiographic evaluation to avoid obscuring the mass by hemorrhage.

When confined to the middle ear and lying behind an intact tympanic membrane, the otoscopic appearance of a glomus tumor may be confused with a high jugular bulb, an ectopic internal carotid artery or with a cholesterol granuloma of the middle ear.

Radiographic Technique

Several radiographic techniques are used to study glomus tumors. These include conventional radiography, tomography, arteriography, retrograde jugular venography and computerized tomography.

Conventional Radiography

Glomus tympanicum tumors cannot be visualized by conventional radiography, since they are confined to the middle ear. Glomus jugulare tumors which have eroded large areas of the bone around the jugular fossa can be diagnosed by Towne-Chamberlain, Stenvers, and modified basal views.

The modified basal view is obtained by elevating the basal plane of the skull anteriorly 20° to 30° from the film plane. This angulation exposes the jugular foramen. An additional view for the study of the jugular foramen area is the Chausse II, an open mouth oblique view of the skull base.

Tomography

Tomography is the method of choice in the study of glomus tumors since this technique demonstrates soft tissue lesions of the middle ear as well as bony erosion.

Coronal, sagittal, and semiaxial sections of the middle ear and petrous pyramid are indicated. The entire undersurface of the petrous pyramid and the adjacent occipital bone should be included in the tomographic sections. When the lesion extends beyond the middle ear, basal tomographic sections are also indicated.

Arteriography

The feeding vessels of a glomus tumor arise from branches of the external carotid, the internal carotid, and the vertebral circulation. Injection should be done in the common carotid to visualize internal and external carotid circulation. The ascending pharyngeal artery is usually the largest feeding vessel. A vertebral arteriogram may also be performed.

Subtraction should be used to delineate the vascular mass and feeding vessels which are otherwise obscured by the density of the surrounding temporal bone.

Retrograde Venography

This study is done by percutaneous puncture of the jugular vein with a Seldinger needle. The stylet is withdrawn and a guide wire is advanced through the needle lumen into the internal jugular vein to the bony roof of the jugular fossa. The needle is removed then, and a radiopaque polyethylene catheter is threaded into the jugular vein over the guide wire which is in turn removed.

Computerized Tomography

Computerized tomography both axial and coronal, will demonstrate bony erosions, and after infusion will demonstrate large vascular masses.

Radiographic Findings

Glomus Tympanicum

In glomus tympanicum the tomographic examination shows a soft tissue mass of variable size usually in the lower portion of the tympanic cavity, Figs. 9.29–9.32. The nature of the soft tissue mass cannot be determined by the tomographs. The otoscopic appearance of a red-purple mass within the middle ear strongly suggests that the lesion is a glomus tumor but biopsy is necessary. When inflammation or serous fluid fills the middle ear and surrounds the tumor the outline of the mass is obscured.

A large glomus tympanicum filling the entire middle ear causes a bulge of the tympanic membrane laterally and a concave erosion of the bone of the promontory. The lesion may also extend posteriorly into the mastoid. In glomus tympanicum the roof of the jugular fossa is intact, and this feature differentiates glomus tympanicum from a glomus jugulare.

Subtraction arteriography demonstrates the vascular mass in the middle ear and the supplying vessels. Jugular venography will be negative.

Glomus Jugulare

The radiographic evaluation of glomus jugulare tumors depends on the size and extension of the lesion. Large lesions produce erosions visible by conventional radiography, but more detailed information is gained by tomography. Smaller lesions may be invisible by conventional studies and are only seen by tomography.

Typical tomographic findings of a glomus jugulare tumor are, Figs. 9.33–9.39:

1. Erosion of the cortical outline and enlargement of the jugular fossa. The size of the jugular fossa is extremely variable and asymmetry of the two jugular fossae is a common finding. A large jugular fossa is not indicative of a glomus tumor unless there is associated cortical erosion.
2. Erosion of the triangular bony septum which devides the jugular fossa from the outer opening of the carotid canal. This finding appears on sagittal tomographs.
3. Erosion of the floor of the middle ear cavity.
4. A soft tissue mass of variable size projecting into the middle ear cavity from the jugular fossa. The mass may extend superiorly to encroach upon the ossicular chain. Further extension may occur into the mastoid. Lateral extension of the mass erodes the tympanic membrane and fills the external canal.
5. Erosion of the posteroinferior aspect of the petrous pyramid. This is typical of medial extension of the glomus. The glomus first undermines the posteroinferior aspect of the petrosa and erodes the external aperture of the cochlear aqueduct. Further enlargement of the lesion leads to partial or complete destruction of the petrous apex. The labyrinth becomes skeletonized, but is seldom invaded.
6. The adjacent aspect of the occipital bone is also involved and gradually eroded in large lesions. Further medial extension involves the hypoglossal canal and reaches the foramen magnum.

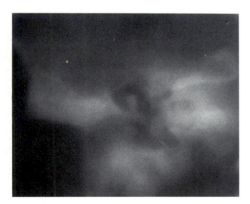

Fig. 9.**29** Glomus tympanicum, semiaxial tomogram, right. A soft tissue mass fills the lower half of the middle ear cavity. The hypotympanic floor is intact.

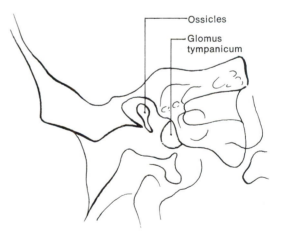

Fig. 9.**30** Diagram of Fig. 9.29

Jugular Venography

Jugular venography shows a filling defect in the lumen of the jugular bulb. Enlargement of the lesion results in partial or complete obstruction of the jugular vein, Fig. 9.41.

Venography is the best method to demonstrate a downward extension of the glomus tumor into the neck along the wall of the jugular vein. The venogram shows narrowing or obstruction of the vein extending inferiorly from the base of the skull.

This information is necessary to outline the inferior radiotherapy ports.

Jugular venography is essential in differentiation of a glomus jugulare tumor from a high but normal jugular bulb.

Arteriography

Subtraction films outline the presence of a vascular mass in the region of the jugular fossa, Fig. 9.42. The mass may extend superiorly into the middle ear cavity, inferiorly into the neck, laterally into the external canal and mastoid, medially toward the petrous apex and foramen magnum and intracranially into the cerebellopontine cistern.

Arteriography exposes the feeding vessels and their origins. This information enables the surgeon to determine which vessels, if any, need to be ligated during surgery. If embolization treatment is used, arteriography will indicate which vessels must be selectively catheterized. Postembolization arteriographic studies are used to determine the effectiveness of the treatment.

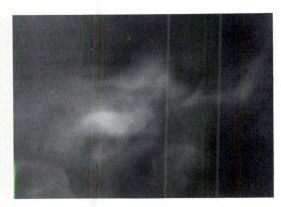

Fig. 9.31   Glomus tympanicum, coronal tomogram, left. The glomus tumor fills the lower half of the tympanic cavity. The hypotympanic floor is slightly eroded.

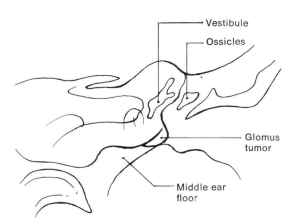

Fig. 9.32   Diagram of Fig. 9.31

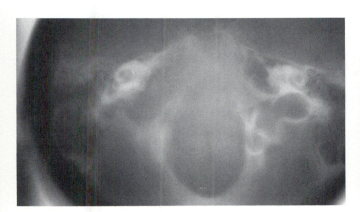

Fig. 9.33   Glomus jugulare, right, horizontal tomogram. The cortex of the right jugular fossa is destroyed and there is erosion of the posterior aspect of the petrous pyramid.

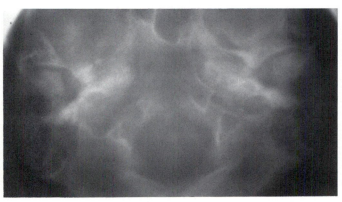

Fig. 9.34   Glomus jugulare, right, horizontal tomogram. The right jugular fossa is enlarged and the hypoglossal canal partially eroded. The left hypoglossal canal is normal.

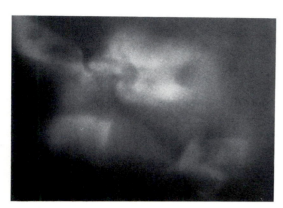

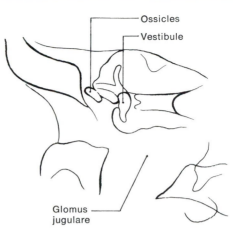

Fig. 9.**35** Glomus jugulare, coronal togram, right. The jugular fossa is enlarged and the floor of the middle ear eroded.

Fig. 9.**36**   Diagram of Fig. 9.35

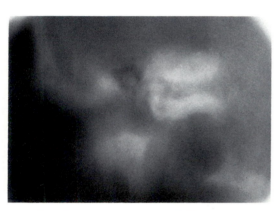

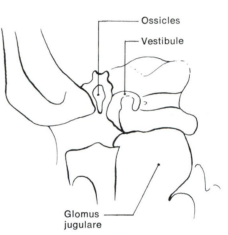

Fig. 9.**37**   Same ear as in Figs. 9.35 and 9.39, semiaxial tomogram. The cortex of the enlarged jugular fossa is eroded. A soft tissue mass protrudes into the middle ear through the eroded hypotympanic floor.

Fig. 9.**38**   Diagram of Fig. 9.37

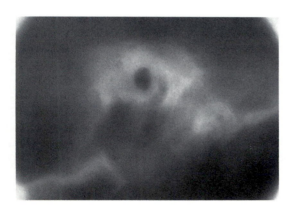

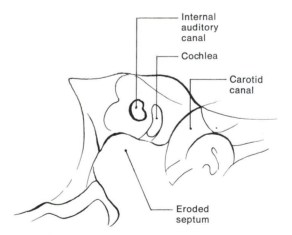

Fig. 9.**39**   Same ear as in Figs. 9.35 and 9.37, sagittal tomogram. There is erosion of the inferior aspect of the petrous pyramid with destruction of the bony septum dividing the jugular fossa from the outer opening of the carotid canal.

Fig. 9.**40**   Diagram of Fig. 9.35

Computerized Tomography

Small vascular masses limited to the jugular fossa and middle ear are not recognizable by computerized tomography.

Computerized tomography is particularly valuable in the study of larger lesions which extend either intracranially or into the neck.

The postinfusion study reveals areas of enhancement at the tumor site. Since the tumor is extradural, intracranial lesions are not surrounded by edema, Figs. 9.43, 9.44. Displacement of the fourth ventricle and other structures is rare.

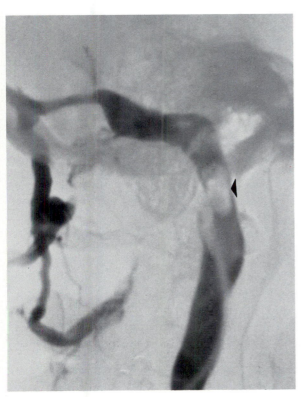

Fig. 9.**41**   Glomus jugulare, right, retrograde jugular venogram. A filling defect is present in the jugular vein 1 cm below the dome of the jugular bulb.

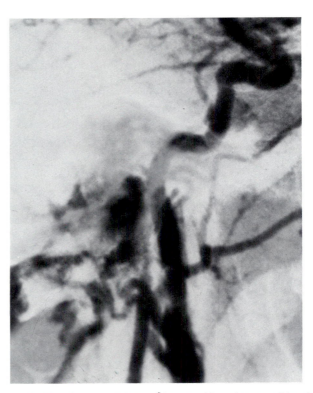

Fig. 9.**42**   Glomus jugulare, right, carotid angiogram with subtraction. A vascular mass lies in relation to the inferior aspect of the petrous pyramid. The ascending pharyngeal artery which feeds the glomus tumor is dilated.

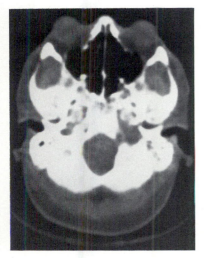

Fig. 9.**43**   Glomus jugulare, computerized tomography, horizontal section. CT section at the level of the base of the skull shows a destructive lesion expanding the left jugular fossa and involving the adjacent aspect of the occipital bone.

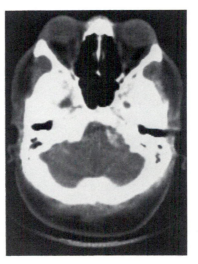

Fig. 9.**44**   Same patient as Fig. 9.43, CT, horizontal section, 1 cm. superior to Fig. 9.43. After infusion the extension of the glomus tumor into the posterior cranial fossa is demonstrated.

Malignant Tumors

Primary Malignancies

Carcinoma

Carcinomas of the temporal bone arise chiefly from the external auditory canal. Primary carcinomas of the middle ear cavity are extremely rare since most middle ear carcinomas actually begin in the external canal at the anulus and infiltrate from there into the middle ear.

Carcinomas of the canal usually do not cause large polypoid lesions of the external canal but infiltrate and spread deep into the surrounding portions of the temporal bone.

The predominant symptoms of carcinomas of the canal are pain and bleeding. There is no subcutaneous tissue between the skin and the periosteum of the external canal. Therefore carcinomas involve the periosteum early and cause severe pain due to periosteal infiltration.

Extension

Carcinomas of the external canal can extend anteriorly into the temporal mandibular joint, posteriorly into the mastoid and facial nerve, inferiorly into the neck and medially into the middle ear. Further medial extension involves the jugular fossa and the petrous pyramid.

Otoscopic Findings

Otoscopically in carcinoma of the external canal there is a granular ulcerating lesion which bleeds easily on contact with an instrument. All such granular lesions of the external and middle ear should be biopsied.

Radiographic Evaluation

The role of radiography in temporal bone carcinomas is twofold; to demonstrate bony erosions characteristic of carcinomas and to delineate the extent of the lesion. This information will enable the surgeon to determine the resectibility of the lesion. When radiotherapy is indicated, the radiographic evaluation will help in establishing the size of the treatment ports.

Tomography should always be used in the evaluation of carcinomas of the external canal and temporal bone. Conventional radiography is of value only in far advanced lesions where there is massive bony destruction. Coronal, sagittal, and horizontal tomographic projections should be obtained.

The sagittal sections should extend laterally to include the entire external auditory canal and mastoid areas. Computerized tomography is the technique of choice when the tumor extends outside the confines of the temporal bone. Axial and coronal sections should be taken, and a sagittal reconstruction should be made to define the lesion.

Findings

In an early lesion, tomography will show erosion and destruction of portions of the bony wall of the external auditory canal, Fig. 9.45. In lesions confined to the cartilagenous portion of the external canal there are no tomographic findings.

Spread of tumor through the anterior canal wall will result in erosion of the temporomandibular fossa and anterior displacement of the condyle, Fig. 9.49.

Extension into the mastoid causes a typical moth-eaten appearance of the bone due to infiltration of the neoplasm.

The vertical segment of the facial canal is involved most commonly in posterior extensions, Figs. 9.49, 9.50.

As the lesion extends medially there will be a soft tissue mass in the middle ear, Figs. 9.47, 9.48. From the middle ear the lesion often extends inferiorly into the jugular fossa or medially into the petrous pyramid. Petrous extension usually results in skeletonization of the labyrinth, since the otic capsule is relatively resistant to infiltration.

Far advanced carcinomas cause massive destruction of the temporal bone and adjacent bony structures. In these cases computerized tomography will demonstrate intracranial and neck extension of the tumor.

Sarcoma

Sarcomas of the temporal bone are extremely rare. They occur chiefly in children and arise from the middle ear or petrous pyramid. Histologically they are rhabdomyosarcoma, fibrosarcoma, lymphosarcoma, osteogenic sarcoma, chondrosarcoma and undifferentiated sarcoma.

Technique

Conventional radiography is useful because these lesions are usually far advanced when diagnosed. Towne-Chamberlain, transorbital, basal, and Stenvers projections are indicated.

Tomographic studies should consist of coronal, sagittal and horizontal projections.

Computerized tomography should be performed as indicated for carcinomas.

Findings

If the lesion originates in the middle ear there will be a soft tissue mass in the middle ear and often lateral bulging of the tympanic membrane. The mastoid air cells are

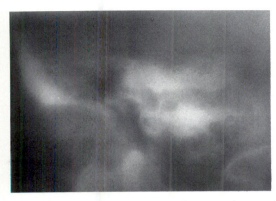

Fig. 9.**45**   Carcinoma, external auditory canal, coronal tomogram, right. The floor of the canal is eroded, and the lumen of the canal narrowed by a concentric soft tissue mass of the carcinoma.

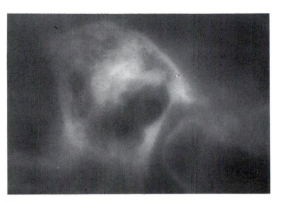

Fig. 9.**46**   Same ear as in Fig. 9.45, sagittal tomogram. The tumor erodes the floor and posterior wall of the external canal. The lesion extends to involve the anterior wall of the facial canal.

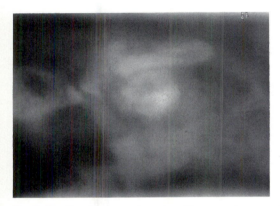

Fig. 9 **47**   Carcinoma, external auditory canal, coronal tomogram, right. The floor of the external canal is destroyed. The carcinomatous mass extends into the middle ear space from the floor of the canal.

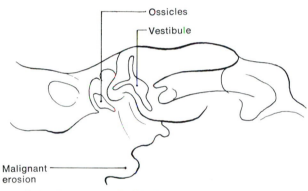

Fig. 9.**48**   Diagram of Fig. 9.47

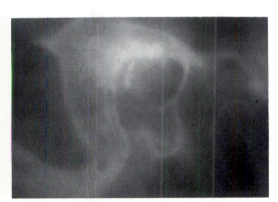

Fig. 9.**49**   Same ear as in Fig. 9.47, sagittal tomogram. The carcinoma extends into the mastoid and involves the vertical segment of the facial canal. The mandible is displaced anteriorly by anterior tumor extension.

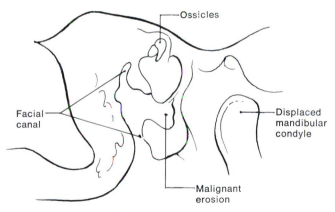

Fig. 9.**50**   Diagram of Fig. 9.49

cloudy. The external auditory canal is usually intact. Sarcomas tend to spread into the eustachian tube. Sarcomas, which arise in the nasopharynx and eustachian tube, extend retrogradely to involve the middle ear and temporal bone.

The pyramid is often completely destroyed either by lesions arising in the petrosa or by extension of the highly malignant tumor from the middle ear.

Computerized tomography will determine intracranial and extracranial extensions.

Secondary Malignancies

Secondary involvement of the temporal bone by malignant tumors occurs by direct extension from lesions in adjacent structures and by metastases.

Direct Extension

The most common lesion which involves the temporal bone by direct extension is carcinoma of the parotid. As the lesion extends upwards from the parotid it involves the base of the skull and the temporal bone. The floor of the external canal and the inferior surface of the mastoid are usually eroded by tumor. The lesion may obstruct the external auditory canal. Involvement of the stylomastoid foramen will cause facial nerve paralysis. These tumors have a tendency to spread from the foramen along the facial nerve and erode and expand the facial nerve canal, Figs. 9.51–9.54.

Computerized tomography will demonstrate the origin and extent of parotid tumors and any involvement of the skull base, Figs. 9.55, 9.56.

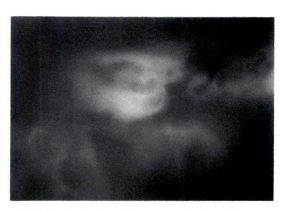

Fig. 9.**51** Parotid carcinoma, extension into temporal bone, coronal tomogram, left. The parotid malignancy infiltrates and erodes the lateral portion of the floor of the external canal.

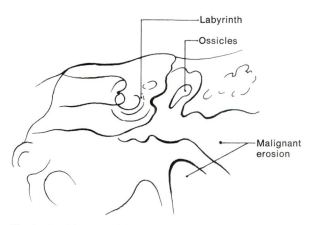

Fig. 9.**52** Diagram of Fig. 9.51

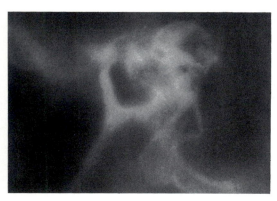

Fig. 9.**53** Same ear as in Fig. 9.51, sagittal tomogram. The tumor erodes the undersurface of the petrous bone and infiltrates into and enlarges the facial canal.

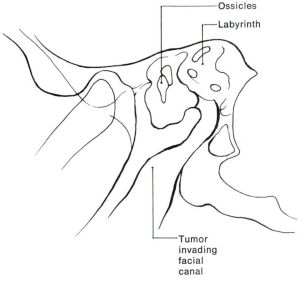

Fig. 9.**54** Diagram of Fig. 9.53

Metastatic Extension

The most common metastatic lesion of the temporal bone is carcinoma of the breast. Lung, prostate, and kidney and other lesions also metastasize to the temporal bone, Fig. 9.57. Any area of the temporal bone may be involved and symptomatology varies depending on the location of the lesion. The lesion may be destructive, as with lung metastasis, osteoblastic as with carcinoma of the prostate, or mixed, destructive and sclerotic, as with breast carcinoma.

Computerized tomography should be performed to rule out intracranial extension of the temporal bone lesion and the presence of other intracranial metastases.

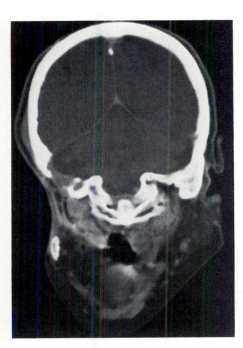

Fig. 9.55   Recurrent parotid carcinoma, computerized tomography, coronal section. There is destruction of the posterior portion of the right mastoid and occipital bone caused by extension of a recurrent parotid tumor.

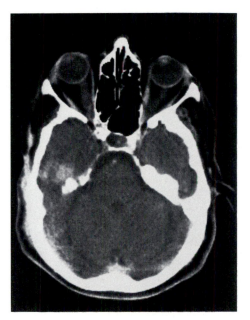

Fig. 9.56   Same patient as Fig. 9.55, CT horizontal section. After infusion an intracranial extension of the tumor is visible in the right middle cranial fossa. The lateral portion of the petrous pyramid is destroyed.

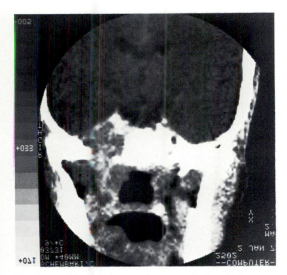

Fig. 9.57   Metastatic carcinoma of the kidney, computerized tomography, coronal section. The metastatic lesion has eroded and destroyed the right petrous pyramid. The enhanced tumor mass bulges into the floor of the middle cranial fossa.

Chapter 10　Internal Auditory Canal and Acoustic Neuroma

Acoustic neuromas are the cause of unilateral sensorineural hearing loss and vestibular function loss in approximately 10% of the patients with these presenting symptoms who are referred to the radiologist.

Acoustic neuromas usually arise within the lumen of the internal auditory meatus and, as they slowly enlarge, erode the bony margins of the meatus. Erosion of the meatus is visible radiographically. Acoustic neuromas account for approximately 10% of all intracranial tumors and 90% of all cerebellopontine angle tumors.

An acoustic neuroma is a benign, encapsulated, slowly growing tumor of one of the branches of the eighth cranial nerve. The lesion arises from proliferation of the neurilemmal or Schwann cells. Histologically the tumors are made up of streams of elongated spindle cells with fairly large nuclei which often are arranged in a palisading pattern. The larger tumors undergo cystic degenerative changes within the tumor mass. The cystic nature of the larger neuromas is apparent in enhanced computerized tomography. Approximately two thirds of acoustic neuromas arise from the vestibular division of the eight nerve and one third from the cochlear division. Most acoustic nerve tumors arise within the lumen of the internal auditory canal at the junction between the neurilemmal sheaths deriving from the peripheral vestibular ganglia and the neuroglial fibers which extend peripherally from the brain steim. Early growth of an acoustic neuroma occurs within the lumen of the internal auditory canal without producing significant symptoms until the perineural subarachnoid space is filled with tumor mass. Once the lesion has expanded to come in contact with the bony margin of the internal auditory

canal, pressure of the growing tumor results in neurological symptomatology of the vestibular and cochlear branches of the eight nerve and erosion of the walls of the internal auditory canal.

Bilateral acoustic neuromas are extremely rare except in patients with neurofibromatosis.

The most common initial symptom of an acoustic neuroma is unilateral sensorineural hearing loss. Vestibular symptoms such as mild dizziness and a sensation of imbalance occasionally occur as the first symptom. The otolaryngologist is usually the first physician to see these patients.

The otolaryngologist uses a series of hearing tests which help in differentiating cochlear from retrocochlear lesions and in selecting patients for referral for radiologic studies. The commonly used tests are: pure tone air and bone conduction audiometry, speech discrimination tests, adaptation tests such as the tone decay test, evoked electrocochleography and brain stem evoked responses. Caloric tests and electronystagmography determine the function of the vestibular portion of the eighth nerve. Vestibular function is abnormal in over 80% of acoustic neuromas. The facial nerve is rarely involved in early neuromas because of the resistance of the motor fibers of the seventh nerve to pressure.

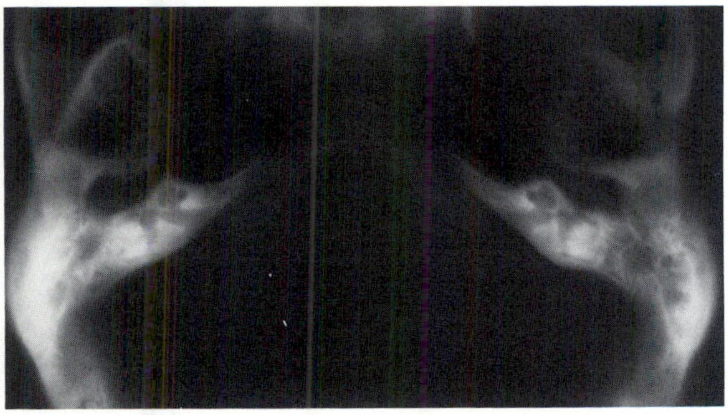

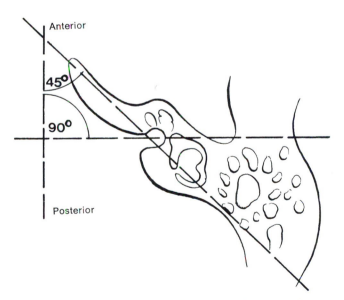

Fig. 10.1 Horizontal tomograph at the level of the internal auditory canal. The long axis of the internal auditory canal forms a right angle to the sagittal plane and an approximately 45° angle with the long axis of the petrous pyramid.

Fig. 10.2 Diagram of internal auditory canal relationship. The long axis of the petrous pyramid forms an approximately 45° angle with the sagittal plane. The internal auditory canal enters the pyramid at an angle of 90° to the sagittal plane.

As the neuromas grow, they extend medially into the cerebellopontine angle. Upward extension of the lesion causes pressure on the fifth cranial nerve. Loss of the corneal reflex on the ipsilateral side may be the first sign of pressure on the fifth nerve.

Further enlargement of the tumor mass will produce encroachment on other cranial nerves with paralytic lesions of fifth through twelfth nerves. Encroachment on the cerebellum and brain stem likewise occurs in larger lesions. Far advanced lesions of this severity fortunately are rarely seen today because of improved methods for early diagnosis.

With early diagnosis increased cerebrospinal fluid pressure and papilledema occur extremely rarely. Cerebrospinal fluid proteins are elevated only in the larger tumors.

Normal Internal Auditory Canal

The petrous pyramids lie in the base of the skull at approximately 45° to the sagittal plane of the skull. The internal auditory canal enters the petrous pyramid from the posteromedial surface at the junction of the anterior two fifths with the posterior three fifths of the long axis of the pyramid. The long axis of the canal forms a right angle with the sagittal plane of the skull and an angle of about 45° with the long axis of the petrous pyramid, Figures 10.1, 10.2.

The opening or porus of the canal is shaped much like the bevel of a needle with the maximum diameter in the same axis as the petrous pyramid. The posterior, superior, and inferior lips of the porus are prominent and are made up of dense bone. The anterior lip is usually poorly demarcated because the anterior wall of the canal blends smoothly with the posteromedial surface of the petrous bone.

The internal auditory canal contains the facial nerve, the nervus intermedius, the acoustic nerve, consisting of cochlear and vestibular portions, and the internal auditory artery. The nerves are enclosed within a common arachnoid sheath.

Radiographic Techniques

Radiographic studies are essential in the diagnosis of acoustic neruomas and other lesions of the cerebellopontine angle.

The radiographic techniques used for the study of the internal auditory canal and cerebellopontine angle cistern are:

1. conventional radiography; 2. multidirectional tomography;
3. computerized tomography; 4. cisternography;
5. arteriography.

Conventional Radiography

Conventional x-ray projections are unsatisfactory except for visualizing gross enlargements of the internal auditory canal. Superimposition of petrous air cells and other structures obscure the details of the internal canals. The transorbital and Towne views of the pyramid demon-

strate the full length of the canal. The Stenvers projection shows the porus of the internal canal, but the canal appears foreshortened.

Tomography

Tomography is the most valuable technique for the study of the internal auditory canal. Multidirection or high definition computerized tomography with 1.5 mm. sections are used.

In order to evaluate the entire contour of the internal canal, two projections should be obtained with each technique. With multidirectional tomography, coronal and sagittal sections, 2 mm. apart are taken through the length of the canal, with high definition CT, coronal and horizontal sections 1.5 mm. apart.

It is important to be able to visualize the walls of the internal auditory canal. The superior and inferior walls can be seen in coronal sections by both methods. The anterior and posterior walls of the canal are visualized in the sagittal projection by multidirectional tomography and in the horizontal sections by CT. The fundus and the porus of the canal are seen in all of these projections.

Both sides should always be examined for comparison. The two internal auditory canals of the same patient normally are symmetrical. But variations of the sizes and shapes of the internal auditory canals of different patients are very common and often quite pronounced. There are several factors to consider in evaluating the internal auditory canal: shape, diameter, length, cortical outline, and position of the crista falciformis. Both internal auditory canals of the same patient must be compared to determine significant differences.

The shape of the normal internal auditory canals viewed on frontal tomography varies considerably from one patient to the next, but must be the same for the two canals of the individual patient. In 50% of the cases the canals are cylindrical, and the vertical diameter is the same throughout the length of the canal. In 25%, the canals have an oval shape and the middle portion is larger than the medial and lateral ends. In the remaining 25%, the canals taper either medially or laterally.

The vertical diameter of the normal internal auditory canal may vary from 2–12 mm. and the mean diameter is about 5 mm. In 95% of normal patients, the difference between the paired internal auditory canals does not exceed 1 mm. Measurement should be obtained in comparable sections at points equidistant from each vestibule.

The length of the canal is the shortest distance between the vestibule and the medial lip of the posterior wall. Figure 10.3–10.5. The length ranges from 4–15 mm with a mean of 8 mm. Again both sides must be compared. In 95% of normal patients there is a 2 mm or less difference in the length of the posterior wall of the two canals.

The normal internal auditory canal is surrounded by a layer of well defined cortical bone which is particularly evident when the canal is surrounded by diploic or pneumatized bone, Figs. 10.6–10.8.

The crista falciformis is a horizontal bony septum dividing the lateral portion of the internal auditory canal into

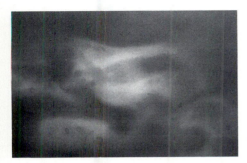

Fig. 10.**3**   Frontal tomograph at level of maximum vertical diameter of internal auditory canal. This frontal section cuts through the horizontal semicircular canal, the oval window, the incus, and the maximum vertical diameter of the internal auditory canal. This canal is slightly larger in its midportion than in the medial end. The crista lies above the midpoint of the vertical diameter.

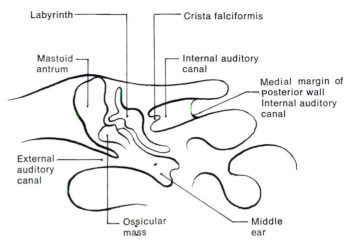

Fig. 10.**4**   Diagram of structures in figures 10.3, and 10.5

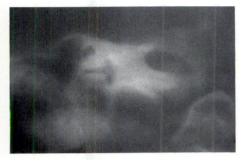

Fig. 10.**5**   Frontal tomograph at level of the posterior wall of the internal auditory canal, 4 mm posterior to figure 10.3. The horizontal semicircular canal extends laterally from the vestibule. The margin of the posterior wall of the canal appears concave medially.

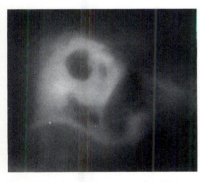

Fig. 10.**6**   Lateral tomograph of internal auditory canal at level of medial portion of cochlea. This lateral tomograph exposes the lateral portion of the internal auditory canal. The crista falciformis anteriorly demarcates the upper and lower compartments of the canal.

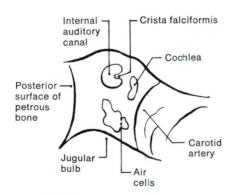

Fig. 10.**7**   Diagram of structures in figures 10.6, and 10.8

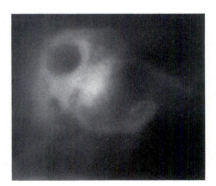

Fig. 10.**8**   Lateral tomograph demonstrating the lip of the posterior wall of the internal auditory canal, 6 mm medial to figure 10.6. At this level the thin, sharp lip of the posterior canal wall forms the posterior margin of the petrous bone.

a smaller upper and larger lower compartment. The position of the crista should be a above the midpoint of the vertical diameter and should be symmetrical in the two canals, Figure 10.3.–10.6.

Abnormal Internal Auditory Canal

Multidirectional tomography or high definition CT of the internal auditory canal is the first step in establishing the definitive diagnosis of acoustic neuromas. Coupled with clinical audiometric and vestibular findings, tomography will detect a high percentage of acoustic neuromas.

When tomography reveals symmetrical internal auditory canals, the presence of a neuroma is unlikely. Variations in the bilateral symmetry of the internal auditory canal suggest pathology.

The value of multidirectional tomography in detecting acoustic neuromas is illustrated in a study of 800 proven cases of acoustic neuromas. Conventional radiology showed evidence of pathology in 50% of the cases, while tomography detected 80% of the lesions. In another 15%, tomographic findings were suggestive of tumor. In only 5% of this series tomographic studies were normal. An accurate analysis of the shape and diameter of the internal auditory canal, the length of the posterior wall, and the position of the crista falciformis is required to detect significant asymmetry of the internal auditory canal. This analysis provides important information for the diagnosis of a tumor and for the location and extent of the lesion.

Shape of Internal Auditory Canal

When similar coronal tomographs of the right and left sides are compared, various abnormalities may be visualized depending on the site of the neuroma. Lesions limited within the lumen of the canal cause bowing of the superior and inferior contour of the internal auditory canal giving the canal an oval shape, Figure 10.11. Lesions arising within the internal auditory canal and extending into the cerebellopontine cistern erode the medial portion of the internal auditory canal and produce a funnel shape contour of the canal, Figure 10.9, 10.17.

Diameter of the Internal Auditory Canal

The vertical and anteroposterior diameters of the internal auditory canal are measured at points equidistant from each vestibule. An expansile mass usually produces a concentric increase in the diameters of the canal, therefore both vertical and anteroposterior diameters must be

evaluated and compared. Occasionally only one diameter may be significantly increased, Figure 10.15.

Widening of 2 mm or more of any portion of one internal auditory canal when compared with the corresponding segment of the opposite canal is very suspicious for the presence of a tumor.

Widening of 1–2 mm of any portion of the canal on the affected, side in comparison with the corresponding segment of the opposite side is considered suggestive but not conclusive for a space-occupying lesion.

Length of the Internal Auditory Canal

Lesions arising within the internal auditory canal and extending into the cerebellopontine cistern produce expansion of the medial portion of the canal and erosion of the medial lip of the posterior canal wall. This erosion is manifested by a shortening of the distance between the vestibule and the medial lip of the posterior wall, Figure 10.13.

Lesions which arise within the cerebellopontine cistern do not expand the diameters of the internal auditory canal, but impinge on the posterior wall and produce a significant shortening of this wall, Figure 10.35.

Shortening of the posterior wall by at least 3 mm in comparison with the opposite side, Figure 10.13, is usually indicative of a tumor while shortening of 2 to 3 mm the posterior wall is a less positive sign of a lesion.

Cortical Outline

Erosion of the cortical outline surrounding the lumen of the canal and porus is often one of the first signs of an intracanalicular mass, Figure 10.15.

Crista Falciformis

A change in the relationship of the crista falciformis to the superior and inferior canal walls on the affected side of more than 1 mm when compared with the normal side may indicate the site of origin of the tumor.

When the distance between the crista and the superior canal wall is increased when compared to the normal side, the origin of the tumor is most likely in the superior vestibular nerve, rarely the facial nerve, Figure 10.11. If the distance between the crista and the inferior wall is increased, the lesion probably arises from the inferior vestibular or cochlear nerves, Figure 10.9.

In small intracanalicular lesions, this information is of practical importance for the surgeon in determining whether to use a middle cranial fossa or translabyrinthine approach. Lesions in the upper compartment are more easily removed via the middle cranial approach.

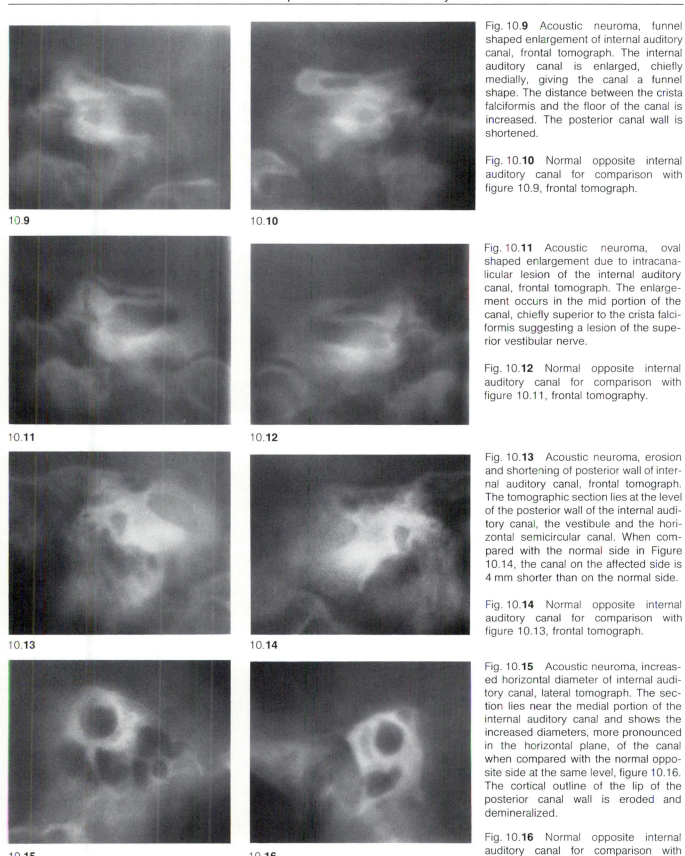

10.9

10.10

Fig. 10.**9** Acoustic neuroma, funnel shaped enlargement of internal auditory canal, frontal tomograph. The internal auditory canal is enlarged, chiefly medially, giving the canal a funnel shape. The distance between the crista falciformis and the floor of the canal is increased. The posterior canal wall is shortened.

Fig. 10.**10** Normal opposite internal auditory canal for comparison with figure 10.9, frontal tomograph.

10.11

10.12

Fig. 10.**11** Acoustic neuroma, oval shaped enlargement due to intracanalicular lesion of the internal auditory canal, frontal tomograph. The enlargement occurs in the mid portion of the canal, chiefly superior to the crista falciformis suggesting a lesion of the superior vestibular nerve.

Fig. 10.**12** Normal opposite internal auditory canal for comparison with figure 10.11, frontal tomography.

10.13

10.14

Fig. 10.**13** Acoustic neuroma, erosion and shortening of posterior wall of internal auditory canal, frontal tomograph. The tomographic section lies at the level of the posterior wall of the internal auditory canal, the vestibule and the horizontal semicircular canal. When compared with the normal side in Figure 10.14, the canal on the affected side is 4 mm shorter than on the normal side.

Fig. 10.**14** Normal opposite internal auditory canal for comparison with figure 10.13, frontal tomograph.

10.15

10.16

Fig. 10.**15** Acoustic neuroma, increased horizontal diameter of internal auditory canal, lateral tomograph. The section lies near the medial portion of the internal auditory canal and shows the increased diameters, more pronounced in the horizontal plane, of the canal when compared with the normal opposite side at the same level, figure 10.16. The cortical outline of the lip of the posterior canal wall is eroded and demineralized.

Fig. 10.**16** Normal opposite internal auditory canal for comparison with figure 10.15, lateral tomograph.

Radiographic Visualization of Acoustic Neuromas

On the basis of the results of the radiographic study of the internal auditory canal we decide whether to perform CT with infusion or cisternography, the final and most conclusive tests for the diagnosis of a cerebellopontine angle tumor. Vertebral arteriography is performed as a supplementary examination in selected cases.

Computerized Tomography

The conventional CT examination consists of two series of scans obtained first before and then after drip infusion or bolus injection of contrast material. The first examination shows indirect signs of the tumor mass such as displacement of the fourth ventricle, narrowing of the opposite cerebellopontine cistern by the displaced brain stem, and, in a large lesion presence of obstructive hydrocephalus. The tumor is usually not recognizable since it is isodense to the surrounding brain structures and is usually not surrounded by edema.

The second, post infusion study demonstrates the actual tumor, mass following enhancement of its density by the contrast material. In large lesions there is a central area of decreased absorption produced by cystic degeneration of the tumor, Figs. 10.18–10.23. CT is particulary useful for medium and large sized tumors, since it allows evaluation of the size of the lesion and of its extension particularly in the region of the tentorial notch more precise than cisternography. It should be remembered that small tumors less than 1.2 cm in diameter are usually not recognizable in the standard 1 cm axial CT sections.

By adding 5 mm axial and coronal sections through the cerebellopontine cistern, we are able to visualize extracanalicular tumors as small as 8 mm in diameter. If the canal is markedly enlarged the intracanalicular portion of the tumor is also visualized.

Another important application of CT is for the evaluation of the postoperative patient. In the immediate postoperative period when intracranial complications occur, CT without infusion can demonstrate intracranial hemorrhage or brain edema and hydrocephalus. In the late postoperative period when there is a suspicion of recurrent tumor or when a subtotal resection was done, CT with infusion is more valuable than cisternography in delineating the size of the recurrent or residual lesion and in evaluating the progression of the tumor, Figure 10.24.

Cerebellopontine Cisternography

The cerebellopontine cisterns are lateral, symmetrical extensions of the pontine cistern. At the porus of the internal auditory canal each cerebellopontine cistern divides into two branches. The main branch extends along the posteromedial aspect of each petrous pyramid at an angle of 45° to the sagittal plane of the skull. This branch is quite variable in size, and it may be so small that it only reaches the posterior wall of the internal

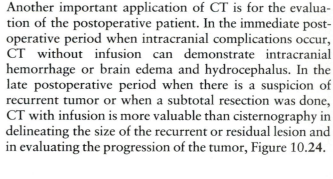

Fig. 10.17 Acoustic neuroma, CT, coronal section. This coronal section demonstrates marked funnel shaped expansion of the left internal auditory canal.

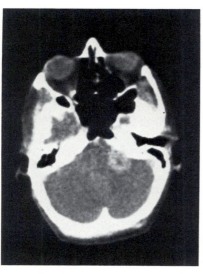

Fig. 10.18 Same patient as Fig. 10.17, CT, horizontal section. This section was obtained using a smaller window after infusion and shows a large mass in the right cerebellopontine cistern. There is an area of decreased absorption in the center of the tumor.

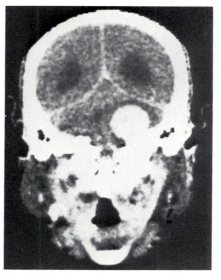

Fig. 10.19 Acoustic neuroma, CT, coronal section. Following infusion a large, solid tumor extends into the cerebellopontine cistern from the porus of the internal auditory canal. The tumor displaces and compresses the fourth ventricle and produces an obstructive hydrocephalus.

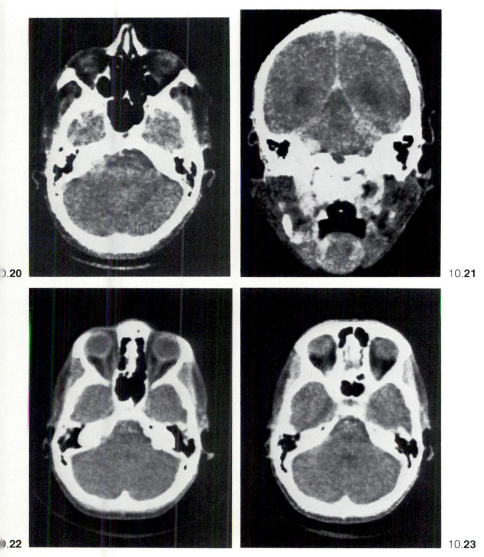

10.20

10.21

10.22

10.23

Fig. 10.20   Acoustic neuroma, CT, horizontal section. A medium sized tumor is visible in the right cerebellopontine cistern following infusion of contrast. The tumor measured 1.5 cm in diameter.

Fig. 10.21   Same patient as Fig. 10.20, CT, coronal section, post-infusion. The contour of the tumor mass is seen better in this coronal section than in the horizontal, Figure 10.20.

Fig. 10.22   Acoustic neuroma, CT, horizontal section, post infusion. There is a small enhanced lesion in the widened porus of the right internal canal.

Fig. 10.23   Same patient as Fig. 10.22, CT horizontal section 5 mm superior to Fig. 10.22. The small tumor protrudes slightly into the cerebellopontine cistern. The tumor at this level measures 7 mm in diameter.

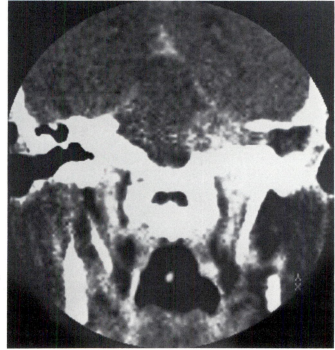

Fig. 10.24   Acoustic neuroma, residual, CT, coronal section. Following partial resection of an acoustic neuroma via the translabyrinthine approach this study was performed to determine the size of the lesion remaining in the cerebellopontine angle. The enhanced residual tumor is seen at the intracranial opening of the surgical defect.

auditory canal. The main branch may also be so large that it extends to the vertical portion of the sigmoid sinus. The average main branch extends as far as a sagittal plane crossing the vestibule.

The smaller cistern branch enters the internal auditory canal and completely lines the wall of the canal. The internal auditory portion of the cistern forms a 90° angle with the sagittal plane of the skull, and hence diverges at an angle of 45° from the main branch of the cistern.

Cerebellopontine cisternography while visualizing lesions well is not capable of differentiating the various types of lesion that may occur in this area such as neuroma, meningioma, cholesteatoma or subarachnoid cyst.

At present there are three methods of cisternography of the cerebellopontine angle: 1. Pantopaque cisternography; 2. CT pneumocisternography; 3. CT opaque cisternography with hydrosoluble metrizamide.

Pantopaque cisternography

The examination is done preferably under fluoroscopic control. About 2–3 ml of Pantopaque are injected into the subarachnoid space via lumbar puncture after 2–3 ml of cerebrospinal fluid are withdrawn for chemical analysis. A 22 gauge spinal needle is used to minimize postspinal headache.

With the patient in the lateral decubitus position and the internal auditory canal being studied dependant, the contrast medium is moved into the posterior cranial fossa. Horizontal x-ray beam views are obtained in the Towne, Caldwell and submental vertex positions. When the internal auditory canal and cerebellopontine cistern are well visualized and appear normal the study is terminated as negative, Figs. 10.25–10.26.

If the internal auditory canal and cerebellopontine cisterns are not visualized in these projections, or if a lesion is demonstrated, the head is rotated first to a Stenvers-like position and then face down. Several spot films are obtained with varying degrees of rotation, flexion and extension of the head.

The patient is then placed in the erect position, and the contrast material flows into the spinal canal. The procedure is then repeated to visualize the opposite, presumably normal side. At the end of the procedure, the contrast material is pooled in the lumbar area where it may be withdrawn.

The contrast material, Pantopaque, has a specific gravity higher than cerebrospinal fluid and fills the internal auditory canal by gravity. The amount of filling is in direct proportion to the size of the canal and the subarachnoid space surrounding the neurovascular bundle. In a small internal auditory canal, measuring less than 2.5 mm in diameter, no filling may occur because the neurovascular bundle occupies the entire lumen of the internal auditory canal and prevents entry of contrast material.

In the Stenvers projection of the normal cerebellopontine cistern the contrast material should form a triangular shaped accumulation bounded medially by the basilar artery. The lateral apex of the triangle lies at the porus of the internal auditory canal. Superiorly two indentations are caused by the fifth nerve laterally and the insertion of the tentorium medially, Figure 10.27, 10.28.

When the head is rotated from the Stenvers position to full face down, contrast material collected in the main branch of cerebellopontine cistern will flow by gravity into the pontine cistern but will be retained within the lumen of the internal auditory canal, Figure 10.29, 10.30. A normal cerebellopontine cisternography will rule out the presence of an acoustic neuroma and other tumors of this area.

In some institutions pantopaque cisternography is performed without fluoroscopy. Following the subarachnoid injection of pantopaque the patient is placed in the Trendelenberg position on the multidirectional tomographic table. Tomograms are taken in several projections.

We prefer to use the fluoroscopic technique because it allows better control of the flow and position of the pantopaque. We use additional tomographic sections only when there is the possibility of a small intracanalicular mass not well outlined in the spot views.

CT Pneumocisternography

CT pneumocisternography is best done with high definition scanner and 1.5 mm sections. Air has the advantage of being the most innocuous contrast material which is rapidly absorbed and does not cause unwanted reactions. Four to five cc of air are injected by lumbar puncture into the subarachnoid space with the patient in the lateral decubitus position lying on the normal side. The patient is instructed to elevate his torso so that he rests on his elbow. At the same time the chin is tilted upward so that the air will rise into the cerebellopontine angle.

After the air has filled the cerebellopontine angle the patient again assumes the lateral decubitus position and scans are obtained. The head is then rotated 180°, the air shifts to the opposite side, and the normal canal is scanned.

When no tumor is present the air will outline the contours of the internal canal and cistern. The seventh and eight cranial nerves, are clearly demonstrated as they stretch from the brain stem into the internal auditory canal, Fig. 10.38.

CT pneumocisternography can demonstrate three patterns of acoustic neuroma.

When the tumor is very small, air outlines the localized swelling of the nerve within the internal auditory canal.

In larger tumors which fill the internal canal completely, CT shows failure of air to enter the canal and the convex medial contour of the tumor at the porus.

When the tumor protrudes into the cerebellar pontine cistern CT shows the contour of the extracanalicular mass and the obstruction of the internal canal, Figure 10.39.

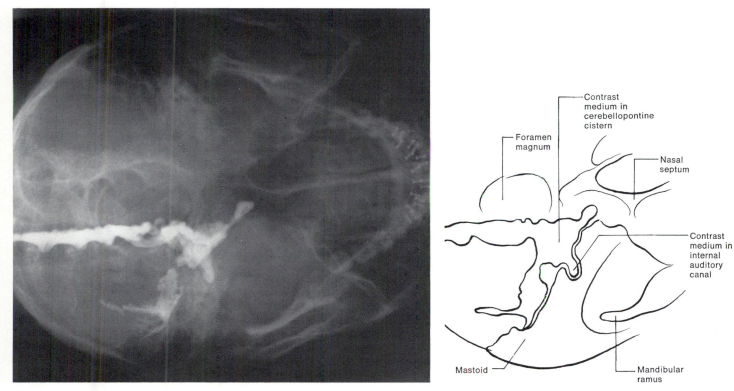

Fig. 10.**25** Normal cisternogram, complete filling of internal auditory canal, basal view, horizontal beam. Contrast medium fills the cerebellopontine cistern and extends into and fills the internal auditory canal.

Fig. 10.**26**   Diagram of cisternography in figure 10.25.

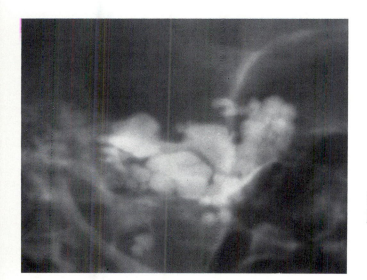

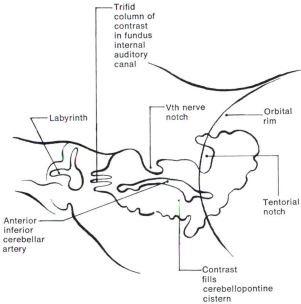

Fig. 10.**27** Normal cisternogram, Stenvers projection. Contrast medium fills the fundus of the internal auditory canal. The nerves of the canal cause the trifid appearance of the lateral portion of the column of contrast in the fundus. The fifth cranial nerve and the tentorum cause the notches on the superior margin of the contrast material. The anterior inferior cerebellar artery stretches across the contrast medium which fills the cerebellopontine cistern.

Fig. 10.**28**   Diagram of cisternography in figure 10.27

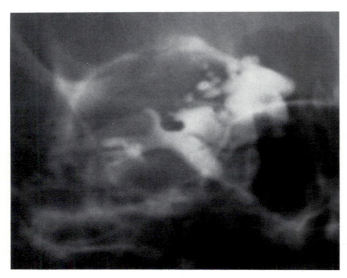

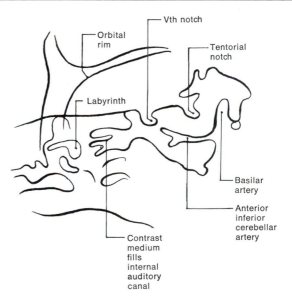

Fig. 10.**29**   Normal cisternogram, face down position. The internal auditory canal, completely filled with contrast medium, appears through the orbit. The trifid appearance of the lateral extent of the column of contrast is due to the nerves of the internal auditory canal. The notches of the fifth cranial nerve and tentorum lie on the superior margin of the contrast medium. The anterior inferior cerebellar artery extends laterally from the basilar artery.

Fig. 10.**30**   Diagram of cisternogram in figure 10.29

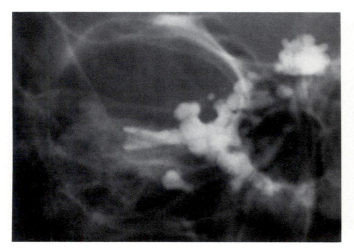

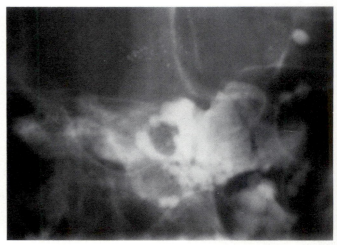

Fig. 10.**31**   Cerebellopontine cisternogram, acoustic neuroma, intracanalicular. A small intracanalicular acoustic neuroma fills the lateral one third of the internal auditory canal and blocks entrance of contrast medium. The lateral end of the contrast medium column is concave laterally due to the medialward convexity of the tumor.

Fig. 10.**32**   Cerebellopontine cisternogram, acoustic neuroma, extension into cerebellopontine cistern. A one cm tumor extends from the internal auditory canal into the cerebellopontine cistern. The circumference of the tumor is outlined in the cistern. The lesion does not extend to the fifth nerve notch.

CT Opaque cisternography

Amipaque, a brand of metrizamide is used for opaque cisternography. This contrast material, while being absorbed rapidly, is a brain irritant at full strength, and, to avoid convulsions, should be used at low concentrations of 170 mgm per ml. We prefer to use air as a contrast to avoid central nervous system complications.

Pathology in Cisternography

There are three possible types of lesions which may be defined by cisternography: 1. an intracanalicular lesion; 2. an intracanalicular lesion which extends into the cerebellopontine cistern in varying degrees; and 3. a lesion limited to the extracanalicular portion of the cistern.

1. Intracanalicular filling defects

Intracanalicular masses may obstruct the internal auditory canal and produce a cutoff of the radio-opaque or air column. The lateral cutoff margin will outline the medial surface of the mass and form a concave contour facing laterally, Figure 10.31. If the tumor is small, some contrast materal may infiltrate laterally beyond the mass and outline the circumference of the lesion.

When the canal being examined for tumor does not fill, it is mandatory to study the opposite canal. If both sides fail to fill the possibility of an intracanalicular lesion in the suspect side cannot be confirmed and follow-up studies are indicated.

Incomplete canal filling may be due to anatomical features of the internal auditory canal. The cochlear division of the acoustic nerve, which occupies the anteroinferior compartment of the canal, is the largest of the five nerves composing the nerve bundle. At approximately 2–3 mm from the fundus of the canal, the cochlear nerve makes a sharp turn forward to reach the cochlea where it fans into the spiral foraminous tract. This anatomic feature is responsible for either incomplete filling or a filling defect in the inferior compartment.

The superior and inferior vestibular nerves are located in the posterior part of the canal above and below the crista falciformis. These nerves flare at the lateral end of the canal in order to reach the foramina in the cribriform plate dividing the internal auditory canal from the vestibule. This flaring narrows the subarachnoid space and causes the typical trifid shape of the lateral aspect of the radio-opaque column, Figure 10.27, 10.29, and 10.30. Finally, the anterior inferior cerebellar artery which may loop within the canal, and the internal auditory canal artery which may follow a tortuous and redundant course around the nerve bundle may account for small linear or round filling defects, depending on the projection.

2. Lesions of the internal auditory canal extending into the cerebellopontine cistern

Typically an acoustic neuroma has a mushroom shape with the stalk within the internal auditory canal. In these cases the contrast material outlines a filling defect of varying size within the cistern. The internal auditory canal does not fill since the stalk of the lesion blocks the canal, Figures 10.32, 10.33, 10.34. With larger lesions the notch of the fifth nerve may be obliterated by tumor. Evaluation of the tumor size by cisternography is precise only if the contrast mateial outlines the medial aspect of the tumor. If the medial surface of the tumor is in contact with the brain stem or cerebellum the medial extent cannot be determined by this technique.

3. Extracanalicular tumors of the cerebellopontine cistern

In lesions confined to the cerebellopontine cistern a defect of varying size is visualized in the cistern, Figs. 10.35–10.37. The internal auditory canal may be filled with contrast medium or may be blocked off by the tumor mass.

Since these lesions do not extend into the canal lumen, the internal auditory canals are not expanded. However, there is often a bevel shaped erosion of the porus of the canal.

Fifty percent of extracanalicular cerebellopontine angle masses are lesions other than acoustic neuromas.

Vertebral Arteriography

Vertebral arteriography is not performed as a primary diagnostic test for cerebellopontine angle lesions. Arteriography is performed when: 1. a vascular lesion is suspected on the basis of history or physical findings; 2. When a large lesion is demonstrated by other techniques; and 3. when cisternography demonstrates large vessels entering or surrounding a tumor mass.

Subtraction technique has improved visualization of the vessels in the cerebellopontine cistern area. The many variations in the course and size of these vessels cause equivocal findings on angiography except in cases of large neoplasms. Visualization of the blood supply of the lesion by arteriography may be helpful to the surgeon. If the anterior inferior cerebellar artery loops within the lumen of the internal auditory canal and should be injured during a translabyrinthine tumor removal, a fatality could result.

Selection of Diagnostic Procedures

The selection of the diagnostic procedure will depend on the availability of a high definition scanner capable of producing 1.5 mm sections.

High Definition Scanner Available

When a high definition scanner is available multidirectional tomography is bypassed and horizontal and coronal CT sections 1.5 mm are taken through the internal auditory canals and cerebellopontine cisterns.

To shorten the procedure a preinfusion scan is not done and sections are obtained following infusion. This permits evaluation of the size of the internal auditory canal simultaneously with the demonstration of a tumor should one be present.

If no mass is demonstrated by the above procedure but there is asymmetry of the internal auditory canals or strong clinical suspicion for a lesion, a CT pneumocisternogram is performed while the patient is still on the table. This procedure will rule out or rule in the presence of a small intracanalicular tumor, Fig. 10.38–10.39.

High definition scanner not available

When the high definition scanner is not available, multidirectional tomography should be performed first to analyze the internal auditory canals.

Depending on the results of the tomographic study, we decide whether or not to perform pantopaque cisternography or conventional computerized tomography. These studies are carried out in the following situations:

1. When the tomographic examination has demonstrated an abnormal internal auditory canal whatever the result of the audiometric and vestibular tests;

2. When the results of the different audiometric and vestibular tests are strongly suggestive of a retrocochlear lesion, whatever the result of the tomographic examination;

3. When the borderline findings of a tomographic study are coupled with questionable audiometric and vestibular test results.

Whether to perform computerized tomography or a cerebellopontine pantopaque cisternography depends on various factors. Lesions less than 1.2 cm in diameter cannot be visualized by horizontal computerized tomography using the older equipment.

Neurological findings, the degree of enlargement of the internal auditory canal, and the age of the patient are factors which help to determine which procedure to use. Findings limited to the eight nerve associated with moderate enlargement of the internal auditory canal tomographically suggest a small lesion and indicate the need for cisternography.

Involvement of the fifth cranial nerve with marked enlargement of the internal auditory canal suggest a large lesion. In these cases computerized tomography will visualize the lesion and define the size and extent of the lesion.

The age and the general physical condition of the patient are factors in determining the selection of the procedure to be used. In old or debilitated patients who are poor surgical risks a negative computerized tomography will assure that the lesion is less than 1.2 cm in diameter. Since acoustic tumors are slow growing, a lesion of this size will probably not foreshorten the patient's life.

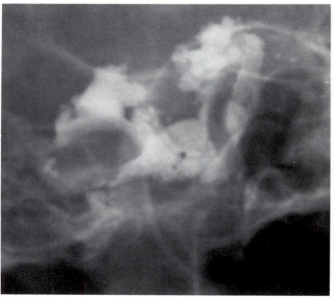

Fig. 10.**33** Cerebellopontine cisternogram, acoustic neuroma, extension into cerebellopontine cistern. This lesion extends from the internal auditory canal into the cerebellopontine cistern and has a diameter of 1.5 cm.

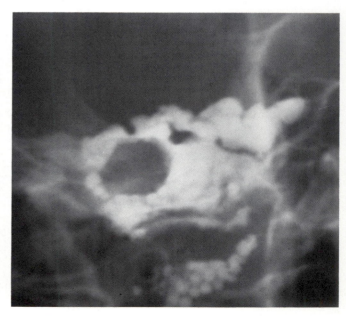

Fig. 10.**34** Cerebellopontine cisternogram, acoustic neuroma, extension into cerebellopontine cistern. The contrast medium surrounds this 1.5 cm tumor in this Stenvers view. The fifth cranial nerve notch is intact and appears on the superior margin of the mass.

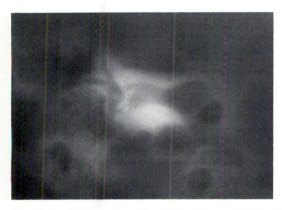

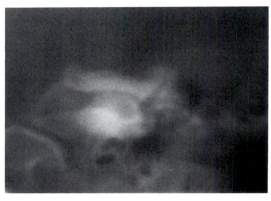

Fig. 10.**35**   Tomogram, acoustic neuroma, extracanalicular lesion. This frontal tomogram shows a bevelled shaped erosion of the internal auditory canal at the porus without enlargement of the canal. These findings suggest erosion of the canal by pressure from a tumor mass arising in the cerebellopontine cistern.

Fig. 10.**36**   Tomogram, normal opposite ear to ear in figure 10.35 for comparison.

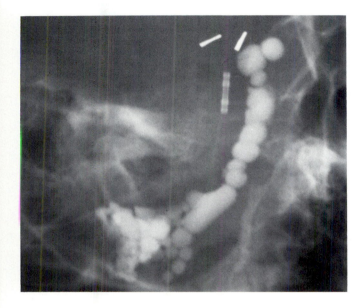

Fig. 10.**37**   Cerebellopontine cisternogram, large extracanalicular tumor. A 3.5 cm mass fills the entire cerebellopontine cistern. The contrast medium outlines the tumor. A shunt tube lies just lateral to the contrast material close to two neurosurgical clips. A shunt was required in this patient to relieve intracranial pressure before the cisternogram.

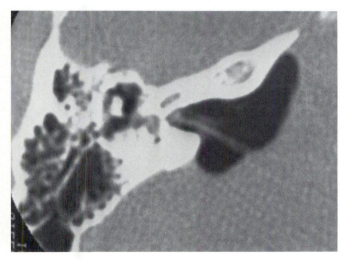

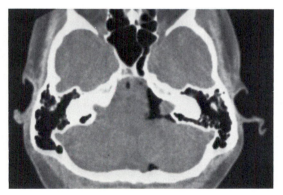

Fig. 10.**38**   Normal CT pneumocisternogram, right. Air fills the cerebellopontine cistern and internal auditory canal. The seventh and eighth cranial nerves extend from the brain stem into the canal.

Fig. 10.**39**   Acoustic neuroma, CT pneumocisternogram, left. The air in the cistern outlines a small tumor which bulges medially from the enlarged internal canal into the cistern.

Chapter 11   Otosclerosis and Bony Dystrophies

Otosclerosis

Otosclerosis is a primary focal disease of the labyrinthine capsule. The otosclerotic foci may be single or multiple and undergo periods of resorption and redeposition of bone at variable intervals. There appears to be an hereditary factor in the etiology. The most common site of a focus is in the labyrinthine capsule just anterior to the oval window. This focus tends to extend posteriorly to fix the stapes footplate, and at times invade and thicken the footplate. Similar foci occur in other areas of the labyrinthine capsule, particularly in the cochlea.

Involvement of the oval window with fixation of the stapes causes conductive deafness. Cochlear foci produce sensorineural deafness by an unknown mechanism.

Histologically the foci which arise in the endochondral layer vary in appearance. In an active focus there is a loose and irregular network of bony trabeculae with numerous blood vessels, osteoblasts and osteoclasts. In a mature focus there is a dense type of bone which is relatively avascular and acellular. These foci may progressively enlarge and extend to the endosteal and periosteal layers of the labyrinthine capsule. Periosteal involvement produces exostotic-like lesions protruding into the lumen of the tympanic cavity.

The progression of otosclerosis is characterized by remission and exacerbation. The disease may be quiescent for relatively long periods of time or there may be rapid progression with deterioration of the hearing.

Clinical Course

Otosclerosis usually begins in young adults as a gradually progressive conductive or mixed type of deafness. The hearing loss which at the onset is usually conductive may stabilize for relatively long periods of time. Progression usually occurs in bouts of exacerbation until there is maximum conductive deafness. Further deafness may then occur due to superimposed sensorineural hearing loss caused by involvement of the cochlea by the otosclerotic process.

In the usual case of otosclerosis, the tympanic membrane and the middle ear appear normal on otoscopy.

When there is severe involvement of the cochlea and promontory by large, active and vascular otosclerotic foci, the mucosa of the promontory becomes hyperemic. This hyperemia is visible through the normal tympanic membrane and causes a blush of the promontory, called the Schwartze sign.

Tomography of the Labyrinthine Windows

Multidirectional tomography must be used to study and diagnose otosclerosis of the labyrinthine windows, the cochlea and the other inner ear structures.

Four projections are used for the study of the labyrinthine windows and cochlear capsule: coronal, semiaxial, axial and Stenvers. The first two projections expose the oval window and the cochlear capsule. The axial demonstrates the cochlear coils, and the Stenvers the round window.

The oval window lies in the medial labyrinthine wall of the middle ear cavity. The long axis of the window measures 3–4 mm and forms an angle of about 20° open posteriorly with the sagittal plane of the skull. The vertical axis of the window measures 1.5 to 2 mm.

Coronal and semiaxial projections demonstrate the oval window. Beginning at the level of the anterior aspect of the cochlea six coronal and semiaxial sections, 1 mm apart are taken that will pass through the oval window area.

The oval window appears as a well defined bony dehiscence in the lateral wall of the vestibule below the ampullated limb of the horizontal semicircular canal.

In the coronal projection the footplate of the normal stapes, which is 0.2 to 0.4 mm thick, is not visible because of its obliquity to the plane of section.

In the semiaxial projection the footplate of the stapes is sectioned at right angles to the long axis. A normal footplate often appears as a fine line extending across the oval window.

The round window closes the scala tympani and is located deep in the round window niche. The round window niche lies on the posteroinferior aspect of the promontory below the oval window.

The Stenvers projection gives the best demonstration of the round window. In this projection the round window appears as a dehiscence in the contour of the posterolateral aspect of the promontory separated from the oval window by a 3–4 mm dense area of the cochlear capsule.

The round window is also visible in coronal tomographic sections as a small radiolucent area superimposed of the lumen of the posterior portion of the basal cochlear coil. The round window should not be confused with the radiolucency of the ampulla of the posterior semicircular canal which lies 2 mm posteriorly.

Computerized Tomography

High definition C. T. with zoom or localized reconstruction capability can demonstrate otosclerotic lesions of the oval window. Horizontal and coronal sections 1.5 mm thick are used.

Radiographic Findings of Fenestral Otosclerosis

The radiographic appearance of otosclerosis of the oval window depends on the degree of maturation and the extent of the pathological process.

In mature otosclerosis the oval window becomes narrowed or closed by calcified foci, Figs. 11.1–11.2.

In active otosclerosis or otospongiosis the poorly calcified foci may not be recognizable. The margin of the oval window becomes decalcified so that the oval window seems larger than normal.

The extent of the involvement varies. When otosclerosis involves the margin only there is narrowing or obliteration of the aperture of the oval window. Occasionally the footplate of the stapes becomes greatly thickened with minimal involvement of the surrounding oval window margin. In these cases tomography shows a thick bony plate within a relatively normal oval window. In diffuse otosclerosis the entire footplate is involved as well as the oval window margin. In these cases the oval window appears completely obliterated by a thick bony plate.

The otosclerotic process may involve the vestibular aspect of the footplate and oval window margin to encroach upon the vestibule.

The round window may be involved by an isolated focus or by extension of a large focus from the oval window area. Tomographically there are areas of demineralization or sclerotic foci surrounding or encroaching the round window. The radiologist cannot predict the functional loss of hearing from round window otosclerosis, since it is known that a minute opening in the round window is sufficient for hydrodynamic function.

Pre- and Postoperative Evaluation of the Labyrinthine Windows

Otosclerosis is diagnosed clinically by the otologist on the basis of otoscopy, audiometry and tuning fork tests. The clinical evaluation cannot determine the extent of the degree of the pathological involvement of the footplate.

Tomography on the other hand can visualize the extent of the pathology of the oval window and footplate.

Tomography can be used in those cases where the clinical diagnosis of otosclerosis is in doubt and in some bilateral cases for selection of the ear to be operated. Tomography is also indicated in patients with pronounced mixed deafness to determine the presence of cochlear otosclerosis.

Poststapedectomy Tomography

Tomography is helpful in determining the cause of immediate and delayed vertigo, poststapedectomy hearing loss and vertigo.

When metallic prosthesis is used a tomographic study allows a precise evaluation of the position of the strut, Fig. 11.3. In cases where a severe sensorineural deafness or vertigo follow immediately after surgery, tomography may demonstrate protrusion of the prosthesis into the vestibule, Figs. 11.10.

When a conductive deafness develops after an initial hearing improvement the cause may be a reobliteration of the oval window with fixation or dislocation of the prosthesis, Figs. 11.4–11.9. If the oval window remains patent, conductive deafness can occur from separation of the lateral end of the prosthesis from the incus or from necrosis of the long process of the incus. At times the lateral end of the strut is attached to the long process but the medial end is dislocated from the oval window. When a radiolucent prosthesis has been used the position of the strut cannot be determined.

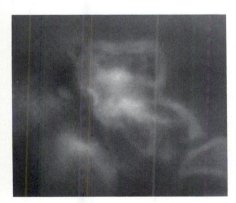

Fig. 11.**1**   Otosclerosis, semiaxial tomogram, right. The oval window is closed by a thick stapes footplate. Small spongiotic foci are present in the capsule of the basal turn of the cochlea.

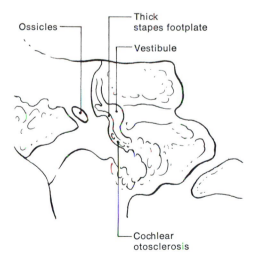

Ossicles

Thick stapes footplate

Vestibule

Cochlear otosclerosis

Fig. 11.**2**   Diagram of Fig. 11.1

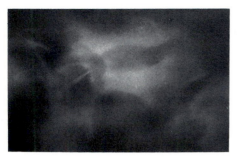

Fig. 11.**3**   Otosclerosis, poststapedectomy, coronal tomogram, right. A metallic prosthesis extends from the long process of the incus to the open oval window.

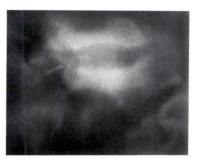

Fig. 11.**4**   Same ear as in Fig. 11.3, four years later, coronal tomogram. Progression of the otosclerosis has reclosed the oval window and fixed the medial end of the prosthesis.

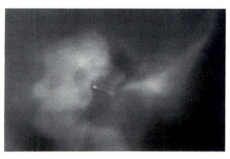

Fig. 11.**5**   Otosclerosis, poststapedectomy, semiaxial tomogram, left. The oval window is reclosed and the medial end of the prosthesis is displaced laterally and inferiorly.

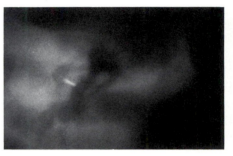

Fig. 11.**6**   Otosclerosis, poststapedectomy, semiaxial tomogram, left. The medial portion of a McGee prosthesis is imbedded and fixed in a large recurrent focus of otosclerosis which obliterates the oval window.

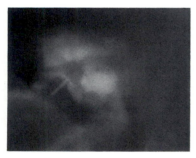

Fig. 11.**7**   Otosclerosis, poststapedectomy, semiaxial tomogram, right. The oval window is reclosed and the medial end of the stapes prosthesis is fixed by the recurrent otosclerosis.

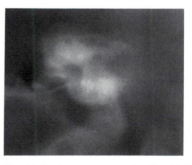

Fig. 11.**8**   Same ear as in Fig. 11.7, one year later, semiaxial tomogram. Following revision of the stapedectomy, the oval window is patent, but the medial end of the prosthesis is displaced inferiorly on the promontory.

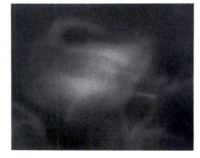

Fig. 11.**9**   Otosclerosis, poststapedectomy, semiaxial tomogram, left. The oval window is reclosed and the medial end of the prosthesis is displaced onto the promontory.

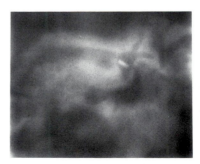

Fig. 11.**10**   Otosclerosis, poststapedectomy, semiaxial tomogram, left. The piston of the McGee prosthesis is displaced into the vestibule.

Tomography in Cochlear Otosclerosis

Tomography visualizes otosclerotic foci within the cochlear capsule.

The normal cochlear capsule appears as a sharply defined dense bony shell outlining the lumen of the cochlear coils. The density of the capsule enhances the contrast between the lumen and the capsule. Because of this optical phenomenon the lumen of the cochlear coil seems more radiolucent.

When the otosclerotic foci affect the cochlear capsule there is a variable disruption of the density and outline of the capsule.

In the interpretation of the radiographic findings of cochlear otosclerosis three factors must be considered:

1. The otosclerotic focus must be 2 mm or larger in diameter to be visible in the tomographs.
2. The density of the otosclerotic focus must be different from the density of the normal otic capsule.
3. Since the normal labyrinthine capsule is very dense, sclerotic foci can only be recognized when they are apposed to the periosteal or endosteal surfaces of the capsule.

The radiographic changes of cochlear otosclerosis are classified according to extension, degree, and stage of maturation of the focus.

The otosclerotic process may be limited to a small portion of the basal turn of the cochlea immediately adjacent to the anterior margin of the oval window or spread into other areas of the basal turn. These foci are seen best in semiaxial sections. When the process involves the middle and apical coils the changes are best demonstrated in the axial projection. Occasionally other areas of the labyrinthine capsule are involved such as the fundus of the internal auditory canal, the semicircular canals and vestibule. These changes are well seen in coronal tomographic sections.

The degree of involvement is classified according to the size and confluence or coalescence of the otosclerotic foci. There may be minimal, moderate or severe degrees of involvement.

Since small foci are only recognizable in the portion of the capsule seen in profile, multiple projections should be obtained to visualize these small foci.

The radiographic appearance of the otosclerotic lesion varies with the stage of maturation of the disease. In the demineralizing or spongiotic stage the normally sharp outline of the capsule becomes interrupted and may disappear completely. The demineralization of the capsule causes loss of the normal differential density between the lumen of the cochlear coils and the capsule. In severe involvement the outline of the capsule becomes indistinguishable from the surrounding bone of the petrosa, Figs. 11.11–11.20.

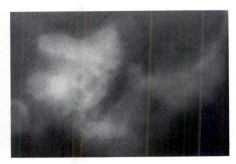

Fig. 11.**11**   Otosclerosis, cochlear, semiaxial tomogram, left. Multiple otospongiotic foci are scattered throughout the cochlear capsule.

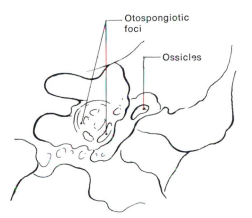

Fig. 11.**12**   Diagram of Fig. 11.11

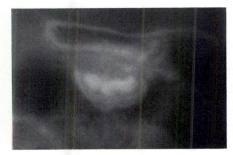

Fig. 11.**13**   Otosclerosis, cochlear, semiaxial tomogram, left. A fine band of demineralization reduplicates the contour of the basal turn of the cochlea.

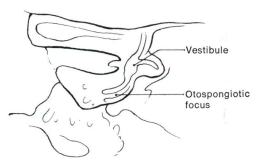

Fig. 11.**14**   Diagram of Fig. 11.13

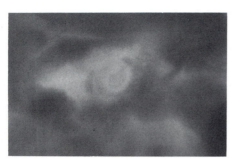

Fig. 11.**15** Otosclerosis, cochlear, coronal tomogram, left. A band of demineralization follows the contour of the lumen of the basal turn of the cochlea. The capsule of the middle coil is demineralized.

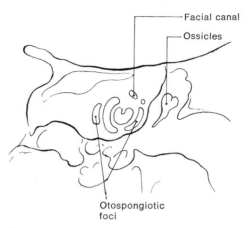

Fig. 11.**16** Diagram of Fig. 11.15

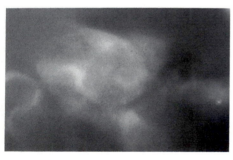

Fig. 11.**17** Same ear as in Fig. 11.15, coronal tomogram, 4 mm posterior. The capsule of the basal turn of the cochlea is irregularly demineralized.

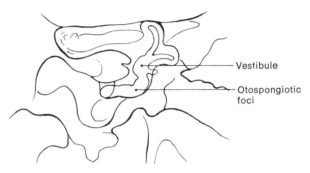

Fig. 11.**18** Diagram of Fig. 11.17

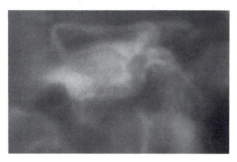

Fig. 11.**19** Otosclerosis, cochlear, semiaxial tomogram, left. There is demineralization of the entire cochlea by a severe otospongiotic process.

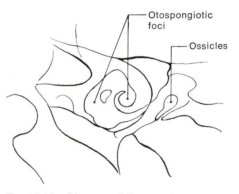

Fig. 11.**20** Diagram of Fig. 11.19

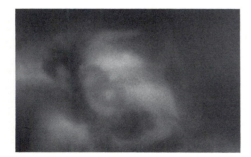

Fig. 11.**21** Otosclerosis, cochlear, semiaxial tomogram, right. Mixed otosclerotic and otospongiotic foci disrupt the capsule of the basal turn of the cochlea.

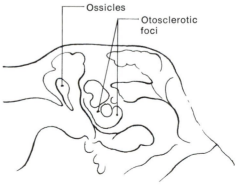

Fig. 11.**22** Diagram of Fig. 11.21

In the mature or sclerotic stage there are localized or diffuse areas of thickening of the capsule due to apposition of new otosclerotic bone. Such foci when seen on end appear as areas of roughening or scalloping of the outer or inner outline of the capsule. These same foci seen on face appear as spotty areas of increased density superimposed on the radiolucency of the cochlear lumen, Figs. 11.23–11.28.

When spongiotic and sclerotic changes occur simultaneously, there is a mosaic pattern characterized by a mixture of areas of decreased density intermingled with areas of increased density, Figs. 11.21–11.22. A similar mosaic pattern occurs as the result of several small spongiotic foci scattered throughout an otherwise normal capsule.

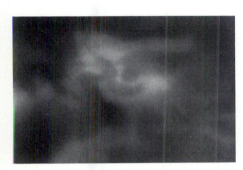

Fig. 11.23   Otosclerosis, cochlear, coronal tomogram, right. Sclerotic foci are present in the capsule of the basal turn of the cochlea. The contour of the promontory appears thickened.

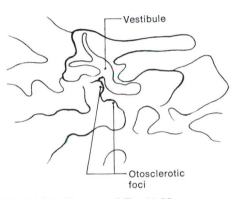

Fig. 11.24   Diagram of Fig. 11.23

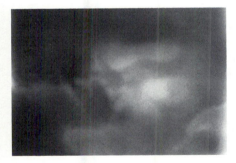

Fig. 11.25   Otoscleros cochlear, semiaxial tomogram, right. A large sclerotic focus thickens the capsule of the basal turn of the cochlea. The footplate of the stapes is thickened.

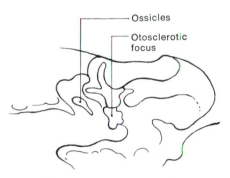

Fig. 11.26   Diagram of Fig. 11.25

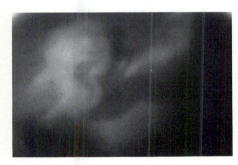

Fig. 11.27   Otosclerosis, cochlear, semiaxial tomogram, left. A large sclerotic foci encroaches upon the narrow round window niche. The oval window is also closed.

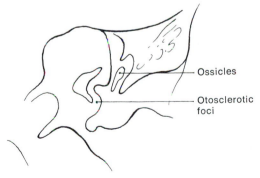

Fig. 11.28   Diagram of Fig. 11.27

Paget's Disease

Paget's disease can affect the calvarium and the base of the skull including the petrous pyramids. When the disease process extends into the otic capsule there will be a mixed or sensorineural hearing loss which is progressive.

Radiographic Findings

Even in the absence of typical changes elsewhere in the skeleton, the diagnosis of Paget's disease can be made by recognition of pathognomonic features in the petrous pyramid.

In Paget's disease there is an active stage with progessive bone resorption followed by a stage of irregular reconstruction leading to a hypertrophied, vascular, irregularly mineralized bone.

The haversian bone of the petrosa is affected first, with spread of the disease from the apex laterally. At first, due to severe demineralization of the petrosa, the labyrinthine capsule becomes more prominent than normal. Involvement of the otic capsule begins at the periosteal surface. Slow demineralization occurs which produces first thinning and finally complete dissolution of the capsule. This results in a washed out appearance of the entire petrous bone characteristic of Paget's disease. The internal auditory canal is usually the first structure involved followed by the cochlea and the vestibular system, Figs. 11.29–11.35.

In the late stage of the disease deposition of irregular mineralized new bone occurs which results in thickening and enlargement of the petrous bone, Figs. 11.36–11.37. The stapes footplate is often affected by the disease process, more rarely the malleus and incus are involved, Fig. 11.37.

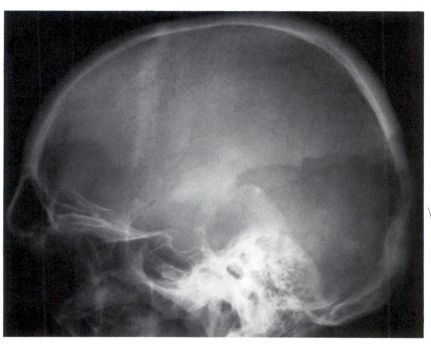

Fig. 11.**29** Paget's disease, skull, lateral view. Two sharply defined areas of demineralization, osteoporosis circumscripta, are present in the occipital and frontal bones.

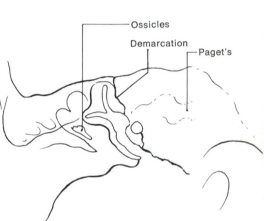

Fig. 11.**30** Diagram of Fig. 11.32

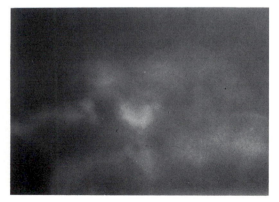

Fig. 11.**31** Same patient as in Fig. 11.29 and 11.32, coronal tomogram, right. The active Paget's disease involves the petrous pyramid and cochlear capsule. Only a remnant of the cochlear capsule is visible.

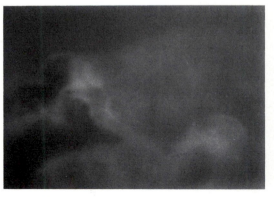

Fig. 11.**32** Same patient as in Figs. 11.29 and 11.31, coronal tomogram, 6 mm posterior to Fig. 11.31. Active Paget's disease is indicated by the sharp demarcation between the diseased petrous pyramid and the uninvolved portion of the labyrinth.

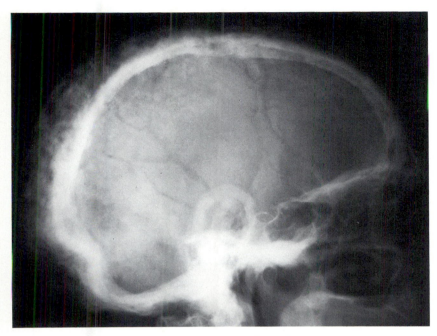

Fig. 11.**33**   Paget's disease, skull, lateral view. The calvarium is markedly thickened. The pathologic remodeling of bone causes an irregular recalcification of the thickened cranial vault.

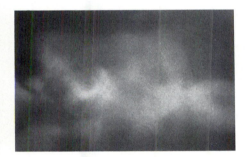

Fig. 11.**34**   Same patient as in Figs. 11.33 and 11.35, coronal tomogram, right. There is severe demineralization of the petrous pyramid and thinning of the cochlear capsule.

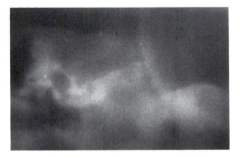

Fig. 11.**35**   Same patient as in Figs. 11.33 and 11.34, coronal tomogram, 6 mm posterior to Fig. 11.34. The contour of the internal auditory canal is poorly defined. The occipital bone in the region of the hypoglossal canal is also affected.

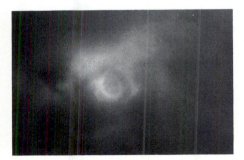

Fig. 11.**36**   Paget's disease, coronal tomogram, right. The petrous pyramid is thickened. The involvement is hyperostotic in the upper portion of the pyramid while demineralization predominates inferiorly.

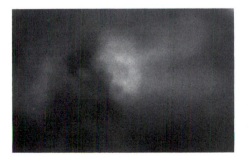

Fig. 11.**37**   Same ear is in Fig. 11.36. The petrous pyramid is thickened, and the contour of the internal auditory canal is poorly defined. A sharp line of demarcation separates the normal from the involved portion of the pyramid. The stapes footplate is thickened by the Paget's disease.

Osteogenesis Imperfecta

Osteogenesis imperfecta or fragilitas osseum is characterized by abnormally thin and fragile long bones with a history of multiple fractures, by a blue color of the sclerae and by severe mixed deafness. In some forms of the disease one or more of the features may be absent. The head is large, the calvarium abnormally thin, and the otic capsules are involved.

The tomographic findings resemble those of active, cochlear otosclerosis, but are much more diffuse and involve the entire otic capsule, Figs. 11.38–11.40.

Osteopetrosis

Osteopetrosis, Albers-Schönberg disease, marble bone disease is a rare bone disease characterized by formation of new bone while resorption of bone is diminished. This results in sclerosis of bone with obliteration of the medullary cavities and diploic spaces and narrowing of the foramina of the skull.

Tomographically the petrous bone shows a complete lack of pneumatization and an homogenous diffuse sclerotic appearance.

Progression of the disease results in narrowing of the internal auditory canals and encroachment of the neurovascular bundles. Facial paralysis may occur on the same basis.

Fibrous Dysplasia

Fibrous dysplasia is an osseous hyperplasia of unknown etiology which may involve the skull. There are two different types of changes which occur in the skull. In the calvarium and mandible there is expansion of the affected portion by multiple cystic lesions. In the base of the skull including the temporal bone proliferation of bone occurs which leads to marked thickening and sclerosis of the affected areas. Involvement by fibrous dysplasia is usually unilateral which leads to asymmetry, Figs. 11.41–11.43.

In the temporal bone the squama becomes thickened and the pneumatic system obliterated. The external auditory canal is often stenosed by new bone formation. As the petrous pyramid becomes thickened and dense, the outline of the labyrinthine capsule becomes poorly distinguishable from the surrounding bone. Further progression may lead to narrowing of the internal auditory canal and obliteration of the lumen of the labyrinth.

Craniometaphyseal Dysplasia

Craniometaphyseal dysplasia is a genetic disorder characterized by alterations in the metaphyses of the long bones and by bone overgrowth of the skull, particularly the face and jaw.

The skull shows marked thickening and increased density of the calvarium with obliteration of the diploic space. The base of the skull, the maxilla and mandible become enlarged, thickened and sclerotic. The paranasal sinuses are obliterated, Fig. 11.46.

In the temporal bone the external auditory canal and middle ear are gradually filled in by new dense bone formation.

The petrous pyramids are thickened and the lumen of the labyrinth becomes obliterated, Fig. 11.44–11.45–11.47. The temporal bone and labyrinthine capsule are also involved in other rare congenital disorders and bony dysplasias such as cleidocranial dysostosis and Hurler's syndrome.

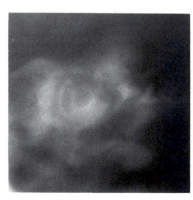

Fig. 11.**38** Osteogenesis imperfecta, coronal tomogram, left. The entire cochlear capsule is demineralized. The double ring appearance of the capsule is produced by a band of demineralization within the thickness of the capsule.

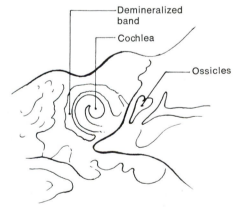

Fig. 11.**39**   Diagram of Fig. 11.38

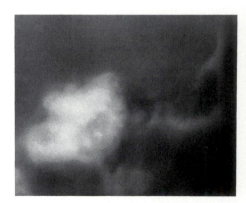

Fig. 11.**40**   Same ear as in Fig. 11.38, semi-axial tomogram. The capsule of the labyrinth is disrupted by the severe and diffuse involvement.

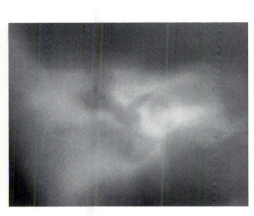

Fig. 11.**41** Fibrous dysplasia, coronal tomogram, right. There is thickening and sclerosis of mastoid and petrous pyramid. The proliferative, hyperostotic process obliterates the air cells and narrows the external auditory canal.

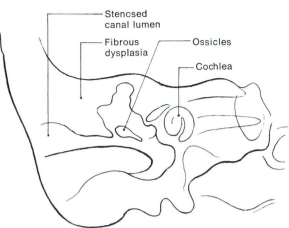

Fig. 11.**42**   Diagram of Fig. 11.41

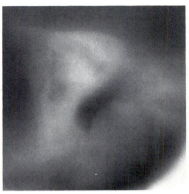

Fig. 11.**43** Same ear as in Fig. 11.41, sagittal tomogram. The hyperostotic process has obliterated most of the air cells of the mastoid. The external auditory canal lumen is narrowed by marked thickening of the anterior wall.

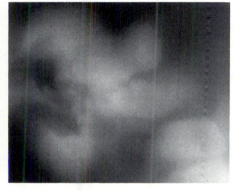

Fig. 11.**44** Craniometaphyseal dysplasia, semiaxial tomogram, right. The petrous pyramid is markedly thickened by dense, sclerotic bone. The process partially obliterates the lumen of the labyrinth and the internal auditory canal. The hypoglossal canal is narrowed.

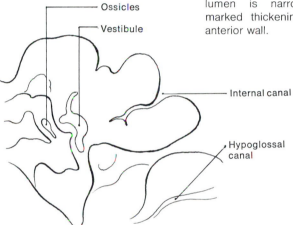

Fig. 11.**45**   Diagram of Fig. 11.44

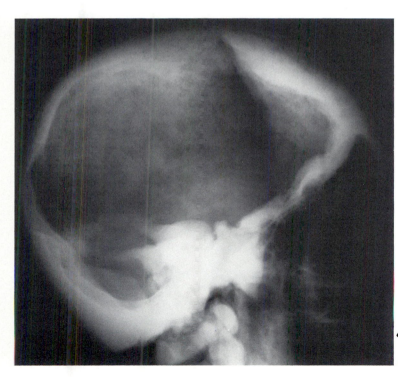

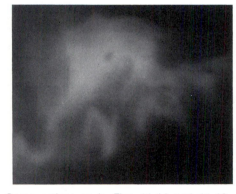

Fig. 11.**47** Same patient as in Figs. 11.44 and 11.46, sagittal tomogram. The petrous pyramid is thickened and sclerotic. The internal auditory canal is markedly constricted.

◄Fig. 11.**46** Same patient as in Figs. 11.44 and 11.47, skull, lateral view. The calvarium and base of skull are thickened by dense sclerotic bone.

Chapter 12   Radiography of the Facial Canal

The bony canal of the facial nerve passes through the temporal bone and can be visualized tomographically. Involvement of the intratemporal portion of the facial nerve may result in facial nerve symptoms such as partial or complete paralysis, tic, hemifacial spasms, alterations in hearing, taste, and tearing.

Conventional radiography is inadequate to study the facial canal and tomography must be employed. The facial nerve itself cannot be visualized, but lesions involving the bony canal are seen in the tomographs.

High definition CT with axial and coronal sections 1.5 mm apart is particularly useful when the facial nerve is involved by extratemporal lesions extending into the temporal bone and facial canal such as parotid tumors and meningiomas.

Tomographic sections are taken 1–2 mm apart and contralateral views are obtained for comparison.

The radiographic projections used in the study of the facial canal depend on the segment being examined. In the temporal bone there are four segments of the facial canal which must be visualized.

1. First or internal auditory canal segment. Coronal and sagittal sections expose this segment. If an intracanalicular mass is suspected on the basis of the tomographs, a posterior fossa cisternogram is required to determine the size and extent of the lesion.
2. Second or petrous segment. This portion of the facial canal extends from the fundus of the internal auditory canal to the geniculate ganglion. The petrous segment is the narrowest part of the facial canal. Coronal and semiaxial projections expose this segment.
3. Third or tympanic segment. This segment extends from the geniculate ganglion along the medial wall of the tympanic cavity to the second or pyramidal turn of the facial nerve. The semiaxial projection is best to expose this segment.
4. Fourth or mastoid segment. This segment stretches from the pyramidal turn to the stylomastoid foramen, and is best visualized by sagittal and Stenvers projections.

Pathological Conditions

Lesions affecting the facial canal can be divided into congenital anomalies, inflammations, fractures and tumors.

Congenital Anomalies

Congenital anomalies of the facial canal involve the size and the course of the canal.

There may be complete or partial agenesis of the facial nerve canal with total paralysis, Figs. 12.1–12.3. Occasionally the facial nerve canal may be unusually narrow and hypoplastic. In these cases, intermittent episodes of facial paresis may occur.

Minor variations of the course of the facial nerve are common and of no clinical or surgical significance. More severe anomalies of the course of the facial nerve occur in the tympanic and vertical portions. Recognition of these anomalies is very important to surgeons planning surgical correction of ear disease. The horizontal segment at times is displaced inferiorly to cover the oval window. If the bony wall of the facial nerve canal is absent the anomaly can not be diagnosed tomographically.

Anomalies of the mastoid segment are common in congenital atresia of the external auditory canal. The facial canal is usually rotated laterally. The rotation varies from a minor obliquity to a true horizontal course.

Since facial nerve anomalies are common in congenital atresia, all such patients should have tomographic assessment preoperatively. Figs. 3.12, 3.13.

Inflammatory Conditions and Cholesteatoma

Bell's palsy is the most common type of facial nerve paralysis of acute onset. The etiology is thought to be a herpes virus polyneuritis, and there are no tomographic changes. All patients initially diagnosed as Bell's palsy but who do not improve should have a tomographic study to rule out other causes of the paralysis.

Facial paralysis may occur as a complication of acute or chronic otitis media.

When paralysis occurs soon after the onset of an acute otitis media, the facial nerve paralysis is usually not due to erosion of the bony canal but to edema and inflammation of the nerve within the bony canal probably similar to Bell's palsy. Recovery of facial nerve function occurs in these cases with conservative treatment.

Facial paralysis occurring two weeks or more after the onset of a persistent acute otitis media usually indicates erosion of the bony facial canal and extension of the infection. Tomographic evaluation is indicated, and surgery is often required in cases of this type.

Chronic Otitis Media with Cholesteatoma

Facial paralysis may occur in patients with chronic otitis media and cholesteatoma. In these cases the paralysis is caused by the expanded mass of the cholesteatoma in the middle ear and mastoid.

The most common site of facial nerve involvement by cholesteatoma is the horizontal portion of the nerve at the pyramidal turn, see Chapter 7.

Congenital Cholesteatoma of the Petrous Pyramid

Facial paralysis may be the first symptom of a congenital cholesteatoma of the petrous pyramid. The nerve is involved in these cases in the intracanalicular or petrous segments, see Chapter 7.

Malignant External Otitis

Facial paralysis due to involvement of the vertical segment in the region of the stylomastoid foramen is common in malignant external otitis, see Chapter 5.

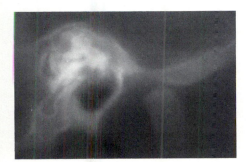

Fig. 12.1   Congenital atresia, facial nerve canal, sagittal tomogram, right. This three year old child has congenital right facial paralysis. The facial canal ends in a blind cul de sac at the midportion of the mastoid segment.

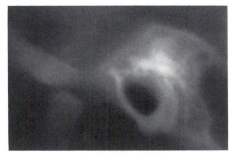

Fig. 12.2   Same patient as in Fig. 12.1, corresponding sagittal tomogram of normal left ear for comparison

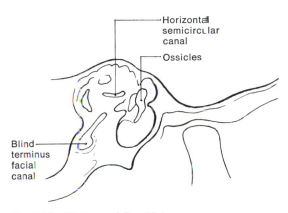

Fig. 12.3   Diagram of Fig. 12.1

Traumatic Facial Nerve Lesions

Traumatic lesions of the intratemporal portion of the facial nerve occur following head injuries of various types, especially with high speed vehicle accidents.

A tomographic study should be performed in these cases to demonstrate the presence of: 1. a temporal bone fracture; 2. the course of the fracture; and 3. the site of involvement of the facial canal.

This information is necessary if surgical decompression of the facial canal is planned.

The radiographic findings are variable:

1. There may be a complete disruption of the contour of a segment of the facial canal;
2. The canal may be transected by the fracture line;
3. There may be separation and depression of a fragment of the canal wall into the facial nerve;
4. The incus may be dislocated and the short process impelled into the facial canal immediately distal to the pyramidal turn.

In some cases the site of the involvement of the facial canal cannot be visualized in the tomographs. However, by evaluation of the course of the fracture line, the site of the lesion can be determined.

Classification of Radiographic Findings

The facial nerve may be injured by transverse or longitudinal fractures, Figs. 12.4–12.10.

While the incidence of transverse fractures is less than that of longitudinal, more than 50% of transverse fractures have an associated lesion of the facial nerve. In these cases the nerve involvement occurs at the geniculate ganglion, the petrous portion or the intracanalicular segment, Figs. 12.9–12.10.

Facial nerve paralysis occurs in approximately 20% of longitudinal temporal bone fractures. About 50% of these lesions are located at or distal to the pyramidal turn, Figs. 4.9, 4.10, 4.12, 4.13, and 50% in the geniculate ganglion region.

When the geniculate ganglion area is involved, the longitudinal fracture crosses the anterior aspect of the mastoid, the external canal and attic and extends into the petrous pyramid anterior to the labyrinth. The fracture involves the facial canal in the region of the superficial and poorly protected anterior genu, Figs. 12.4–12.8.

Bullet Wounds

Facial paralysis may occur in comminuted fractures of the temporal bone caused by bullet wounds.

Iatrogenic Lesions

Facial nerve injury may occur following mastoid surgery. In these cases the most common lesion occurs at the pyramidal turn. Radiographically the facial canal in this area is absent and often there is an associated defect in the horizontal semicircular canal.

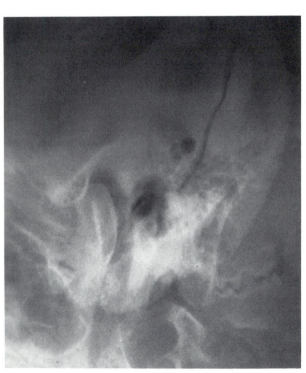

Fig. 12.**4** Longitudinal fracture, temporal bone, Schüller view, left. A longitudinal fracture line extends from the temporal squama, through the mastoid, into the external auditory canal.

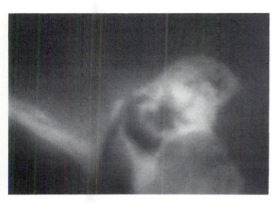

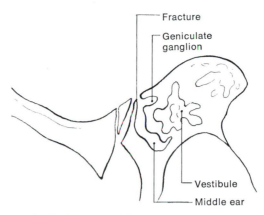

Fig. 12.**5**   Same ear as in Fig. 12.4, sagittal tomogram. The longitudinal fracture crosses the anterior aspect of the epitympanum and extends into the petrous pyramid anterior to the labyrinth. The fracture traverses the anterior portion of the facial nerve canal at the geniculate ganglion area.

Fig. 12.**6**   Diagram of Fig. 12.5

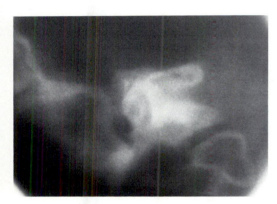

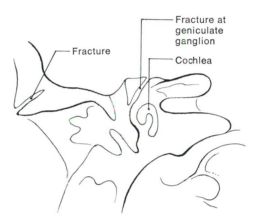

Fig. 12.**7**   Longitudinal fracture, temporal bone, semiaxial tomogram, right. A longitudinal fracture extends from the temporal squama into the petrous pyramid through the geniculate ganglion area.

Fig. 12.**8**   Diagram of Fig. 12.7

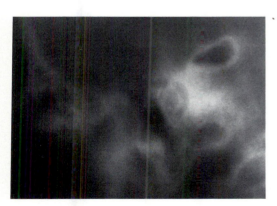

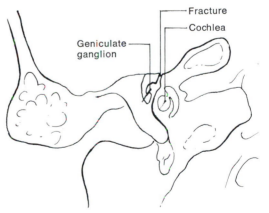

Fig. 12.**9**   Transverse fracture, temporal bone, semiaxial tomogram, right. A transverse fracture extends from the superior petrous ridge into the labyrinth and involves the facial nerve canal at the geniculate ganglion area.

Fig. 12.**10**   Diagram of Fig. 12.9

Neuromas of the Facial Nerve

Intratemporal neuromas or neurilemomas of the facial nerve occur rarely.

The clinical findings depend on the site of origin and size of the lesion. Lesions arising within the internal auditory canal may present symptoms mimicking an acoustic neuroma. Neuromas which arise within the facial canal usually cause a peripheral facial paralysis or tic. When a neuroma arises within the tympanic portion of the facial nerve canal the first symptom may be a conductive deafness due to encroachment of the tumor on the ossicular chain.

In our series of twenty-two cases of facial nerve neuromas, fourteen involved the internal auditory canal and petrous portion of the facial nerve while five were located in the tympanic portion and three in the mastoid segment, Figs. 12.11–12.20.

Radiographic Findings

Initially facial nerve neuromas cause expansion of the lumen of the bony facial nerve canal. To detect early changes it is necessary to compare the affected and normal sides. Enlargement of the lesion results in erosion of the bony canal and involvement of adjacent structures of the petrous pyramid, middle ear and mastoid.

When the tumor extends into the middle ear a well defined soft tissue mass appears.

Lesions arising in the internal auditory canal cause enlargement of the canal. Cerebellopontine angle cisternography or computerized tomography are indicated in these cases to diagnose the presence of a mass and to determine the size of the lesion.

A facial nerve neuroma limited to the internal auditory canal cannot be differentiated from a acoustic neuroma by cisternography. Tomography at times can be used for differentiation. Tomographically with facial nerve neuromas there is often enlargement and erosion of the petrous segment of the facial nerve canal.

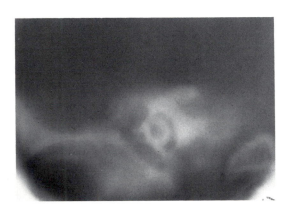

Fig. 12.**11**   Neuroma, facial nerve, coronal tomogram, right. The facial nerve canal in the region of the anterior genu is enlarged by a neuroma of the nerve.

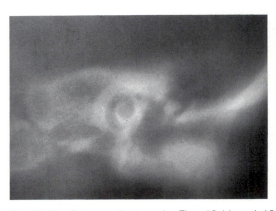

Fig. 12.**12**   Same patient as in Figs. 12.11 and 12.13, corresponding coronal section of normal left ear for comparison

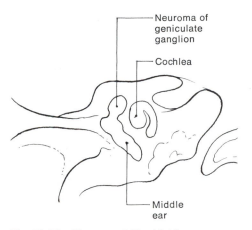

Fig. 12.**13**   Same ear as in Fig. 12.11, semiaxial tomogram. In this projection the expansion of the facial canal is better exposed.

Fig. 12.**14**   Diagram of Fig. 12.13

Neuroma of geniculate ganglion

Cochlea

Middle ear

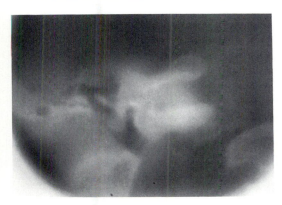

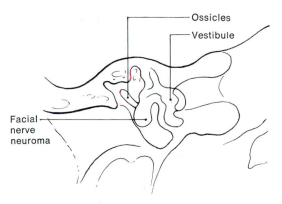

Fig. 12.**15**   Neuroma, facial nerve, semiaxial tomogram, right. A neuroma of the tympanic segment of the facial nerve lies within the lumen of the middle ear and erodes the long process of the incus.

Fig. 12.**16**   Diagram of Fig. 12.15

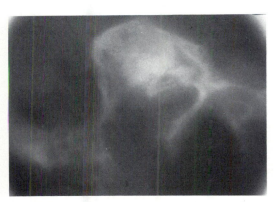

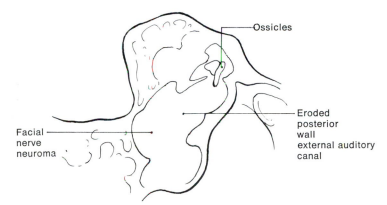

Fig. 12.**17**   Neuroma, facial nerve, sagittal tomogram, right. A very large neuroma of the facial nerve, arising from the mastoid segment, produces a gross dilatation of the facial canal. The lesion erodes the posterior wall of the external auditory canal.

Fig. 12.**18**   Diagram of Fig. 12.17

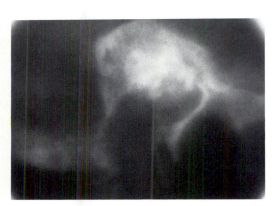

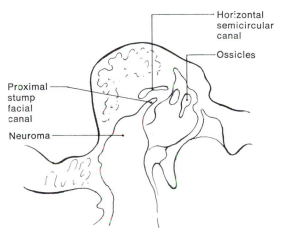

Fig. 12.**19**   Same ear as in Fig. 12.17, sagittal tomogram 2 mm medial. In this section the proximal stump of the facial canal lies under the horizontal semicircular canal. The posterior wall of the middle ear is eroded.

Fig. 12.**20**   Diagram of Fig. 12.19

Chapter 13   Vestibular Aqueduct Abnormalities

The vestibular aqueduct is a small bony canal which extends from the posteromedial wall of the vestibule to the posterior surface of the petrous pyramid. In the adult the shape of the aqueduct forms an inverted J. The proximal segment, the isthmus, which arches medial to the common crus, is the narrowest segment of the aqueduct and measures 0.3 mm in diameter, Figs. 13.1–13.3.

As the aqueduct extends inferiorly it widens and forms a triangular slit parallel to the posterior surface of the pyramid. The outer aperture of the aqueduct measures approximately 2.0–6.0 mm in the larger diameter and 1.0 mm in the shorter.

The aqueduct contains the endolymphatic duct which enlarges to end blindly in the endolymphatic sac lying on the posterior surface of the petrous bone.

Tomography must be used to visualize the vestibular aqueduct. The postisthmic segment appears in more than 90% of normal ears, but the isthmic segment is seen in less than 50% because of the overlying radiolucency of the common crus.

To visualize the postisthmic segment the outer opening of the aqueduct and the common crus should be aligned in the same plane of section. Correct alignment is obtained by varying the projection from the sagittal through 45° towards the axial. In practice we obtain a test section in a plane intermediate between the sagittal and axial. If the aqueduct is not well visualized, the position is changed in the appropriate direction, Fig. 13.3.

Abnormal Aqueducts

Radiographic evaluation is limited to the postisthmic segment. We measure the anteroposterior diameter midway between the outer aperture and the common crus. An aqueduct is considered abnormal when it is: 1. not visualized; 2. obliterated segmentally; or 3. narrow, the diameter is less than 0.5 mm.

Radiographic studies indicate that narrowing or obliteration of the vestibular aqueduct is frequently associated with cochleovestibular disorders of the Menière's type, Figs. 13.2, 13.4, 13.5.

Visualization of a normal-sized aqueduct does not rule out Menière's type otic pathology, since patients with this disorder often have a normal aqueduct.

Enlargement and shortening of the aqueduct occur as a congenital malformation often associated with the Mondini anomaly. This condition is discussed in Chapter 3.

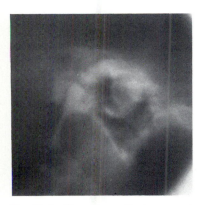

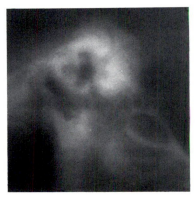

Fig. 13.**1** Normal vestibular aqueduct, modified sagittal tomogram, right.

Fig. 13.**2** Menière-like disorder, modified sagittal tomogram, left. The vestibular aqueduct is visualized but has a filiform diameter and is narrower than on the normal right side.

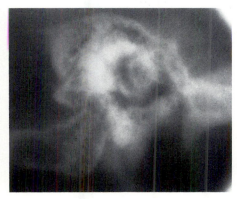

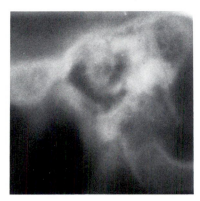

Fig. 13.**3** Normal vestibular aqueduct, modified sagittal tomogram, right.

Fig. 13.**4** Menière-like disorder, modified sagittal tomogram, left. The vestibular aqueduct is barely recognizable because of the filiform diameter. This aqueduct must be compared with the opposite normal ear in Figure 13.3.

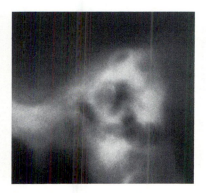

Fig. 13.**5** Obliterated vestibular aqueduct, Menière-like disorder, modified sagittal tomogram, left. Only a short segment of the aqueduct adjacent to the common crus is visible.

Chapter 14 Computerized Tomographic Evaluation of Vertebrobasilar Vascular Insufficiency

Reduction of blood flow to certain areas of the hind brain can cause dizziness and less often sensorineural hearing loss. This reduced blood flow is caused by narrowing or obstruction of the vertebral and basilar arteries. When the carotid circulation is insufficient, stealing from the vertebral arteries occurs with resultant decreased circulation in the hind brain.

The circulation of the blood to the hind brain is often evaluated angiographically. Angiography demonstrates pathology of the major blood vessels but does not show the status of the small vessels of the brain nor of the perfusion of blood to the brain.

Recently, fast rotational CT has been utilized in the study of the blood circulation of the brain. After a preliminary standard study, a 10 mm section of the brain is selected for the evaluation. A bolus of 30–45 ml of contrast material is injected rapidly into a vein in the arm. Six to twelve images of the selected brain section are obtained during a 30 s period. The first image exposes the brain before the contrast arrives. Subsequent images demonstrate the perfusion of the contrast through the section of the brain selected for the study, Fig. 14.1.

A graphic plot of the absorption changes for each cubic centimeter of brain during the 30 s interval is obtained, Fig. 14.2. The density of the contrast material, measured in CT numbers is displayed on the y axis and time on the x axis.

The normal graphic study is seen in Figure 14.2. The peak concentration of contrast material perfusing through the brain tissue is reached in 15–20 s following the injection. The concentration of contrast material reaches an amplitude of 3 to 7 CT numbers. The concentration is usually higher in the temporal and occipital lobes.

The peak concentration of the contrast material perfusing the brain occurs at the end of the wash-in phase. Contrast is eliminated during the wash-out phase. Transit time and concentration during the wash-in and wash-out phases are measured on the graphic plot.

Vascular insufficiency produces characteristic changes in the graphic plot, Fig. 14.3. These changes can be summarized as:

1. Low peak amplitude,
2. prolonged wash-in phase with delayed peak concentration,
3. plateau of the curve of the wash-out phase caused by collateral circulation.

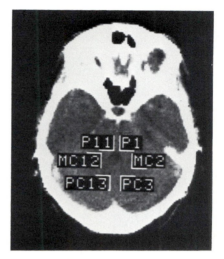

Fig. 14.1 Cubic centimeters of brain from which graphic plot of absorption changes is obtained. MC 2 represents 1 cm of brain tissue in the middle portion of the cerebellum, MC 12 the corresponding area on the opposite side.

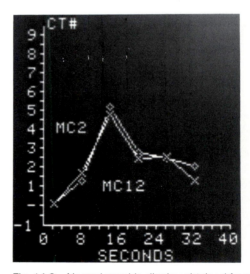

Fig. 14.2 Normal graphic display obtained from six computerized scans of areas MC 2 and MC 12 during a 30 s period. The peak is 5 CT numbers in 16 s.

Fig. 14.3 Vertebrobasilar insufficiency. Abnormal graphic display ▶ demonstrating low peak amplitude and delayed peak bilaterally. The peak is only 2 CT numbers in 22 s.

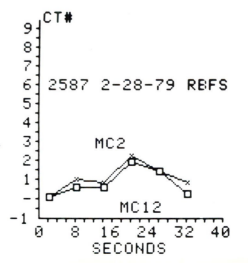

References

1. Anson BJ, Donaldson JA: The surgical anatomy of the temporal bone and ear. Saunders, Philadelphia 1967
2. Bast TH, Anson BJ: The temporal bone and the ear Thomas, Springfield 1949
3. Buckingham RA, Valvassori GE: Tomographic and surgical pathology of cholesteatoma. Arch Otolaryngol 91: 464–469, 1970
4. Carter Bl, Hammerschlag SB, Wolpert SM: Computerized scanning in otorhinolaryngology. Adv Otorhinolaryngol 24: 21–31, 1978
5. Clemis JD, Valvassori GE: Recent radiographic and clinical observations on the vestibular aqueduct (A preliminary report). Otolaryngol Clin North Am: 339–346, October, 1968
6. Dubois PH, Drayer BP, Bank WO, Deeb ZL, et al: An evaluation of current diagnostic radiologic modalities in the investigation of acoustic neurilemmomas. Radiology 125: 173–179, 1978
7. Dulac GL, Claus E, Barrois J: Otoradiology. X-Ray Bull Special Issue. Agfa-Gevaert, Lille 1973
8. Hanafee WN, Mancuso AA, Jenkins HA, Winter J: Computerized tomography scanning of the temporal bone. Ann Otol Rhinol Laryngol 88: 721–728, 1979
9. Hanafee WN, Mancuso A, Winter J, Jenkins H, Bergstrom, LaVonne: Edge enhancement computed tomography scanning in inflammatory lesions of the middle ear. Radiology 136: 771–775, 1980
10. Kricheff II, Pinto RS, Bergeron RT, Cohen N: Air – CT cisternography and canalography for small acoustic neuromas. Am J Neurorad 1: 57–63, 1980
11. Maniglia AJ: Intra and extracranial meningiomas involving the temporal bone. Laryngoscope Suppl 12, 1978
12. Rosenbaum AE, Drayer BP, Dubois PJ, et al: Visualization of small extracanalicular neurilemmomas. Arch Otolaryngol 104: 239–243, 1978
13. Rosenwasser H: Carotid body-like tumor of the middle ear and mastoid bone. Arch Otolaryngol 41: 54–67, 1945
14. Rosenwasser H: Glomus jugulare tumors. Arch Otolaryngol 1968 (monograph)
15. Sackett JF, Strother CM, Quaglieri CE, et al: Metrizamide – CSF contrast medium. Radiology 123: 779–782, 1977
16. Shaffer KA, Haughton VM, Wilson ChR: High resolution computed tomography of the temporal bone. Radiology 134: 409–414, 1980
17. Shambaugh GE Jr: Surgery of the ear, second edition. Saunders, Philadelphia 1967
18. Schuknecht HF: Pathology of the ear. Harvard University Press, Cambridge 1974
19. Spalteholz W, (trans. by) Barker LF: Hand atlas of human anatomy, Vol. III. Lippincott, Philadelphia 1943
20. Valvassori GE, Pierce RH: The normal internal auditory canal. Am J Roentgenol 92: 1232–2141, 1964
21. Valvassori GE: Otosclerosis: A new challenge to roentgenology. Am J Roentgenol Radiol Ther 94: 566–575, 1965
22. Valvassori GE: The interpretation of the radiographic findings in cochlear otosclerosis. Ann Otol (St. Louis) 75: 572–578, 1966
23. Valvassori GE, Naunton RF, Lindsay JR: Inner ear anomalies: Clinical and histopathological considerations. Ann Otol (St. Louis) 78: 929–938, 1969b
24. Valvassori GE: The abnormal internal auditory canal: The diagnosis of acoustic neuroma. Radiology 92: 449–459, 1969
25. Valvassori GE: Myelography of the internal auditory canal. Am J Roentgenol Radium Ther Nucl Med 115: 578–586, 1972
26. Valvassori GE: In: Radiography of the temporal bone in otolaryngology, Vol. 1. ed. by Paparella MM, Shumrick DA. Saunders, Philadelphia 1973
27. Valvassori GE: Benign tumors of the temporal bone. Radiol Clin North Am 12: 533–542, 1974
28. Valvassori GE, Clemis JD: Abnormal vestibular aqueduct in cochleovestibular disorders. Adv Otorhinolaryngol 24: 100–105, 1978
29. Valvassori GE, Dobben GD: Vestibular basilar insufficiency. Ann Otol (St. Louis) 88: 689–692, 1979
30. Valvassori GE, Buckingham RA: Tomography and Cross Sections of the Ear. W. B. Saunders, Philadelphia. Thieme, Stuttgart, 1975

Part II

Radiology of the Paranasal Sinuses and Facial Bones

Guy D. Potter

Chapter 1 Radiographic Anatomy on Routine Views

A request for a radiographic examination of the paranasal sinuses is complete only if all the paranasal sinuses are visualized:

 the frontal sinuses
 the ethmoid sinuses
 the maxillary sinuses
 the sphenoid sinuses

Generally all these sinuses can be visualized on four views:

 the Caldwell view
 the Waters view
 the lateral view
 the base view

An additional oblique projection, the optic canal or Rhese view, is sometimes helpful.

Certainly these four views should be part of every adequate examination of the paranasal sinuses with the optional addition of the optic canal view.

Caldwell View (Inclined Posteroanterior)

The Caldwell view is made with the tragocanthal line perpendicular to the plane of the film and the central ray directed 23 degrees caudad to the tragocanthal line (Fig. 1.1). The central ray enters the skull about 3 cm above the external occipital protuberance and exits at the glabella. More important than the exact angulation of the tube or the entrance or exit point of the x-ray beam from the head is the usefulness of the final image.

Premier Orbit View

The Caldwell view is the premier orbit view, the view which should show the details of the orbits including the margins of the orbits, the linea innominata, the superior orbital fissure, the lacrimal gland fossa, and the lesser and greater wings of the sphenoid. Therefore the ideal Caldwell view is that image which shows all of these orbital structures best.

The image which shows all of these orbital structures best is one in which the crest of the petrous pyramid is immediately inferior to the floor of the orbit.

Improper Angulation

Less caudad angulation of the beam results in projecting the petrous pyramids on the lower part of the orbit, thus obscuring the floor of the orbit in this premier orbital view. Greater caudad angulation of the tube than is needed superimposes the crest of the petrous pyramid on the maxillary sinus more inferiorly.

The result of this mistake is poorer visualization of the structure within the orbits such as the superior orbital fissure and the greater and lesser wings of the sphenoid. Also those structures of the sphenoid which are seen uniquely on the Caldwell view such as the floor of the sella turcica and the planum sphenoidale are less well visualized when the caudad angulation of the tube is too great.

Proper Angulation

In short, the ideal Caldwell projection produces an image of the facial bones in which the top of the petrous pyramid is immediately beneath the floor of the orbit. The extent to which the image of the petrous pyramid is superimposed on the inferior portion of the orbit is an indication of the degree of insufficient caudad angulation of the tube used in making that image.

On the other hand, the extent to which the crest of the petrous pyramid on the Caldwell view is inferior to the floor of the orbit and is superimposed on the maxillary sinus inferiorly is an indication of the degree of excess caudad angulation of the tube.

How to Make the Correction

When the physician is presented with a Caldwell view in which the tube angulation and position of the head are not correct, that is, where the crest of the petrous pyramid is not just inferior to the floor of the orbit, and he desires to obtain a more informative image, the correction is easy. When the petrous pyramid is superimposed superior to the floor of the orbit, the caudad angulation of the tube should be increased. When the image of the petrous pyramid is superimposed inferior to the floor of the orbit, the caudad angulation of the tube should be decreased.

Diagnostic Importance

The frontal sinus and ethmoid sinus are best seen on the Caldwell view. In addition, the Caldwell view demonstrates the nasal fossa to the best advantage.

The Caldwell view is uniquely valuable for demonstrating the midline structures of the face. Therefore in examining a Caldwell view obtained for a paranasal sinus examination the frontal sinus should be carefully evaluated, the ethmoid sinus evaluated, the nasal fossa, the rim of the orbit and the structures within the orbit. This is what the Caldwell view is good for. Therefore these structures should be carefully evaluated on the Caldwell view.

Size of the Frontal Sinus

The frontal sinuses are normally extremely variable in size and may be completely absent. The frontal sinus may be absent on one side while the other side may be normal in size or even larger.

At times it is difficult to differentiate between an aplastic frontal sinus and a frontal sinus with chronic sinusitis and complete opacification especially if the involved frontal sinus is small.

Margin of the Frontal Sinus

The superior margin of the frontal sinus is generally scalloped but occasionally it may be normally smooth. However, the presence of a smooth margin to the frontal sinus suggests the presence of a frontal mucocele.

The margin between the frontal sinus and the orbit is seen best on the Caldwell view and should be evaluated on this view. Displacement or absence of this portion of the common wall between the orbit and the frontal sinus

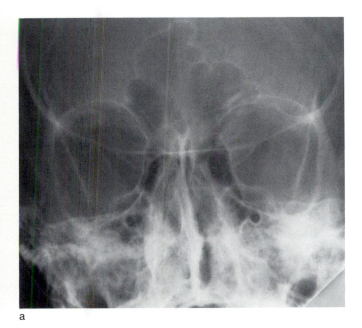

a

Fig. 1.**1**

a) Caldwell view. The head is positioned so that the tragocanthal line is perpendicular to the film. The central ray is directed 23 degrees caudad to the tragocanthal line; it enters the skull about 3 cm above the external occipital protuberance and exits at the glabella.

b) Line drawing of Caldwell view and legend. 1. Alveolar ridge of maxilla, 2. anterior portion of lamina papyracea, 3. anterior portion of orbital floor, 4. body of zygoma, 5. crista galli, 6. ethmoid air cells, 7. ethmomaxillary plate, 8. floor of sella turcica, 9. foramen rotundum, 10. frontal process of zygoma, 11. frontal sinus, 12. frontozygomatic suture, 13. greater wing of sphenoid, 14. hard palate, 15. lateral wall of maxilla, 16. lesser wing of sphenoid, 17. linea innominata, 18. maxillary sinus (antrum), 19. medial wall of maxillary sinus (lateral wall of nasal fossa), 20. nasal fossa, 21. nasal septum, 22. petrous ridge, 23. planum (jugum) sphenoidale, 24. posterior portion of infraorbital groove, 25. posterior portion of lamina papyracea, 26. posterior portion of orbital floor, 27. roof of ethmoid sinus, 28. roof of orbit, 29. superior orbital fissure, 30. superior recess of nasal fossa, 31. temporal line of frontal bone, 32. zygomatic process of frontal bone.

c) Drawing of positioning for Caldwell view showing the position of the patient and the central ray with respect to the plane of the film.

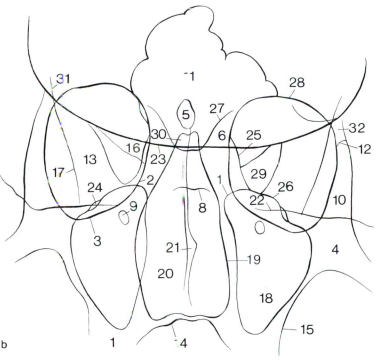

b

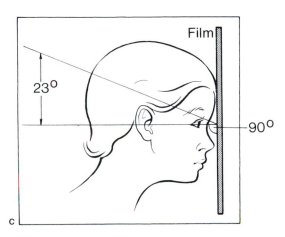

c

indicates a pathological process, either a tumor, infection or a mucocele.

Ethmoid Sinus

On the Caldwell view the ethmoid sinuses or air cells lie between the orbits superimposed upon the sphenoid sinuses. Any line that crosses the midline in the area between the orbits must be produced by a structure in the sphenoid, for example, the planum sphenoidale or the floor of the sella turcica.

We know that any line crossing the midline in the area between the orbits as seen on the Caldwell view must come from the sphenoid because there is no structure in the ethmoid which crosses the midline, and on the Caldwell view, the only bones that are seen between the orbits are the sphenoid and the ethmoid. No structure in the ethmoid crosses the midline because the right and left ethmoid sinuses or air cells are separated one from the other by the vertical ethmoid plate which forms the superior portion of the bony nasal septum.

Medial Wall of the Orbit

The medial wall of the orbit goes from medial to lateral as it proceeds from anterior to posterior. This formation of the medial wall of the orbit is logical if one considers that the anterior portion of the orbit, the aditus, is larger than is the orbital apex and therefore the medial wall of the orbit must deviate laterally as one proceeds posteriorly.

This anatomical configuration produces two lines representing the medial wall of the orbit as seen on the Caldwell view:

1. The more medial line represents the anterior portion of the medial wall of the orbit.
2. The more lateral line represents the posterior portion of the medial wall of the orbit.

Posterior Portion of Lamina Papyracea

The more lateral line of the medial wall of the orbit which is the most obviously visible on the Caldwell view is slightly oblique, running from medial to lateral as it goes from superior to inferior. This line represents the posterior portion of the lamina papyracea or the lateral plate of the ethmoids and thus the lateral wall of the posterior ethmoid air cells.

The more medial line represents the anterior portion of the lamina papyracea and therefore the lateral wall of the anterior ethmoid air cells.

The more lateral line, that is the more posterior portion of the lamina papyracea, should always be seen on the Caldwell view. If it is not seen, this is an indication of an abnormality.

Anterior Portion of Lamina Papyracea

The more medial line, which is the anterior portion of the lamina papyracea, is sometimes seen on the Caldwell view. However it may be invisible due to the fact that it is superimposed on the lucency produced by the posterior ethmoid air cells and the sphenoid sinus. The anterior portion of the lamina papyracea is not always seen on the Caldwell view and is better evaluated on the Waters projection.

Confirmation of the fact that the lateral line demarcating the medial wall of the orbit is actually the posterior portion of the lamina papyracea is the fact that this line produced by the posterior portion of the medial wall of the orbit smoothly joins the posterior portion of the floor of the orbit as seen on the Caldwell view.

Conversely, the anterior portion of the lamina papyracea or the medial line joins the anterior portion of the floor of the orbit.

The Party Wall

One should always remember that there is a party wall between the maxillary sinus and the floor of the orbit; thus the roof of the maxillary sinus is the floor of the orbit. Since the posterior portion of the lamina papyracea joins the posterior portion of the floor of the orbit it is also joining the posterior portion of the roof of the maxillary sinus.

Any changes in this posterior portion of the roof of the maxillary sinus are seen best on the Caldwell view, changes produced by inflammation, trauma or neoplasm.

Maxillary Sinus

The maxillary sinuses are covered by the superimposed petrous pyramids on the Caldwell view. However certain portions of the maxillary sinus are seen well on the Caldwell view. These are the roof of the maxillary sinus which is the floor of the orbit, especially its posterior portion; the ethmomaxillary plate, the curvilinear plate of bone forming the superomedial border of the maxillary sinus, separating the ethmoid air cells from the maxillary sinus; and the medial wall of the maxillary sinus which is the lateral wall of the nasal fossa.

Another Party Wall

Just as the roof of the maxillary sinus and the floor of the orbit are one and the same, a party wall between these two structures, so the medial wall of the maxillary sinus and the lateral wall of the nasal fossa are also a party wall.

Lateral Wall of the Nasal Fossa

The lateral wall of the nasal fossa is best seen on the Caldwell view. The lateral wall of the nasal fossa is approximately 5 cm long. Therefore small areas of bone destruction will not appear as a sharply demarcated radiolucency as is the usual manifestation of bone destruction in other bones of the body, but rather will be manifest as a slight decrease in visualization, the appearance of demineralization.

Since the lateral wall of the nasal fossa is 5 cm long, 1 to 2 cm of bone can be destroyed but there will still be 3 cm of intact bone to cast a shadow, albeit that this shadow will be somewhat less distinct than on the normal side. So the nasal fossa should be carefully evaluated on the Caldwell view where it is seen best.

Ethmomaxillary Plate

The ethmomaxillary plate, the curvilinear plate of bone separating the maxillary sinus from the ethmoids, is seen best on the Caldwell view.

The ethmomaxillary plate is often the first area that is affected by either an expanding lesion such as an ethmoid mucocele displacing the ethmomaxillary plate or a neoplasm in either the ethmoids or the maxillary sinuses producing destruction and nonvisualization of this plate.

Sphenoid Sinus

The sphenoid sinuses cannot be evaluated on the Caldwell view because of the superimposition of the ethmoids. However the roof of the sphenoid sinuses, the planum sphenoidale, is seen best on the Caldwell view.

Superior Orbital Fissure

The orbits are often affected by paranasal sinus disease or abnormalities. For example, the superior orbital fissure, since it is adjacent to the ethmoid sinuses, is often affected by an ethmoid sinus abnormality. It is also adjacent and close to the sphenoid sinuses and any abnormality of the sphenoid sinuses may involve the superior orbital fissure.

Since the superior orbital fissure serves to transmit the nerves of the extraocular muscles, an abnormality of the superior orbital fissure might be suspected in a patient who has ophthalmoplegia or some other abnormality of the function of the extraocular muscles manifest as diplopia. The superior orbital fissure separates the lesser wing of the sphenoid from the greater wing of the sphenoid.

The Caldwell view shows the orbital structures the best, including the lesser wing of the sphenoid, the planum sphenoidale, the sphenoid ridge, the greater wing of the sphenoid and the superior orbital fissure.

Sella Turcica

The floor of the sella turcica can usually be seen on the Caldwell view. In looking for the floor of the sella turcica, one should look for a horizontal line of approximately 1 to 2 cm in width running parallel to, and inferior to, the planum sphenoidale.

The amount of separation between the floor of the sella turcica and the planum sphenoidale is always greater on the Caldwell view than the distance between those two structures as seen on the lateral view.

The reason that the distance between the floor of the sella turcica and the planum sphenoidale is greater on the Caldwell view than on the lateral view is the caudad angulation of the tube used in obtaining the Caldwell view which produces a relative displacement downward of posterior structures in relation to more anterior structures. Thus the floor of the sella turcica which is posterior to the planum sphenoidale will be displaced inferiorly in relation to the planum sphenoidale, making the distance between these two structures on the Caldwell view greater than is seen on the lateral view. It is the lateral view which shows the true anatomic relation of these structures.

Keeping in mind the effect of projection may prevent one from misinterpreting an angled accessory septum in the sphenoid sinus on the Caldwell view for an abnormally slanted floor of the sella turcica.

One should also keep in mind that this floor of the sella turcica is not always seen on the Caldwell view. If it is not seen, the most that can be said is that it is not seen. No statement can be made as to whether it is normal or abnormal.

Waters View

The Waters (inclined posteroanterior) view is made with the midsagittal plane of the skull and the central ray perpendicular to the plane of the film (Fig. 1.2). The head is extended so that the tragocanthal line forms an angle of 37 degrees with the central ray, which enters the skull about 3 cm above the external occipital protuberance and exits through the tip of the nose.

Maxillary Sinus

The Waters view is the best view for visualizing the maxillary sinuses and the anterior ethmoid air cells. Generally the Waters view is most useful when the head is extended just sufficient to have petrous pyramids superimposed over the most inferior portion of the maxillary sinuses.

While it is true that this positioning sacrifices the optimal

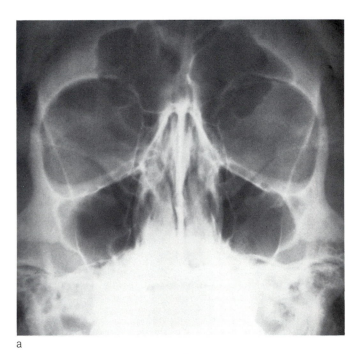

a

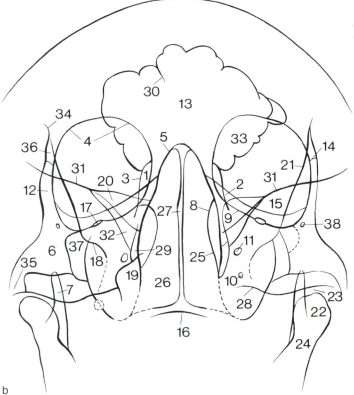

b

Fig. 1.2

a) Waters view. The head is positioned with the midsagittal plane perpendicular to the film, and the head is extended so that the tragocanthal line forms an angle of 37 degrees with the central ray, which is perpendicular to the film. The central ray enters the skull about 3 cm above the external occipital protuberance and exits through the tip of the nose.

b) Line drawing of Waters view and legend. 1. anterior ethmoid air cells, 2. anterior margin of orbital floor, 3. anterior portion of lamina papyracea, 4. anterior portion of orbital roof, 5. arch of nose, 6. body of zygoma, 7. coronoid process of mandible, 8. ethmo-maxillary plate, 9. floor of orbit about 1 cm posterior to anterior margin of orbit, 10. foramen of Vesalius, 11. foramen rotundum, 12. frontal process of zygoma, 13. frontal sinus, 14. frontozygomatic suture, 15. greater wing of sphenoid, 16. hard palate, 17. infraorbital foramen, 18. infratemporal extension of linea innominata, 19. lateral extension of sphenoid sinus, 20. lesser wing of sphenoid, 21. linea innominata, 22. mandibular condyle, 23. mandibular (glenoid) fossa, 24. mandibular neck, 25. medial wall of maxillary sinus (lateral wall of nasal fossa), 26. nasal fossa and conchae (turbinates), 27. nasal septum, 28. petrous ridge, 29. posterior ethmoid air cells, 30. septum of frontal sinus, 31. sphenoid ridge (posteriormost portion of orbital roof), 32. superior orbital fissure, 33. supraorbital recess of frontal sinus, 34. temporal line of frontal bone, 35. zygomatic arch, 36. zygomatic process of frontal bone, 37. zygomatic recess of maxillary sinus, 38. zygomaticofacial foramen.

c) Drawing of positioning for Waters view showing the position of the patient and the central ray with respect to the plane of the film.

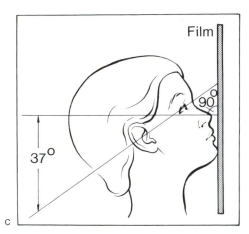

c

visualization of the most inferior portion of the maxillary sinus, this positioning produces a much better view of the floor of the orbit (which is the roof of the maxillary sinus). Significant abnormalities are much more common in the floor of the orbit than in the most inferior portion of the maxillary sinus. By superimposing the petrous pyramid upon the most inferior portion of the maxillary sinus, we give up a little to gain a lot.

As with the Caldwell view, more important than the exact extension of the head that is used in positioning the patient in taking the Waters view, is the final result.

Improper Positioning

If the head is not extended enough, too much of the maxillary sinus will be covered by the petrous pyramid and significant maxillary pathology may be overlooked. On the other hand, if the head is extended too much, producing an image which places the petrous pyramid inferior to the maxillary sinus, the floor of the orbit will be poorly visualized, thus negating one of the primary reasons for obtaining the Waters film, which was the visualization of the orbit floor (the roof of the maxillary sinus).

In short, the ideal Waters view produces an image of the facial bones in which the top of the petrous pyramid is superimposed upon the most inferior portion of the maxillary sinus.

How to Make the Correction

If too much of the maxillary sinus is obscured by the petrous pyramid, then the film should be repeated with the patient's head more extended. If the crest of the petrous pyramid is projected inferior to the maxillary sinus, such that the floor of the orbit is not visualized on the view, then the film should be repeated with the patient's head more flexed.

Frontal Sinus

The Caldwell view is the primary view for evaluating the frontal sinuses. However evaluating the frontal sinuses on the Waters view in conjunction with the Caldwell may help to confirm the findings as seen on the Caldwell view.

For example, a thick anterior wall of a frontal sinus may make that frontal sinus appear opacified on the Caldwell view. But on the Waters film, because the head is more extended than it is for the Caldwell view, the anterior wall of the frontal sinus is viewed more obliquely, less en face, and thus the thick wall of the frontal sinus will have less effect on the image of the sinus on the Waters film than on the Caldwell.

In other words on the Waters view we are looking up underneath the anterior wall of the frontal sinus and not superimposing the image of the anterior wall on the sinus itself.

Orbital Border of Frontal Sinus

A caveat is that because of the angulation of projection, the common wall between the frontal sinus and the orbit is not visualized on the Waters view. The nonvisualiza-tion of that portion of the orbital margin adjacent to the frontal sinus due to projection should not be confused with bone destruction. The portion of the orbital margin adjacent to the frontal sinuses should be evaluated only on the Caldwell view.

Ethmoid Sinus

The Waters film is an inclined projection with anterior structures thrown upward and well visualized and all the posterior structures thrown downward and seen less well. Therefore what we see as ethmoid air cells (the ethmoid sinuses) on the Waters projection are actually the anterior ethmoid air cells. If there is opacification in the ethmoid region on the Waters film but not on the Caldwell film, this indicates that the anterior ethmoid air cells are opacified.

Because of the inclination of the projection, the anterior ethmoid air cells and the posterior ethmoid air cells are seen as separate structures on the Waters film. However because the nasal fossa is superimposed on the posterior ethmoid air cells on the Waters, the posterior ethmoid air cells are not well visualized on this view.

Medial Wall of the Orbit

That portion of the medial wall of the orbit seen on the Waters projection is the anterior portion of the medial wall of the orbit (the lateral plate of the lamina papyracea). In fact it is only on the Waters projection that the anterior portion of the lamina papyracea can be seen well.

Maxillary Structures

The main area of interest in the Waters view is the maxillary sinuses. If the Caldwell view is mainly an orbit view, the Waters is mainly a maxillary sinus view.

The air content and size of the maxillary sinuses can best be seen on the Waters view.

Other maxillary structures which can be evaluated are the anterior portion of the roof of the maxillary sinus which is the floor of the orbit, the medial and lateral walls of the maxillary sinus and the maxillary alveolar ridge.

The ethmomaxillary plate can sometimes be seen on the Waters view but the visualization of this structure is usually better on the Caldwell.

Roof of the Maxillary Sinus

The roof of the maxillary sinus on the Waters film is represented by two lines. The upper line is the most anterior portion of the floor of the orbit which is the inferior rim of the orbit. The more inferior line is produced by the floor of the orbit more posterior than the rim.

On a properly positioned Waters film the more inferior line should represent the floor of the orbit approximately 1 cm posterior to the rim of the orbit.

As the head is extended more and more, the portion of the floor of the orbit which produces the inferior line is more and more posterior in the floor of the orbit. This is reflected in the fact that the distance between these two lines, the upper line representing the rim of the orbit and the lower line representing the more posterior portion of the floor of the orbit, is greater as the head is extended. On any given film the distance from the rim of the orbit to the floor of the orbit should be the same on the two sides.

Blowout Fractures

This fact is particularly important for diagnosing blowout fractures of the floor of the orbit. Since a blowout fracture is by definition a depressed fracture of the floor of the orbit without a fracture of the rim of the orbit, it follows that the floor of the orbit represented by the more inferior line will be more separated from the rim of the orbit on the affected side than the unaffected side.

Medial Wall of the Maxillary Sinus

The medial wall of the maxillary sinus which is the lateral wall of the nasal fossa is also seen on the Waters view. That portion of the lateral wall of the nasal fossa seen on the Waters is different than the portion seen on the Caldwell. The portion seen on the Waters is the anterior portion of the medial wall of the maxillary sinus.

If there is bone destruction visualized in the lateral wall of the nasal fossa seen on the Waters view, this finding indicates that the lesion is in the anterior portion of the lateral wall of the nasal fossa.

If there is destruction of the medial wall of the maxillary sinus, it will not appear as a clear cut radiolucency but rather a decrease in visualization of this area. The reason that this bone will still be seen even though there is bone destruction is the same for the Waters as for the Caldwell. Because this bone is 5 cm long, a portion of it can be destroyed and still the remaining portion will cast a shadow, albeit a different appearing shadow than the normal side.

Lateral Wall of the Maxillary Sinus

The lateral wall of the maxillary sinus is well seen on the Waters view. The lateral wall of the maxillary sinus on the Waters view should make a smooth curve with the zygomatic arch and extending down to the maxillary alveolar ridge.

Fracture of the lateral wall of the maxillary sinus will produce angulation of this line. Also, following this line downward to the alveolar ridge will bring out an abnormality in the alveolar ridge.

Zygomatic Arch

The zygomatic arch should always be perused on the Waters view, since the Waters is the best view of the zygomatic arch one obtains on routine sinus films without taking specific zygomatic arch views. An abnormality of the zygomatic arch can be seen on the Waters view without special views.

Sphenoid Sinus

If the sphenoid sinus is well developed, then the lateral recess of the sphenoid sinus can be seen on the Waters view superimposed on the maxillary sinuses. In this view, an air fluid level or opacification of the lateral recess of the sphenoid sinus can be diagnosed.

Orbit

In addition to visualizing the anterior portion of the floor of the orbit and the inferior rim of the orbit, the Waters view shows the lateral wall of the orbit, made up of the frontal process of the zygomatic bone and the zygomatic process of the frontal bone. Therefore the Waters view can be used to evaluate the frontozygomatic suture for diastasis of that suture after trauma to the face. However, diastasis of this suture is usually seen better on the Caldwell view than on the Waters.

Because of the angulation of the Waters view, the orbit is visualized on this view like a cone tilted upward at a 30° angle.

As a result of this angulation the orbital apex is superimposed on the lower portion of the maxillary sinus and the superior orbital fissures are superimposed on the maxillary sinuses, producing a paired linear radiolucency extending laterally as it goes from inferior to superior. This normal anatomical structure should not be confused with a fracture of the maxillary sinus.

One should always keep in mind that it is the anterior facial structures that are well demonstrated on the Waters view, namely, the anterior portion of the lamina papyracea, the anterior portion of the floor of the orbit, and the anterior portion of the nasal fossa.

Base View (Submentovertical or Axial)

The base view is made with the tragocanthal line parallel to the film. The central ray is directed perpendicular to the film. The central ray enters the skull in the midline midway between the mandibular angles (Fig. 1.3).

Base of the Skull

The base view is uniquely valuable for visualization of the structures in the base of the skull and those structures of the skull which are oriented in a caudocephalad direction. Among the structures oriented in a caudocephalad

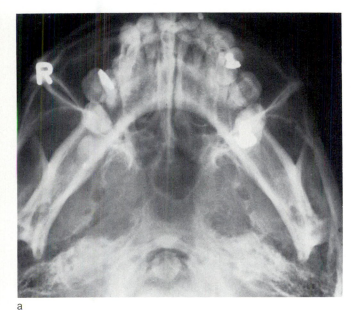

a

Fig. 1.3
a) Base view. The head is positioned so that the tragocanthal line is parallel to the film. The central ray is perpendicular to the tragocanthal line; it enters the skull in the midline between the mandibular angles.
b) Line drawing of base view and legend. 1. anterior arch of C-1, 2. anterior wall of middle cranial fossa, 3. body of zygoma, 4. clivus, 5. coronoid process of mandible, 6. ethmoid air cells and nasal fossa, 7. eustachian tube, 8. external auditory canal, 9. foramen magnum, 10. foramen ovale, 11. foramen spinosum, 12. greater palatine foramen, 13. incus, 14. inferior portion of lateral pterygoid plate, 15. infraorbital foramen, 16. inner table of frontal bone, 17. internal auditory canal, 18. lateral wall of maxillary sinus, 19. lateral wall of orbit, 20. malleus, 21. mandibular angle, 22. mandibular body, 23. mandibular condyle, 24. mandibular symphysis, 25. mastoid air cells, 26. maxillary sinus (antrum), 27. medial pterygoid plate, 28. medial wall of maxillary sinus (lateral wall of nasal fossa), 29. nasal septum, 30. nasopharynx, 31. odontoid process (dens), 32. outer table of frontal bone, 33. petrooccipital fissure, 34. petrosphenoid fissure, 35. posterior border of vomer, 36. sphenoid sinus, 37. superior portion of lateral pterygoid plate.
c) Drawing of positioning for base view showing the position of the patient and the central ray with respect to the plane of the film

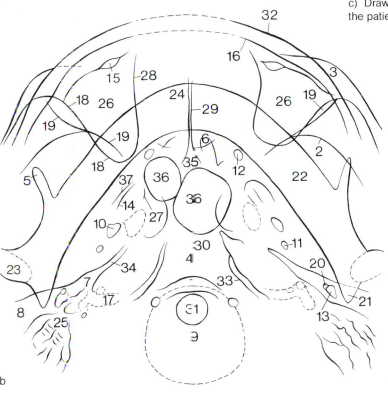

b

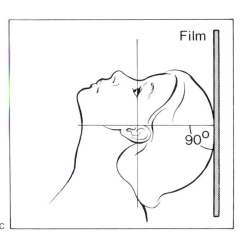

c

direction are the anterior wall of the middle cranial fossa, the lateral wall of the orbit and the lateral wall of the maxillary sinus.

Lateral Wall of the Orbit

The anterior wall, or margin, of the middle cranial fossa joins the lateral wall of the orbit. This is not surprising since both the lateral wall of the orbit and the anterior margin of the middle cranial fossa are derived from and are made up of the greater wing of the sphenoid.

Lateral Wall of the Maxillary Sinus

The lateral wall of the maxillary sinus, which is superimposed on the lateral wall of the orbit on the base view, has a curvilinear, S-shaped contour. Because the S-shaped line represents the lateral wall of a structure beginning with the letter "S" (the sinus), a mnemonic for identifying this wall is S-and-S.

Three Diagnostic Curvilinear Lines

In summary the anterolateral portion of the skull as seen on the base view contains three more or less superimposed curvilinear lines:
1. An "S"-shaped line representing the lateral wall of the maxillary sinus;
2. a straighter line with a slight posterior concavity representing the lateral wall of the orbit which is joined by
3. an anteriorly bowed curvilinear line representing the anterior wall of the middle cranial fossa.

If one keeps in mind the relationship of these lines one can then be able to differentiate the site of bone destruction when either the lateral wall of the maxillary sinus is destroyed or the lateral wall of the orbit is destroyed. This information can also be used to analyze displacement of the lateral wall of the maxillary sinus or orbit.

Caudocephalically Oriented Structures

All structures which are oriented in a caudocephalic direction are well seen on the base view. Amongst the caudocephalically oriented structures are the pterygoid plates, medial and lateral; the pterygopalatine fossa; and the foramina in the base of the skull that are oriented caudocephalically, such as the foramen ovale and the foramen spinosum.

On the other hand, the basal foramina that are oriented anteroposteriorly such as the foramen rotundum are not visualized on the base view. The foramen rotundum is seen better on the Caldwell view (Fig. 1.1) and sometimes even on the Waters view (Fig. 1.2).

Lateral Pterygoid Plate

The lateral pterygoid plate can always be seen on the base view. It points posterolaterally toward the foramen ovale.

The lateral pterygoid plate is represented by two lines pointing posterolaterally. The lateral pterygoid plate produces two lines on the base view because the lateral pterygoid plate flares laterally in its inferior portion.

Thus of the two lines produced by the lateral pterygoid plate, the more medial is the superior part of the lateral pterygoid plate and the more lateral is produced by the more inferior part of the lateral pterygoid plate. Both of these lines produced by the lateral pterygoid plate extend posterolateral and point in the general direction of the foramen ovale.

Because the lateral pterygoid plate is usually quite visible on the base view, its absence produced by bone destruction can be appreciated.

Medial Pterygoid Plate

The medial pterygoid plate extends posteriorly parasagittally almost as a continuation of the lateral wall of the nasal fossa. The medial pterygoid plate is a short structure often superimposed upon the sphenoid sinus and the air in the nasopharynx and thus it is often not seen on the base view. However if it is going to be seen on any view, it is going to be seen on the base view.

Pterygopalatine Fossa

The image of the pterygopalatine fossa in the base view produces a short horizontal canal just posterior to the posterior wall of the maxillary sinus (which is the posteromedial end of the "S"-shaped line mentioned above) and the anterior margin of the junction of the pterygoid plates.

This short horizontal canal produced by the pterygopalatine fossa has an opening medially to the nose which is the sphenopalatine foramen. It has an opening laterally to the infratemporal fossa which is the sphenomaxillary fissure.

The pterygopalatine fossa can usually be seen in the base view. Therefore either enlargement of the pterygopalatine fossa by infiltration by a benign lesion, such as a juvenile angiofibroma, or destruction by a more aggressive tumor can be seen on the base view.

The pterygopalatine fossa can be visualized best if the head is fully extended when the film is obtained. If the head is allowed to flex, the pterygopalatine fossa will not be seen.

Frontal Sinus

The frontal sinuses are not seen well on the base view because the mandible is superimposed on the frontal sinuses in the base view. Occasionally, however, an "overshot" view of the base can show the anterior and posterior walls of the frontal sinus.

The "overshot" view is obtained by having the tragocanthal line parallel to the film with a cephalad angulation of the tube. However, when it is desirable to see the posterior wall of the frontal sinus, it is generally easier and more informative to get lateral tomograms.

Ethmoid Sinus

The area of the ethmoids is seen well on a properly extended base view. If the head is allowed to flex when the film is obtained, the mandible will be superimposed on the ethmoid region. Even though the ethmoid area may be well visualized, it can still be difficult to evaluate the status of the ethmoid air cells on the base view because of the sausage-shaped shadow produced by the inferior turbinate (concha).

Inferior Turbinate

The base view can still be used to help in the evaluation of the ethmoid air cells as long as one keeps in mind the presence of the superimposition of the inferior turbinate and checks the Caldwell view for the presence of asymmetry of the turbinates.

If one inferior turbinate is larger than the other, the larger inferior turbinate will produce a more prominent shadow in the ethmoid region in the base view, resulting in spurious appearance of opacification of the underlying ethmoid region.

Lamina Papyracea

The lamina papyracea is so thin and delicate that the superimposed denser medial wall of the maxillary sinus (lateral wall of the nasal fossa) obscures it.

Maxillary Sinus

As was stated above, the posterolateral wall of the maxillary sinus is represented by the "S"-shaped line. The posterior wall is the anterior wall of the pterygopalatine fossa discussed above. The medial wall is also the lateral wall of the nasal fossa.

The medial wall of the maxillary sinus and the medial wall of the orbit (lamina papyracea of the ethmoid) are superimposed upon one another. However, the medial wall of the orbit is so thin and delicate that it could be completely destroyed and not affect the appearance of the line produced by the two structures.

If there is any difference in the appearance of the lateral wall of the nasal fossa on the two sides, it is due to an abnormality of the medial wall of the maxillary sinus.

Sphenoid Sinus

The base view is the premier view for the sphenoid sinus. The combined shadow of the two sphenoid sinuses can be seen on the lateral view but the sphenoid sinuses can be analyzed as separate structures only on the base view. The corticated margin of the sphenoid sinus should be traced on every base view to rule out bone destruction involving a wall of the sphenoid.

The sphenoid sinus varies enormously in size from virtually absent to a huge air cavity extending anterolaterally into the greater wing of the sphenoid and the lateral wall of the orbit.

Ear

The base view is the only view that demonstrates the bony eustachian tube. It is also the only view that shows two of the three auditory ossicles – the incus and the malleus – as separate structures.

Since the malleus and incus are in the attic of the middle ear, identifying these ossicles on the base view identifies the middle ear. Thus clouding of the middle ear can be identified on the base view.

Lateral View

In the lateral view, the head is positioned so that the midsagittal plane is parallel to the film. The central ray is perpendicular to the film (Fig. 1.4). The central ray enters the skull 2 cm anterior and 2 cm above the external auditory canal.

Structures Visualized

The lateral view presents a good view of the pterygopalatine fossa, the hard palate, and the posterior nasopharyngeal soft tissue shadow. It is the only view that shows the length and depth of the sella turcica.

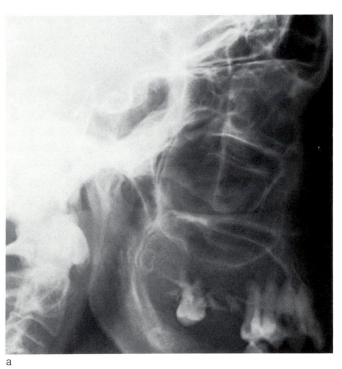

a

Fig. 1.**4**
a) Lateral view. The head is positioned so that the midsagittal plane is parallel to the film. The central ray is perpendicular to the midsagittal plane; it enters the skull 2 cm anterior to and 2 cm above the external auditory canal.
b) Line drawing of lateral view and legend. 1. Alveolar ridge of maxilla, 2. anterior arch of C1, 3. anterior border of pterygoid process, 4. anterior edge of frontal process of zygoma, 5. anterior nasal spine, 6. anterior wall of frontal sinus, 7. anterior wall of maxillary sinus (antrum), 8. anterior wall of middle cranial fossa, 9. apophyseal joint, 10. body of C2, 11. body of zygoma, 12. cerebral surface of orbital roof, 13. clivus, 14. coronoid process of mandible, 15. cribriform plate, 16. ethmoid air cells, 17. floor of maxillary sinus, 18. floor of sella turcica, 19. frontal sinus, 20. hard palate, 21. lateral mass of C1, 22. lateral portion of orbital floor, 23. mandibular angle, 24. mandibular body, 25. mandibular canal, 26. mandibular condyle, 27. mandibular neck, 28. mandibular notch, 29. mandibular ramus, 30. medial pterygoid plate, 31. nasal bone, 32. nasion, 33. nasopharyngeal soft tissues, 34. odontoid process (dens), 35. orbital surface of orbital roof, 36. petroclinoid ligament, 37. planum (jugum) sphenoidale, 38. posterior arch of C1, 39. posterior border of pterygoid plate, 40. posterior edge of frontal process of zygoma, 41. posterior wall of frontal sinus, 42. posterior wall of maxillary sinus, 43. premaxilla, 44. prevertebral soft tissues, 45. pterygoid hamulus, 46. pterygopalatine fossa, 47. roof of maxillary sinus (medial portion of orbital floor), 48. sphenoid sinus, 49. zygomatic recess of maxillary sinus.
c) Drawing of positioning for lateral view showing the position of the patient and the central ray with respect to the plane of the film.

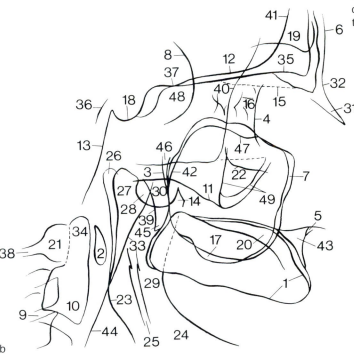

b

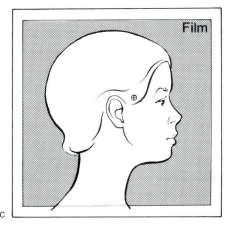

c

Pterygopalatine Fossa

The pterygopalatine fossa is a "V"-shaped lucency open superiorly. The anterior wall of the pterygopalatine fossa is the posterior wall of the maxillary sinus. The posterior wall of the pterygopalatine fossa is produced by the anterior margin of the pterygoid process.

The pterygoid processes posterior to the pterygopalatine fossa often cannot be seen. However, abnormalities of the pterygoid plates can be inferred by abnormalities of the pterygopalatine fossa. For example, disruption of the sides of the "V"-shaped lucency of the pterygopalatine fossa infers pterygoid plate fracture and thus a LeFort type facial fracture.

Also tumor destruction or enlargement of the pterygopalatine fossa by the tumor can be seen on the lateral view.

Nasopharynx

The nasopharyngeal soft tissues of the posterior wall of the nasopharynx are seen best on the lateral view. The curve of the posterior wall of the nasopharynx should always be concave. If the curve is convex, it is abnormal. If the posterior wall of the nasopharynx of a child has a convex curve, hypertrophied tonsils are usually responsible. In an adult, however, a mass in the nasopharynx should be considered a tumor until proven otherwise.

Sella Turcica

The lateral view is the only of the skull that shows the shape, length and depth of the sella turcica.

When the length and the depth of the sella turcica measured on the lateral view are combined with the width of this structure determined from the right-angle view of its floor on the Caldwell view, the volume of the sella turcica can be calculated. The width of the sella turcica multiplied by one half of the product of the length times the depth equals the volume. The volume of the sella turcica calculated this way should not be greater than 1100 mm^3.

Hard Palate

The lateral is the only view that shows a good view of the hard palate. The hard palate is represented by a horizontal corticated line superimposed upon the inferior portion of the maxillary sinus. The cortical bone that outlines the hard palate should extend from the pterygopalatine fossa posteriorly to the premaxilla anteriorly.

If the hard palate is completely destroyed, there is no horizontal line at all superimposed on the maxillary sinus.

If the corticated line does not extend as far posteriorly as the pterygopalatine fossa, this indicates destruction of the posterior portion of the hard palate.

With destruction of the anterior portion of the hard palate, the premaxilla – the double corticated line characterizing the premaxilla – is absent.

Frontal Sinus

The anterior and posterior walls of the frontal sinus can be seen on the lateral view.

When the anterior walls of the frontal sinus are of equal thickness, only two lines are present – one line for the anterior cortex and one line for the posterior cortex.

The anterior wall of the frontal sinus may be thick on one side and thinner on the other.

When such an asymmetry of the thickness of the anterior wall of the frontal sinus is present, it can be appreciated on the lateral skull view because the anterior wall of the frontal sinus will appear as three lines:

1. The anterior line produced by the anterior wall of the frontal sinus is the anterior cortex of the frontal wall of both frontal sinuses.
2. The second line more or less parallel to the first represents the posterior cortex of the anterior wall of the sinus with the thinner anterior wall.
3. The third and most posterior line represents the posterior cortex of the anterior wall of the sinus with the thicker anterior wall.

Which Frontal Sinus Has the Thick Wall?

In examining the lateral view, we can tell that one sinus has a thick wall because one extends more superiorly or more inferiorly. But being a lateral view, we cannot identify which one it is, the left or the right frontal sinus.

However, if we combine the knowledge we have from the lateral view that one frontal sinus has a thick wall with the knowledge we have from the Caldwell view, we can make an assumption as to which sinus it is.

For example, the Caldwell view can show that the upper cortex of the right frontal sinus does not extend as high as the upper cortex of the left frontal sinus, and we know from the lateral that the sinus with the thick anterior wall does not extend as high on the lateral as does the sinus with the thinner wall, therefore the sinus with the thick wall on the lateral is the right frontal sinus. One can identify, even on the lateral view, to which sinus the thick wall belongs by comparing the most superior extent of the frontal sinus as seen on the Caldwell and the height of the sinus to which the thick wall belongs on the lateral skull view.

Significance of Asymmetry in Thickness

The significance of the asymmetry in thickness of the anterior walls of the frontal sinus is that the sinus with the thicker wall will appear opacified in the Caldwell view.

Unilateral opacification of the frontal sinus seen on the Caldwell view may be produced by sinusitis. However, unilateral opacification of the frontal sinus on the Caldwell view may also be produced by a frontal sinus which has a thicker anterior wall – a normal variant. The only view in which the relative thickness of the anterior walls of the frontal sinus can be analyzed is the lateral view.

If on the Caldwell one frontal sinus appears opacified, the explanation for the opacification is not necessarily due to sinusitis but rather may be due to the superimposition of this thick anterior wall of the sinus.

Only with the lateral view can one ascertain that there is in fact a frontal sinus with a thick wall. This fact cannot be ascertained from the Caldwell.

Pneumatization

Often the frontal sinus will be quite extensive and pneumatize not only the vertical plate of the frontal bone but also the horizontal plate of the frontal bone (which is the roof of the orbit). In such cases the cerebral surface of the orbital roof can be differentiated from the orbital surface of the orbital roof.

Ethmoid Sinus

The ethmoid sinuses are superimposed on the orbits on the lateral view.

Since there are normally 8 to 14 ethmoid air cells on each side and both sides are superimposed one on the other in the lateral view, there are thus 16 to 28 ethmoid air cells and their component walls seen on the lateral view. This produces a multilocular almost bubbly appearance of the ethmoid region as seen on the lateral view.

When the air cell walls of the ethmoid air cells are not seen at all on the lateral view, this is an indication of bilateral ethmoid sinus opacification.

Maxillary Sinus

The maxillary sinuses are also superimposed on one another on the lateral view. Therefore if one sinus is opacified, one may not be able to appreciate this fact from the lateral view alone. A clear maxillary sinus on a lateral view does not rule out unilateral maxillary sinus opacification.

The anterior and posterior walls of the maxillary sinus can be analyzed on the lateral view. The posterior wall of the maxillary sinus is the anterior wall of the pterygopalatine fossa.

The anterior wall of the maxillary sinus can be seen but it is not seen well. Extensive destruction of the anterior wall of the maxillary antrum can be present but may not be seen on the lateral view. Lateral tomograms will be necessary to demonstrate the anterior wall of the maxillary sinus wall.

Destruction of the anterior wall of the maxillary sinus is difficult to see. However expansion can usually be visualized.

Malar Eminence

On the lateral view, a triangle is superimposed on the anterosuperior portion of the image of the maxillary sinus. This triangle is produced by the cortex of the body of the zygomatic bone, the malar eminence. This triangle often contains air representing the zygomatic or malar extension of the maxillary sinus.

Alveolar Extension

The alveolar extension of the maxillary sinus inferiorly into the alveolar process of the maxilla may be quite extensive and in such cases the contour of the inferior cortex of the maxillary sinus is quite irregular and might be mistaken for an abnormality.

Sphenoid Sinus

The sphenoid sinuses are superimposed upon one another and therefore unilateral opacification cannot be evaluated. However a mass in the sphenoid sinus can be seen on the lateral view.

The roof of the sphenoid sinus is made up of the planum sphenoidale and the anterior wall and floor of the sella turcica. Changes of the planum sphenoidale such as those produced by meningioma can be seen on the lateral view.

One should keep in mind that the cortex of the sella turcica is always denser and brighter over the aerated portion of the sphenoid bone than over the nonaerated cancellous bone.

Destruction of the walls of the sella turcica and invasion of the sphenoid sinus are seen best on the lateral view.

Optic Canal (Rhese) View

This projection is obtained in a posteroanterior position with the patient's head rotated 40 degrees to the contralateral side. The head is extended so that the tragocanthal line forms an angle of 20 degrees with the central ray.

Positioning

This projection was originally designed to demonstrate the optic foramen or optic canal and this explains the need for rotation of the head and the extension of the head when taking this projection.

The head is rotated 40 degrees because the optic canal forms an angle of 40 degrees with the midsagittal plane going from medial to lateral as it goes from posterior to anterior. Also the optic canal has a downward angulation of 20 degrees to the tragocanthal line, so that in order to place the optic canal perpendicular to the film the head must be rotated 40 degrees to the contralateral side and the head must be extended 20 degrees.

Another way to estimate the proper extension of the head for this view is to remember that the downward inclination of the optic canal is approximately parallel to the occlusal plane of the teeth which is also approximately parallel to the lower edge of the body of the mandible.

The head should be rotated 40 degrees to the contralateral side and the head should be extended so that the inferior edge of the body of the mandible is parallel to the beam.

Usefulness of the View

This view is valuable for the paranasal sinuses because it gives us a chance to visualize the frontal sinuses separately and also gives another visualization of the ethmoid air cells and of the ipsilateral sphenoid sinus.

Chapter 2   Normal Tomographic Anatomy

The most commonly used tomographic projections are the coronal or frontal, lateral or sagittal, and axial projections. An adequate tomographic examination should always include at least two of these projections and occasionally all three are necessary to delineate the areas of abnormality or to demonstrate the absence of pathology. I will illustrate the normal tomographic anatomy by means of anatomic sections one millimeter thick obtained from cadaver heads, a labeled line drawing of each anatomic section and tomograms which were obtained at every millimeter when the heads were intact.

I will analyze the coronal projection proceeding from anterior to posterior, the lateral projection from lateral to medial, and the axial projection proceeding from superior to inferior.

Coronal Tomographic Projection

The coronal projection is usually obtained with the orbitomeatal line, that is a line drawn between the infraorbital rim and the tragus of the ear, perpendicular to the table top. However no effort should be made to strictly adhere to this positioning. It is preferable that the patient be comfortable even though the orbitomeatal line is not quite perpendicular to the table top.

Sections at every 5 mm are usually adequate for a tomographic examination of the paranasal sinuses in the coronal projection.

Patient Comfort

If a patient is not comfortable he will tend to move his head at some time during the examination. The tendency is for older patients who have relatively rigid necks and a dorsal kyphosis to extend their head too much so they must be encouraged to flex their head perhaps slightly more than comfort would dictate. They can be aided in this by placing angled sponges beneath a plastic box holding the head in position. With children the opposite tendency is manifest; that is children tend to flex the head more than is desirable to get ideal tomograms of the paranasal sinuses. Usually children have to be encouraged to extend their head more than is their wont.

Positioning of the Head

It is important that the head be perfectly straight; that is the midsagittal plane should be perpendicular to the table top as well as the orbitomeatal line being perpen-

dicular to the table top. If the head is rotated there may be the impression of factitious abnormalities created by the bad positioning and not by any pathological process.

Coronal Section Through the Nasolacrimal Canal

Adequate diagnosis of abnormalities depends very much on a thorough familiarity with the normal tomographic anatomy. Therefore I will first discuss the normal tomographic anatomy.

The first section is the coronal section through the frontal sinuses, the most anterior portion of the maxillary sinuses and the nasolacrimal canal (Fig. 2.1).

Normal Nasolacrimal Canal

The entire length of the nasolacrimal canal and lacrimal sac fossa is seen with the canal extending from the lacrimal sac fossa above to the inferior meatus below. The lateral wall of the nasolacrimal canal is formed by a groove in the medial wall of the maxilla, and the medial wall of the nasolacrimal canal is formed superiorly by the descending process of the lacrimal bone and inferiorly by the lacrimal process of the inferior turbinate bone.

Medial Wall of the Orbit

There is a slight medial curvature of the medial wall of the orbit produced by the nasolacrimal sac fossa. The slight medial curvature should not be confused with displacement medially of the medial wall of the orbit. This is a normal curvilinear bowing of the medial wall of the orbit in the region of the nasolacrimal sac fossa.

Ethmoid Air Cells

In this first section there are three anterior ethmoid air cells on the right and two on the left. These anterior ethmoid air cells open into the frontal recess which is the most superoanterior extent of the middle meatus lateral to the middle turbinate.

Abnormal Nasolacrimal Apparatus

This section is the most important coronal section to analyze when the patient presents with epiphora and an abnormality is suspected in the nasolacrimal apparatus such as enlargement of the lacrimal fossa by an obstructed and enlarged lacrimal sac with medial displacement of the medial wall of the lacrimal sac fossa, or destruction by tumor of the nasolacrimal canal, or fractures of the nasolacrimal canal after trauma.

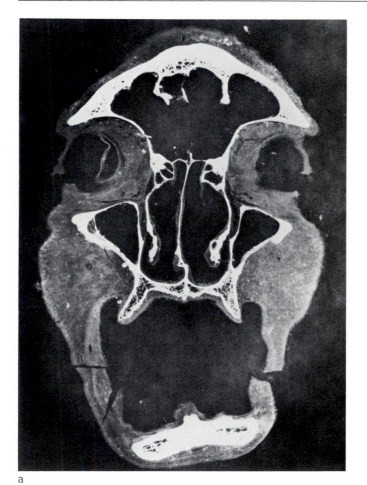

a

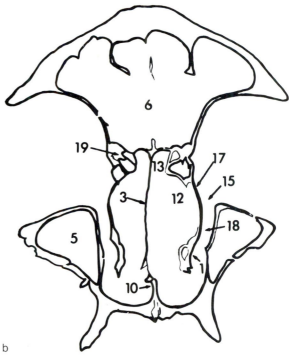

b

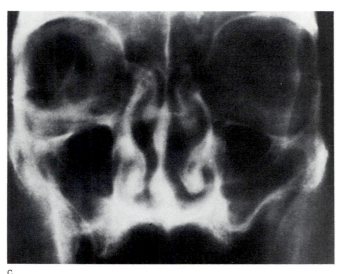

c

Fig. 2.**1**
a) Coronal anatomic section through the nasolacrimal canal.
b) Line drawing and legend. 1. Inferior meatus, inferior turbinate
(arrow), 3. perpendicular plate of the ethmoid, 5. maxillary sinus,
6. frontal sinus, 10. vomer, 12. nasal atrium, 13. olfactory sulcus,
15. lacrimal sac fossa, 17. lacrimal bone, 18. nasolacrimal canal,
19. anterior ethmoid cell.
c) Normal coronal tomogram of a).

Coronal Section – Encroachment on Frontal Sinus

The next coronal section (Fig. 2.2) is 4 mm posterior to Figure 2.1. The anterior cranial fossa encroaches on the frontal sinus. Only the supraorbital extensions of the frontal sinus, that portion pneumatizing the roof of the orbit, are still present.

Anterior Cranial Fossa and Frontal Sinus

The most striking feature of this section is the way the supraorbital extensions of the frontal sinus are virtually wrapped around the most anterior extent of the anterior cranial fossa, emphasizing the intimate nature of the relationship between the frontal sinuses and the anterior cra-

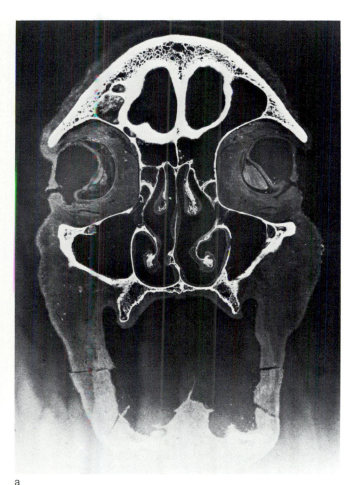

a

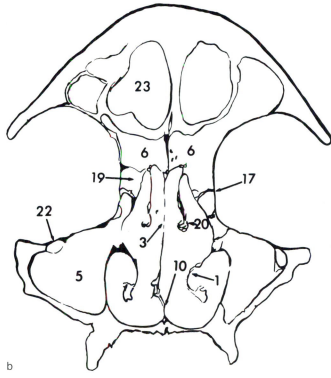

b

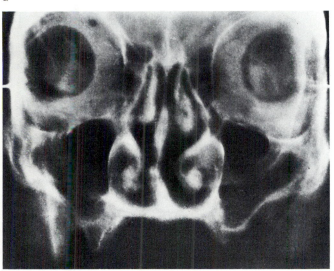

c

Fig. 2. **2**
a) Coronal anatomic section showing supraorbital extension of the frontal sinus.
b) Line drawing and legend. 1. Inferior meatus, inferior turbinate (arrow), 3. perpendicular plate of the ethmoid, 5. maxillary sinus, 6. frontal sinus, 10. vomer, 17. lacrimal bone, 19. anterior ethmoid cell, 20. middle meatus, middle turbinate (arrow), 22. infraorbital canal, 23. anterior cranial fossa.
c) Normal coronal tomogram of a).

nial fossa. It is not merely a relationship of the frontal sinuses being anterior to the anterior cranial fossa but rather that the most anterior portion of the anterior cranial fossa is almost completely encased in frontal sinus.

Infraorbital Canal

The right infraorbital canal has its definitive shape, that is a horizontal oval. On the left, however, the section through the infraorbital canal is more anterior. The section is through the portion of the infraorbital canal as it descends from the floor of the orbit to the infraorbital foramen which is approximately a centimeter inferior.

A coronal section, through this obliquely descending canal, produces on section a vertical oval as opposed to the true shape of the infraorbital canal which is a horizontal oval.

Lateral Crest of the Nasal Septum

At the articulation of the vomer and the perpendicular plate of the ethmoid is a bony ridge, the lateral crest of the nasal septum. This lateral crest can often be of sizeable proportions. If there is a deviation of the septum in addition to the presence of a lateral crest, there can be marked encroachment on the space of the nasal fossa.

The presence of such a crest may give the nasal septum the appearance of being deviated when in fact it is relatively sagittal in position but the clinical effect of a large lateral crest has the same effect as a deviated septum, that is encroachment on the space of the ipsilateral nasal fossa.

Medial Wall of the Orbit

In contradistinction to Figure 2.1, which was a coronal section through the nasolacrimal sac, the medial wall of the orbit is now straight up and down. It is now perpendicular because this section is now posterior to the nasolacrimal fossa. The medial wall of the orbit here is formed by the lamina papyracea of the ethmoid.

Coronal Section Posterior

The next coronal section (Fig. 2.3) is 4 mm posterior to Figure 2.2. This section is now almost completely posterior to the frontal sinuses. Just a small portion of the supraorbital extension of the left frontal sinus is still present.

Ostium of Maxillary Sinus

The ostium of the left maxillary sinus is well visualized. The ostium of the sinus is seen at the lower end of the ethmoid infundibulum. The walls of the infundibulum are formed superiorly by the ethmoid bulla and inferiorly by the uncinate process of the ethmoid.

Hiatus Semilunaris

The superior opening of the ethmoid infundibulum is the hiatus semilunaris. The length of the uncinate process determines the depth of the ethmoid infundibulum and therefore the distance of the maxillary ostium from the nasal fossa. The depth of the ethmoid infundibulum or the length of the uncinate process varies from virtually nothing to 10 mm.

The depth of the ethmoid infundibulum and the width of the hiatus semilunaris determine the accessibility of the maxillary ostium to probing.

Olfactory Plate

The olfactory plate is visualized only faintly because it is pierced by many holes carrying the olfactory nerves into the nasal fossa from the olfactory lobe of the brain above.

The average maximal width of the olfactory plate is 5 mm. This is why it is difficult to visualize the olfactory plate on tomograms. First it is very narrow, only 5 mm. Secondly it is not solid. It is pierced by multiple holes. Thus if there is not a very marked change, neither very extensive destruction by tumor or marked posttraumatic distraction, an abnormality of the olfactory plate may be invisible on tomography.

If there is a cerebrospinal fluid rhinorrhea the presence of an apparently normal olfactory plate on tomography does not rule out this plate as the site of the leak.

Turbinate

In this particular section the crista galli is pneumatized. There is also an air cell in the left middle turbinate. Such pneumatization of the middle turbinate may be quite extensive and on occasion may expand the middle turbinate such that it completely fills the ipsilateral nasal fossa.

One should note the absence of bone immediately superior to the attachment of the inferior turbinate. This absence of bone or membranous portion of the medial maxillary antrum is normal.

Maxillary Hiatus

The membranous portion of the medial wall of the maxillary sinus is formed by the maxillary hiatus.

The maxillary hiatus is a large opening in the medial wall of the maxilla. This large opening is partially covered by bony processes from the ethmoid, inferior turbinate, palatine and lacrimal bones.

The remainder of the maxillary hiatus is not covered by bone but is covered by membrane. This membranous portion of the lateral nasal wall is C-shaped. The top of the C is above the attachment of the inferior turbinate. The bottom of the C is below and the back of the C is posterior to the uncinate process. The gaps in the bone seen in this section represent the top of the C, above the attachment of the inferior turbinate.

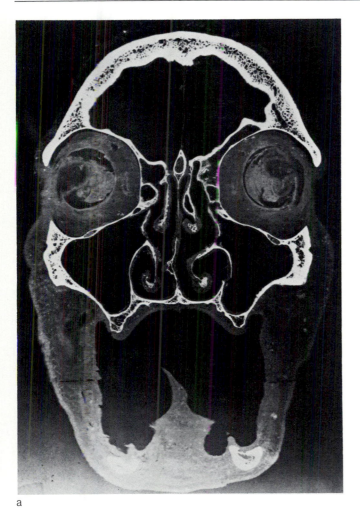

a

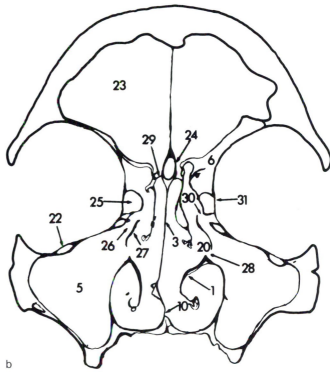

b

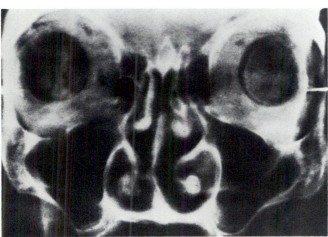

c

Fig. 2.**3**
a) Coronal anatomic section showing maxillary sinus ostium and the olfactory plate.
b) Line drawing and legend. 1. Inferior meatus, inferior turbinate (arrow), 3. perpendicular plate of the ethmoid, 5. maxillary sinus, 6. frontal sinus, 10. vomer, 20. middle meatus, 22. infraorbital canal, 23. anterior cranial fossa, 24. crista galli, 25. ethmoid bulla, 26. ethmoid infundibulum and ostium of the maxillary sinus, 27. uncinate process of the ethmoid, 28. membranous portion of the wall of the nasal fossa, 29. olfactory plate, 30. hiatus semi-lunaris, 31. lamina papyracea.
c) Normal coronal tomogram of a).

Diagnostic Importance

The importance of these membranous portions of the maxillary sinus tomographically is that they should not be confused with abnormal bone destruction. Small areas of absent bone immediately superior or inferior to the attachment of the inferior turbinate should be interpreted as normal.

This section is the section that is most valuable for drainage problems of the maxillary sinus, destruction of the medial wall of the orbit, and destruction of the olfactory plate.

Coronal Section Posterior to Frontal Sinus

The next section (Fig. 2.4) is 4 mm posterior to Figure 2.3. This section is completely posterior to the frontal sinuses.

Anterior Cranial Fossa and Ethmoid Sinus

In this instance we see the intimate relationship of the anterior cranial fossa to the ethmoid sinuses. In seeing the relationship of the ethmoid sinuses and in the previous sections the frontal sinuses to the anterior cranial

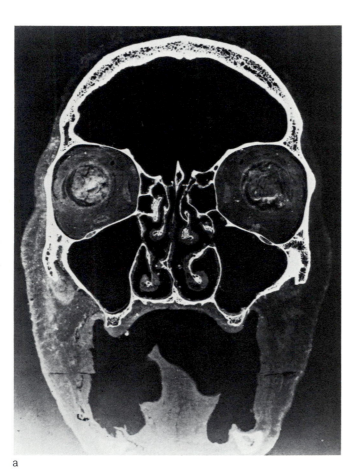

a

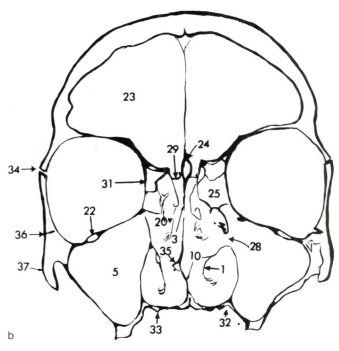

b

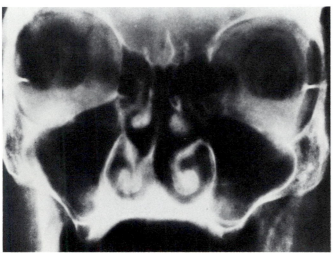

c

Fig. 2.4
a) Coronal anatomic section through the lamina papyracea showing the relationship of the roof of the ethmoid sinus to the anterior cranial fossa.
b) Line drawing and legend. 1. inferior meatus, inferior turbinate (arrow), 3. perpendicular plate of the ethmoid, 5. maxillary sinus, 10. vomer, 20. middle meatus, middle turbinate (arrow), 22. infraorbital canal, 23. anterior cranial fossa, 24. crista galli, 25. ethmoid bulla, 28. membranous portion of the wall of the nasal fossa, 29. olfactory plate, 31. lamina papyracea, 32. palatine groove, 33. palatine spine, 34. frontozygomatic suture, 35. lateral crest of the bony septum, 36. zygomaticotemporal canal, 37. zygomatic arch.
c) Normal coronal tomogram of a).

fossa and the frontal lobe, it is easy to appreciate the reason for frequent intracranial complications of infections of the paranasal sinuses.

Again there is an absence of bone in the medial wall of the maxillary sinus immediately superior to the attachment of the inferior turbinates.

The crista galli and the olfactory plates are again visualized.

This section is important when there is suspected intracranial involvement by an ethmoid condition.

Coronal Section: The Medial Wall of the Orbit

The next section (Fig. 2.5) is 6 mm posterior to Figure 2.4.

The medial wall of the orbit is no longer vertical, but rather oblique, going from medial to lateral as it descends from superior to inferior with the result that the orbit no longer has a circular shape but almost a pyramidal shape or triangular shape. This tendency toward a triangular cross-section becomes more pronounced as one proceeds posteriorly in the orbit.

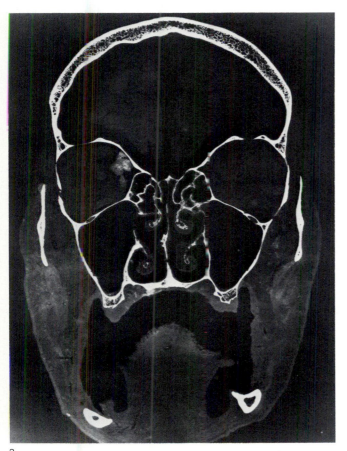

a

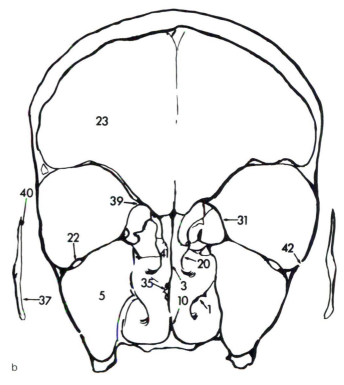

b

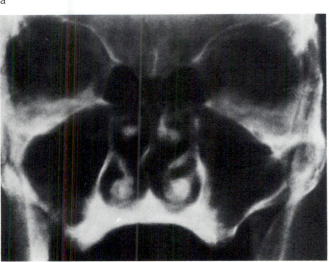

c

Fig. 2.**5**
a) Coronal anatomic section through the ethmomaxillary plate and the ethmoid canal.
b) Line drawing and legend. 1. Inferior meatus, inferior turbinate (arrow), 3. perpendicular plate of the ethmoid, 5. maxillary sinus, 10. vomer, 20. middle meatus, middle turbinate (arrow), 22. infraorbital canal, 23. anterior cranial fossa, 31. lamina papyracea, 35. lateral crest of the bony septum, 37. zygomatic arch, 39. anterior ethmoid foramen, 40. marginal process of the zygomatic bone, 41. superior turbinate, 42. inferior orbital fissure.
c) Normal coronal tomogram of a).

Anterior Ethmoid Canal

Between the superior edge of of the lamina papyracea and the medial edge of the orbital plate of the frontal bone is the orbital end of the anterior ethmoid canal, (the anterior ethmoid foramen).

Roof of the Orbit

The roof of the orbit is markedly indented and thinned by gyri of the frontal lobe of the brain. These thin areas of bone, the depths of these gyral indentations, will be poorly visualized on a tomogram and may often appear as an absence of bone in the roof of the orbit which in reality is merely very thin bone beneath the impressions made by the gyri of the frontal lobe of the brain.

Ethmomaxillary Plate

Separating the ethmoid sinuses from the maxillary antrum is a curvilinear plate of bone, the ethmomaxillary plate. The ethmomaxillary plate is often the first section of the wall of the maxillary sinus altered or destroyed by pathological conditions involving the ethmoid or maxillary sinus. The curvilinear ethmomaxillary plate is visualized on the Caldwell view (Fig. 1.1).

This coronal section is the most important for analyzing the ethmomaxillary plate for destruction by a tumor or displacement by a benign lesion such as an ethmoid mucocele.

Ethmoid Canal

Destruction of the medial wall of the orbit can be localized by means of an anatomic marker, the ethmoid canal, which is visualized on this section.

Coronal Section: Infraorbital Sulcus

The next section (Fig. 2.6) is 6 mm posterior to Figure 2.5. This section is posterior to the most posterior extent of the right infraorbital canal. Instead of a canal there is a slight groove in the floor of the right orbit. This is the infraorbital sulcus.

The second division or maxillary division of the fifth cranial nerve leaves the intracranial compartment via the foramen rotundum. It then crosses the pterygopalatine fossa and the inferior orbital fissure to enter a groove in the floor of the orbit which is the infraorbital sulcus. A variable distance anterior to the inferior orbital fissure, this sulcus becomes roofed such that the sulcus is turned into a canal at which point it is called the infraorbital canal.

In this particular coronal section on the right, we see the infraorbital sulcus but on the left the infraorbital sulcus has been roofed to form the infraorbital canal. Lateral both to the infraorbital sulcus and the infraorbital canal we can see the gap in the lateral wall of the orbit formed by the inferior orbital fissure.

Medial Wall of the Orbit

The medial wall of the orbit has a pronounced obliquity extending laterally from superior to inferior. This obliquity of the medial wall of the orbit in this section is so pronounced that the medial wall and the floor make one single plane. The result is that the orbit is triangular in cross section rather than round as it was in the more anterior section such as in Figure 2.4.

Abnormal Comparisons

This section is important because by comparing tomograms taken at the same level to it, we can demonstrate destruction in the area of the inferior orbital fissure and of the posterior portion of the lamina papyracea.

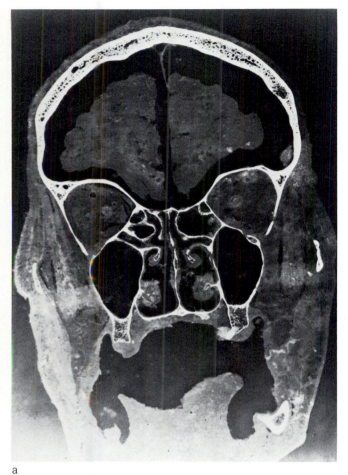

a

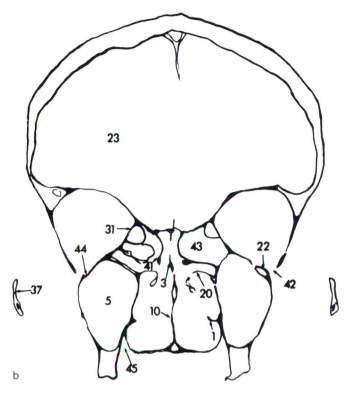

b

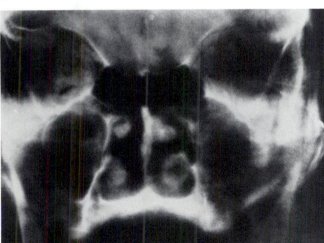

c

Fig. 2.**6**
a) Coronal anatomic section through the posterior part of the lamina papyracea and inferior orbital fissure.
b) Line drawing and legend. 1. Inferior meatus, inferior turbinate (arrow), 3. perpendicular plate of the ethmoid, 5. maxillary sinus, 10. vomer, 20. middle meatus, middle turbinate (arrow), 22. infra-orbital canal, 23. anterior cranial fossa, 31. lamina papyracea, 37. zygomatic arch, 41. superior meatus, superior turbinate (arrow), 42. inferior orbital fissure, 43. posterior ethmoid air cell, 44. infraorbital sulcus, 45. greater palatine foramen.
c) Normal coronal tomogram of a).

Coronal Section Through the Pterygoid Plates

The next section (Fig. 2.7) is 12 mm posterior to Figure 2.6. This section is through the pterygoid plates, the most anterior portion of the pterygopalatine fossa and the superior orbital fissure and the sphenoid sinuses.

Superior Orbital Fissure

The close approximation of the sphenoid sinuses to the superior orbital fissure gives an anatomical explanation for this close relationship of the sphenoid sinuses to the structures of the superior orbital fissure, namely the

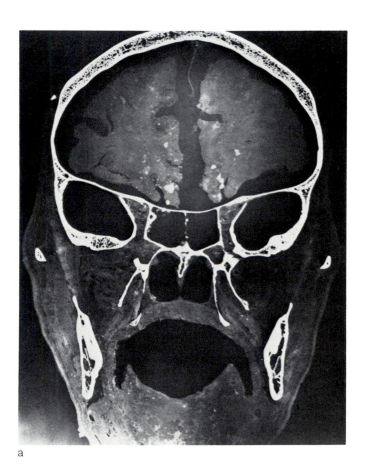

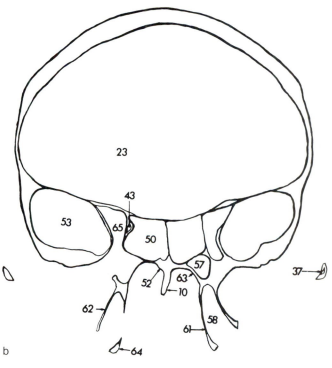

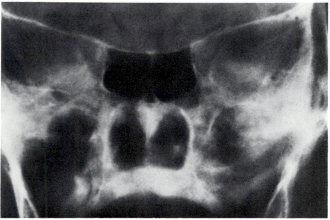

Fig. 2.7
a) Coronal anatomic section through the sphenoid sinuses, the superior orbital fissure and the pterygoid plate.
b) Line drawing and legend. 10. vomer, 23. anterior cranial fossa, 37. zygomatic arch, 43. posterior ethmoid air cell, 50. sphenoid sinus, 52. sphenoid rostrum and alae of the vomer, 53. middle cranial fossa, 57. pterygopalatine fossa, 58. pterygoid fossa, 61. medial pterygoid plate, 62. lateral pterygoid plate, 63. sphenoidal process of the palatine, 64. hamulus of the medial pterygoid plate, 65. superior orbital fissure.
c) Normal coronal tomogram of a).

nerves of the extraocular muscles including the 3rd, 4th and 6th nerves, the venous return from the orbit represented by the superior and inferior ophthalmic veins and the first division or ophthalmic division of the fifth cranial nerve. From this close approximation of the sphenoid sinus to the superior orbital fissure it is easily appreciated why diplopia often occurs with sphenoid sinus afflictions.

Pterygopalatine Fossa

The most anterior portion of the right pterygopalatine fossa is in wide communication with the inferior portion of the superior orbital fissure and this demonstrates how a tumor invading the pterygopalatine fossa can easily invade upward into the superior orbital fissure and then subsequently posteriorly into the middle cranial fossa or laterally into the infratemporal fossa.

Abnormalities of other Structures

This section is important for showing abnormalities affecting the superior orbital fissure, the pterygoid plate, and the sphenoid sinus.

Coronal Section Through the Middle Cranial Fossa

The next section (Fig. 2.8) is 12 mm posterior to Figure 2.7. This coronal section is through the middle cranial fossa, the sphenoid sinuses, the very posterior edge of the pterygoid plates and the cranial end of the optic canals.

Sphenoid Sinus

The groove formed by the second division of the left fifth cranial nerve is shown.
In the floor of the sphenoid sinus is seen the pterygoid canal.
The relationship of these nerves to the sphenoid sinus demonstrates how sphenoid sinus affections can produce decreased vision by affecting the optic nerve, facial numbness and pain due to impingement on the second division of the fifth cranial nerve

Maxillary Nerve

This illustrates the importance of looking at all the areas through which the maxillary nerve traverses. In other words if there is numbness or pain in the cheek it is not sufficient to look in the maxillary sinus in the floor of the orbit in the region of the infraorbital canal. The same symptoms can be produced by pathology in the sphenoid sinus affecting the second division of the fifth nerve and the middle cranial fossa or in the foramen rotundum.

Pterygoid Canal

A dry eye may be explained by a sphenoid sinus pathology affecting the pterygoid canal which runs in the floor of the sphenoid sinus.

The pterygoid canal carries the pterygoid or Vidian nerve which contains the presynaptic, parasympathetic fibers of the motor nerve of lacrimation.

Ala of the Vomer

The bulge in the pharyngeal surface of the floor of the sphenoid sinus is formed by the ala of the vomer and should not be confused with an abnormal excrescence of bone such as an osteoma.
This section is important to show an abnormality of the pterygoid canal especially in a patient with a dry eye and to show destruction of the floor of the sphenoid sinus (roof of the nasopharynx) in patients with a nasopharyngeal carcinoma.

Lateral Tomographic Projection

Lateral tomograms of the paranasal sinuses may be obtained on a field the size of one quarter of a 10 inch by 12 inch x-ray film.

Small Field

In other words the lateral tomographic image of the paranasal sinuses can be performed by placing four images on a 10 inch by 12 inch film. It is extremely important to use as small a field as possible when making tomograms of any anatomic area. Therefore if one quarter of a 10 inch by 12 inch film is sufficient to adequately cover the lateral projection of the paranasal sinuses no larger field should be used for this purpose.

Positioning of the Head

It is important when positioning the head for lateral tomograms of the paranasal sinuses that the midsagittal plane be parallel to the table top (perpendicular to the central beam). The midsagittal plane should be parallel to the table top so that the two sides of the head are comparable in projection.

Comparision of the Two Sides

Comparability of the two sides of the head is useful when one suspects an abnormality and would desire a normal comparison. If the head is allowed to rotate so that the midsagittal plane is not parallel to the table top the resulting lateral tomographic section will be oblique and the two sides of the head will not be comparable on the tomogram.
Sections at every 5 mm are usually adequate for an examination of the paranasal sinuses in the lateral projection.

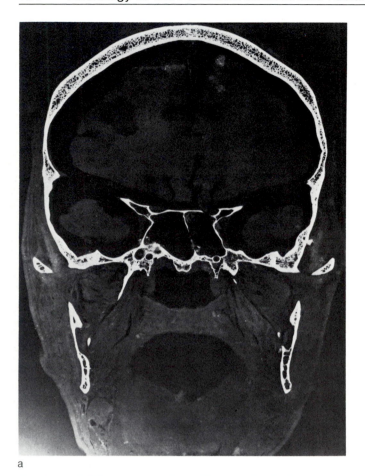

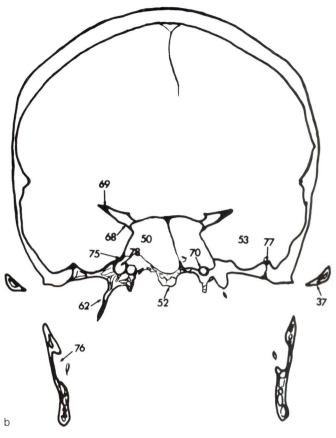

b

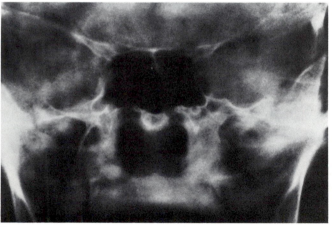

c

Fig. 2.**8**

a) Coronal anatomic section through the sphenoid sinus, the optic canal, and the pterygoid canal.

b) Line drawing and legend. 37. Zygomatic arch, 50. sphenoid sinus, 52. sphenoid rostrum and alae of the vomer, 53. middle cranial fossa, 62. lateral pterygoid plate, 68. optic canal floor, 69. lesser wing of the sphenoid, 70. pterygoid canal, 75. maxillary nerve groove, 76. mandibular foramen, 77. sphenosquamous suture, 78. lateral recess of the sphenoid sinus.

c) Normal coronal tomogram of a).

Lateral Section

This section demonstrates the frontal sinus above the orbit and the maxillary sinus below the orbit (Fig. 2.9). In the floor of the orbit very faintly seen is the infraorbital canal, posterior is the inferior orbital fissure and inferior to it the sphenomaxillary fissure.

Petrous Pyramid

Posteriorly in the petrous pyramid are seen the internal auditory canal, the jugular fossa, the carotid canal and the carotid ridge, the widow's peak of bone which separates the carotid foramen from the jugular foramen. Just anterior to the carotid canal is the angular spine of the sphenoid which in turn is just posterior to the foramen spinosum.

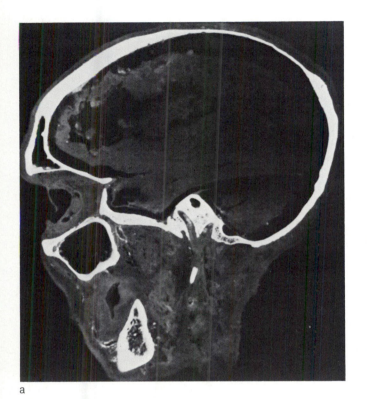

a

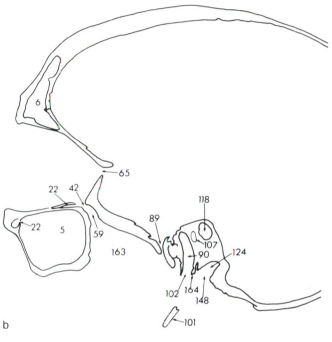

b

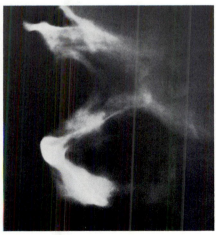

c

Fig. 2.9
a) Lateral anatomic section through the maxillary sinus and the orbit with the infraorbital canal in the floor of the orbit.
b) Line drawing and legend. 5. Maxillary sinus, 6. frontal sinus, 22. infraorbital canal, 42. inferior orbital fissure, 59. sphenomaxillary fissure, 65. superior orbital fissure, 89. foramen spinosum, 90. carotid canal, 101. styloid process, 102. carotid foramen, 107. cochlea, basilar turn, 118. internal auditory canal, 124. jugular fossa, 148. jugular foramen, 163. infratemporal fossa, 164. carotid ridge.
c) Normal lateral tomogram of a).

Superior Orbital Fissure

The gap between the posterior wall and the roof of the orbit represents the lateral portion of the superior orbital fissure. The angular spine is in the posterolateral corner of the greater wing of the sphenoid.

Inferior Orbital Fissure

The gap between the floor of the orbit and the greater wing of the sphenoid is formed by the inferior orbital fissure.

Infraorbital Canal

This section is important to show abnormalities of the infraorbital canal either by a fracture or a tumor.

Proptosis

Also in patients whose symptom is proptosis this section will demonstrate an abnormality of the greater wing of the sphenoid forming the posterior wall of the orbit.

Lateral Section through the Maxillary Sinus

The next section (Fig. 2.10) is 8 mm medial to Figure 2.9. We now see the maximum diameter of the maxillary sinus.

Frontal Sinus

The frontal sinus is seen pneumatizing both the vertical plate of the frontal bone and the orbital plate of the frontal bone (which is the roof of the orbit), a supra-orbital extension of the frontal sinus. The upper part of the pterygopalatine fossa is demonstrated.

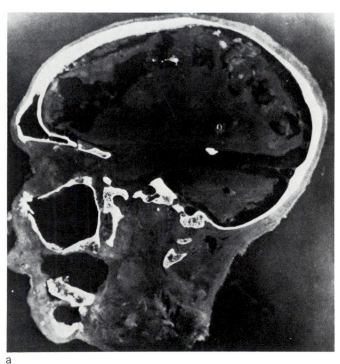

a

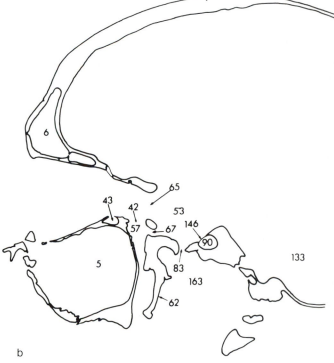

b

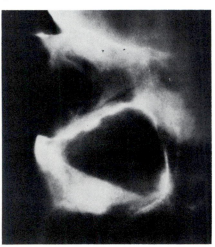

c

Fig. 2.**10**
a) Lateral anatomic section through the pterygopalatine fossa and the foramen rotundum.
b) Line drawing and legend. 5. Maxillary sinus, 6. frontal sinus, 42. inferior orbital fissure, 43. posterior ethmoid air cell, 53. middle cranial fossa, 57. pterygopalatine fossa, 62. lateral pterygoid plate, 65. superior orbital fissure, 67. foramen rotundum, 83. foramen ovale, 90. carotid canal, 133. posterior cranial fossa, 146. trigeminal impression, 163. infratemporal fossa.
c) Normal lateral tomogram of a).

Foramen Rotundum

The foramen rotundum is seen extending from the middle cranial fossa posteriorly to the pterygopalatine fossa anteriorly. Separating the foramen rotundum from the superior orbital fissure is a small piece of bone which can routinely be seen on lateral tomograms.

Petrous Pyramid

Posteriorly in the petrous pyramid is the horizontal portion of the carotid artery canal and anterior to the petrous pyramid the foramen ovale.

Pterygopalatine Fossa

This section is important to show changes in the pterygopalatine fossa either traumatic or by tumor destruction.

Foramen Rotundum Destruction

This section also shows the superior orbital fissure and the foramen rotundum. In this section one can locate destruction or enlargement of the foramen rotundum to explain numbness or pain in the cheek.

Lateral Section: The Pterygopalatine Fossa

This section (Fig. 2.11) is 4 mm medial to Figure 2.10. We can see almost the entire extent of the pterygopalatine fossa. The anterior wall of the pterygopalatine fossa bulges anteriorly and this bulge represents the sphenopalatine foramen.

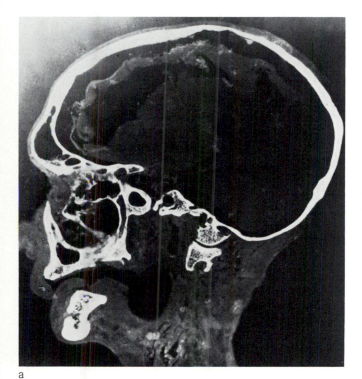

a

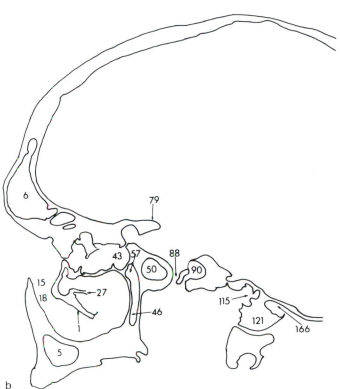

b

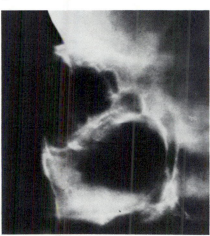

c

Fig. 2.**11**

a) Lateral anatomic section through the frontal sinus, the lacrimal sac fossa, the nasolacrimal canal and the lateral extension of the sphenoid sinus.
b) Line drawing and legend. 1. Inferior meatus, inferior turbinate (arrow), 5. maxillary sinus, 6. frontal sinus, 15. lacrimal sac fossa, 18. nasolacrimal canal, 27. uncinate process, ethmoid, 43. posterior ethmoid air cell, 46. pterygopalatine canal, 50. sphenoid sinus, 57. pterygopalatine fossa, 79. anterior clinoid process, 88. foramen lacerum, 90. carotid canal, 115. hypoglossal canal, 121. occipital condyle, 166. condyloid fossa.
c) Normal lateral tomogram of a).

Extension of the Sphenoid Sinus

Posterior to the pterygopalatine fossa is an air cell. This air cell is an inferolateral extension of the sphenoid sinus pneumatizing the base of the pterygoids. This is a common finding.

Lacrimal Apparatus

Anteriorly you can see the nasolacrimal fossa, the anterior lacrimal spine, and the direction and size and shape of the nasolacrimal canal.

Abnormalities of the Pterygopalatine Fossa

This section is important for showing abnormalities of the pterygopalatine fossa.

Abnormalities of Lacrimal Apparatus

Anteriorly, abnormalities of the nasolacrimal sac fossa, especially the anterior lacrimal spine and the nasolacrimal canal, can be seen on this section.

Lateral Section: Sphenoid Sinus

This section (Fig. 2.12) is 6 mm more medial than Figure 2.11. It demonstrates the sphenoid sinus bordering on the ethmoid sinuses and the frontal sinus.

Nasofrontal Canal

Descending inferiorly from the frontal sinus is a canal, the nasofrontal canal, which is an important structure especially after trauma and fracture of the frontal sinus.

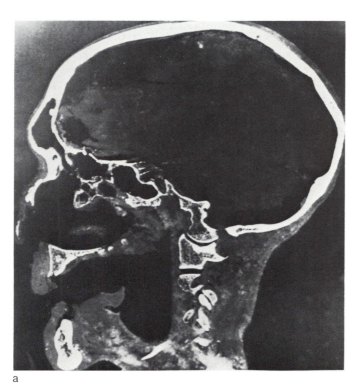

a

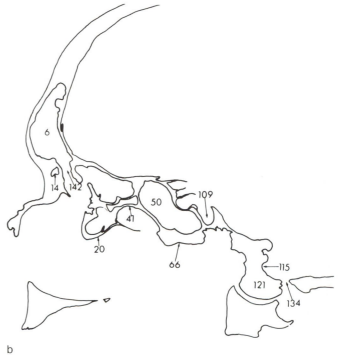

b

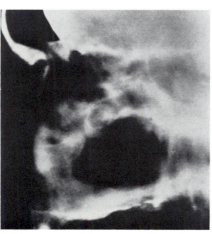

c

Fig. 2.**12**
a) Lateral anatomic section through the frontal sinus, the nasofrontal duct and the sphenoid sinus.
b) Line drawing and legend. 6. Frontal sinus, 14. agger nasi cell, 20. middle turbinate, 41. superior turbinate, 50. sphenoid sinus, 66. vaginal process, medial pterygoid plate, 109. carotid sulcus, 115. hypoglossal canal, 121. occipital condyle, 134. foramen magnum, 142. nasofrontal duct.
c) Normal lateral tomogram of a).

It is important to demonstrate damage to the nasofrontal canal because damage to this canal will interfere with the drainage of the frontal sinus which may produce a mucocele at some time in the future if it is not corrected.

It is important to inform the referring physician who is contemplating surgical correction of a frontal sinus fracture if the nasofrontal canal is injured. Abnormalities of the nasofrontal duct such as a fracture and the relation of the ethmoid sinuses to the sphenoid sinus can be seen on this section.

Axial Tomographic Projection

Axial (which is the same as basal or submentovertical) tomograms are obtained with the patient supine. The head is extended to its maximum excursion so that the tragocanthal line is as parallel to the table top as possible. To encompass both sides of the paranasal sinuses it is usually necessary to use one half of a 10 by 12 inch film.

Sections at every 5 mm are usually adequate for an examination of the paranasal sinuses in the axial projection.

Axial Section Through Ethmoid Sinus

The first axial section is through the lower portion of the ethmoid sinuses and visualizes the sphenoid sinuses, the inferior orbital fissure, the foramina rotunda, and the most superior portion of the pterygopalatine fossa (Fig. 2.13).

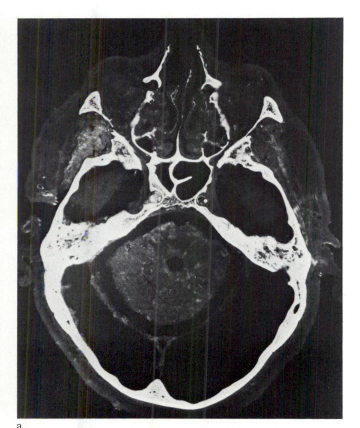

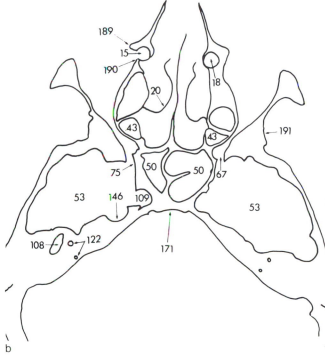

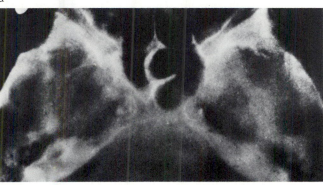

Fig. 2.**13**
a) Axial anatomic section through the orbit, ethmoid sinuses, sphenoid sinuses and the foramen rotundum.
b) Line drawing and legend. 15. Lacrimal sac fossa, 18. nasolacrimal canal, 20. middle turbinate, 43. posterior ethmoid air cell, 50. sphenoid sinus, 53. middle cranial fossa, 67. foramen rotundum, 75. maxillary nerve groove, 108. tympanic cavity, attic, 109. carotid sulcus, 122. superior semicircular canal, 146. trigeminal impression, 171. clivus, 189. anterior lacrimal spine, 190. posterior lacrimal spine, 191. sphenoid, greater wing, temporal surface (linea innominata).
c) Normal axial tomogram of a).

Lacrimal Apparatus

The left nasolacrimal canal is visualized. The right lacrimal sac fossa is demonstrated. The anterior margin of the lacrimal sac fossa is formed by the anterior lacrimal spine, part of the frontal process of the maxilla. The posterior margin is formed by the posterior lacrimal spine, part of the lacrimal bone.

Greater Wing of the Sphenoid

At the junction of the two portions of the greater wing of the sphenoid, the portion forming the anterior margin of the middle cranial fossa and the portion forming the lateral wall of the orbit, the bone is thick.

It is this thick buttress of bone that makes possible the classic approach to the orbit by the ophthalmologist (the Kronlein procedure). In the Kronlein procedure, a saw cut is made in the lateral wall of the orbit through the frontal process of the zygomatic bone near the floor of the orbit and another saw cut is made more superior in the lateral wall of the orbit through the upper part of the frontal process of the zygomatic bone or through the lower part of the zygomatic process of the frontal bone. The portion of the lateral wall of the orbit between these two saw cuts is fractured out. This portion of the lateral wall of the orbit can be fractured out without danger of fracturing posteriorly into the middle cranial fossa because of the buttress of bone between the greater wing of the sphenoid and the lateral wall of the orbit.

Innominate Line

Also one should note the lateral cortex of this buttress of bone, this strong triangular buttress. The lateral cortex forms the innominate line seen on the routine Caldwell view of the paranasal sinuses (see Fig. 1.1).

Orbit

This section also shows an important configuration of the orbit which is also seen on computerized axial tomograms.

The contour of the medial wall of the orbit is different according to the level at which the computerized axial tomogram is obtained. In the more superior sections, the lamina papyracea or the lateral plate of the ethmoids is more or less straight with a slight lateral bulge in its center.

In more inferior sections, such as this one, there is a marked lateral bulge in the posterior portion of the lamina papyracea as it approaches the orbital apex. This configuration produces the marked curvilinear contour of the medial wall of the orbit and of course a similar appearance will be produced on a computerized scan at the same level in the orbit.

Pterygopalatine Fossa

There is a close approximation of the inferior orbital fissure, pterygopalatine fossa and the foramen rotundum. Coronal tomograms showed that there was a free communication between the pterygopalatine fossa, the inferior orbital fissure and the infratemporal fossa.

On this axial section one can see that there is a free communication between the pterygopalatine fossa and inferior orbital fissure and the middle cranial fossa through the foramen rotundum, thus explaining how a tumor invading the pterygopalatine fossa such as a juvenile angiofibroma may go into the orbit superiorly or into the middle cranial fossa posteriorly.

Accessory Sphenoid Sinus Septum

In this section also there is an accessory septum in the sphenoid sinus. Incomplete septa, in fact multiple incomplete septa, are not uncommon in the sphenoid sinus and should not be confused with an abnormality. Note also the close approximation of the carotid artery to the sphenoid sinus.

Abnormalities

This axial section is important to show abnormalities of the lateral wall of the orbit and the foramen rotundum.

Axial Section Through the Pterygopalatine Fossa

This section (Fig. 2.14) is 4 mm inferior to Figure 2.13. This is a section through the uppermost portion of the maxillary sinus and the pterygopalatine fossa. In fact only the medial portion of the maxillary sinus is seen.

Lateral Floor of the Orbit

The lateral portion of the floor of the orbit slopes downward as it goes from medial to lateral, so in one axial cut it is not surprising to have a portion of the maxillary sinus medially and a portion of the floor of the orbit laterally.

Communication of Pterygopalatine Fossa

The pterygopalatine fossae are well demonstrated. In this section the pterygopalatine fossa communicates laterally with the infratemporal fossa through the sphenomaxillary fissure and communicates with the nasal fossa medially through the sphenopalatine foramen. Both nasolacrimal canals are clearly demonstrated.

Ear Structures

Posteriorly are the internal auditory canal, vestibule, basilar turn of the cochlea and the lateral semicircular canal. The middle ear cavity and the mastoid sinus and the aditus ad antrum are also shown.

Pterygopalatine Fossa: Five Connections

This section shows well why a malignant tumor which has invaded the pterygopalatine fossa is considered inoperable. The section shows two of the five connections that the pterygopalatine fossa has with the other cavities in the skull.

The pterygopalatine fossa communicates:

1. with the infratemporal fossa through the sphenomaxillary fissure.
2. with the nose through the sphenopalatine foramen,
3. with the mouth through the pterygopalatine canal,
4. with the orbit through the inferior orbital fissure, and
5. with the middle cranial fossa through the pterygoid canal and the foramen rotundum.

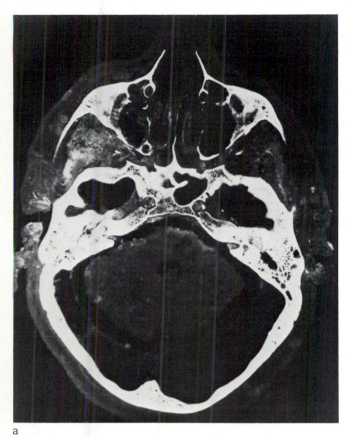

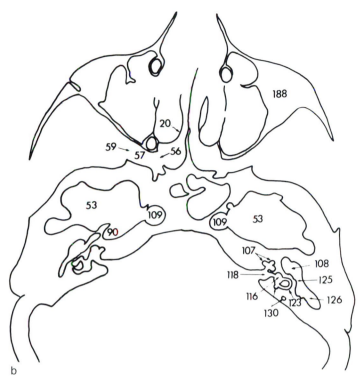

a

b

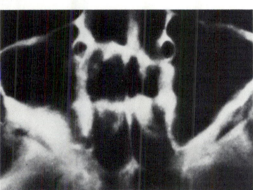

c

Fig. 2.**14**
a) Axial anatomic section through the maxillary sinus and the pterygopalatine fossa.
b) Line drawing and legend. 20. Middle turbinate, 53. middle cranial fossa, 56. sphenopalatine foramen, 57. pterygopalatine fossa, 59. sphenomaxillary fissure, 90. carotid canal, 107. cochlea, basilar and second turns, 108. tympanic cavity, attic, 109. carotid sulcus, 116. vestibule, 118. internal auditory canal, 123. lateral semicircular canal, 125. aditus ad antrum, 126. mastoid antrum, 130. posterior semicircular canal, 188. orbit floor.
c) Normal axial tomogram of a).

Thus any tumor which has broken through from the maxillary sinus posteriorly into the pterygopalatine fossa is probably inoperable because there are so many areas to which it can extend from this point.

Fracture or Tumor of Pterygopalatine Fossa

This section is most important for the demonstration of abnormalities of the pterygopalatine fossa by fracture or by tumor. A benign tumor may expand the fossa or a malignant tumor may destroy the fossa.

Axial Section Inferior to Previous Section

This section (Fig. 2.15) is 8 mm inferior to Figure 2.14. The pterygopalatine fossa is still seen but this section is inferior to the sphenopalatine foramen and therefore the medial border of the pterygopalatine fossa is closed off from the nasal fossa. The lateral portion of the pterygopalatine fossa still opens to the infratemporal fossa through the sphenomaxillary fissure.

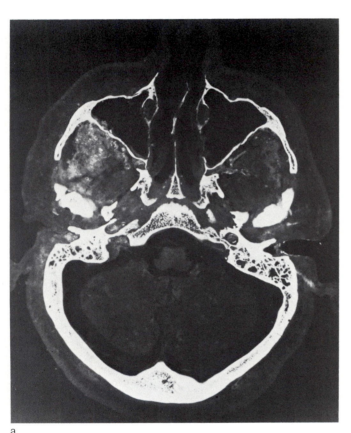

a

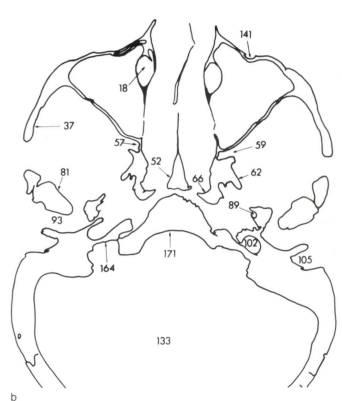

b

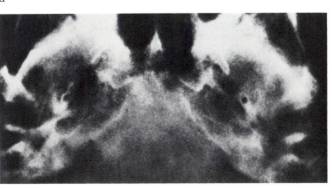

c

Fig. 2.15
a) Axial anatomic section through the maxillary sinus, nasolacrimal canal and inferior portion of the pterygopalatine fossa.
b) Line drawing and legend. 18. Nasolacrimal canal, 37. zygomatic arch, 52. sphenoid rostrum and alae of the vomer, 57. pterygopalatine fossa, 59. sphenomaxillary fissure, 62. lateral pterygoid plate, 66. vaginal process, medial pterygoid plate, 81. temporomandibular joint, articular eminence, 89. foramen spinosum, 93. temporomandibular joint, glenoid fossa, 102. carotid foramen, 105. external auditory canal, 133. posterior cranial fossa, 141. infraorbital foramen, 164. carotid ridge, 171. clivus.
c) Normal axial tomogram of a).

Nasolacrimal Canal

The nasolacrimal canal is still visible. The inferior portion of the nasolacrimal canal is considerably larger than the more superior sections.

Carotid Artery

The left carotid foramen is demonstrated and on the right the carotid artery has just made its turn from the vertical portion of the carotid canal to the horizontal portion. On the right just posterior to the carotid artery is seen the jugular fossa separated from the carotid artery canal by the carotid ridge.

Axial Section: Inferior Turbinate

This section (Fig. 2.16) is 10 mm inferior to Figure 2.15 and demonstrates well the relationship of the inferior turbinate to the medial wall of the maxillary sinus. It also shows that the medial wall of the maxillary sinus is slightly bowed laterally away from the nasal fossa.

Pterygoid Plate

This section is also a good demonstration of the relationship of the lateral and medial pterygoid plates to one another and also to the maxillary sinus anteriorly.

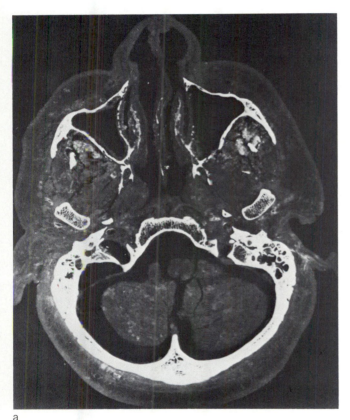

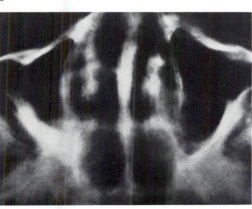

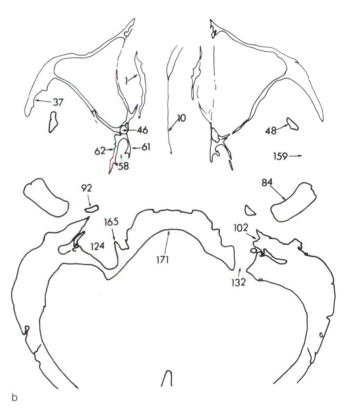

Fig. 2.**16**
a) Axial anatomic section through the pterygoid plate.
b) Line drawing and legend. 1. Inferior turbinate, 10. vomer, 37. zygomatic arch, 46. pterygopalatine canal, 48. coronoid process of the mandible, 58. pterygoid fossa, 61. medial pterygoid plate, 62. lateral pterygoid plate, 84. mandibular condyle, 92. sphenoid, angular spine, 102. carotid foramen, 124. jugular fossa, 132. sigmoid sinus, 159. coronoid notch, 165. intrajugular process, 171. clivus.
c) Normal axial tomogram of a).

Maxillary Sinus

In addition there is a good example of the S-shaped line which forms the lateral wall of the maxillary sinus and was seen on the base view (Fig. 1.3).

Pterygopalatine Fossa

Just anterior to the pterygoid plates we see the ptery-gopalatine canal carrying the pterygopalatine artery and nerve from the pterygopalatine fossa superiorly to the roof of the mouth inferiorly.

Jugular Fossa

Posteriorly one can see the right jugular fossa and on the left the lowermost portion of the left jugular fossa with the entry of the sigmoid sinus into the jugular fossa on the left.

Sphenoid Spine

Note the spine of the sphenoid from which the foramen spinosum gets its name. Since the sphenoid spine extends inferiorly on this axial section it appears detached from any other bone. In actuality, though, this fragment of bone is attached superiorly to the greater wing of the sphenoid and is part of this greater wing of the sphenoid, the most posterior part of the greater wing of the sphenoid immediately posterior to the foramen spinosum.

It should be noted that the angular spine of the sphenoid, seen on the lateral section as a continuous piece of bone (Fig. 2.9) is seen on the axial section as a detached piece of bone.

Abnormalities

This section is most important for showing abnormalities of the pterygoid plate and the anterior and lateral wall of the maxillary sinus.

Axial Section Through the Maxillary Sinus

This section (Fig. 2.17) is 12 mm inferior to Figure 2.16. This section is through the lowermost portion of the maxillary sinus (which is the alveolar recess of the maxillary sinus).

Hard Palate

In the midline we see the hard palate.

Incisive Canal

Anteriorly in the premaxilla we see the paired incisive canals.

Medial and Lateral Pterygoid Plates

This section is inferior to the inferiormost portion of the medial pterygoid plate and therefore the medial pterygoid plate is not seen but the lateral pterygoid plate is still visible. An axial tomogram or a computerized axial tomographic cut would demonstrate the lateral pterygoid plate at this level.

One should not mistake this normal difference in the inferior extent of the lateral and medial pterygoid plates for destruction of the medial pterygoid plate.

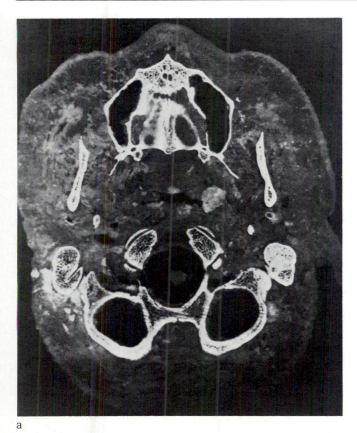

a

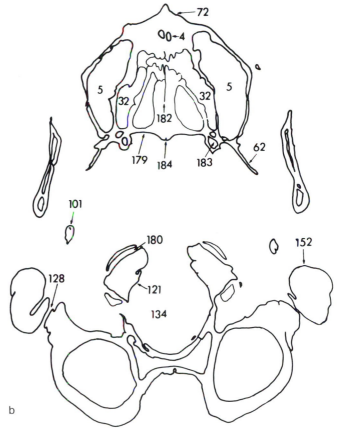

b

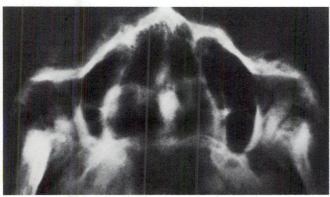

c

Fig. 2.**17**
a) Axial anatomic section through the maxillary alveolar recesses and the premaxillary process containing the incisive canal.
b) Line drawing and legend. 4. Incisive canal, 5. maxillary sinus, alveolar recess, 32. palatine groove, 62. lateral pterygoid plate, 72. premaxilla, 101. styloid process, 121. occipital condyle, 128. digastric (mastoid) notch, 134. foramen magnum, 152. mastoid process, temporal bone, 179. hard palate, 180. atlantocondylar joint, 182. intermaxillary suture, 183. lesser palatine canal, 184. posterior nasal spine.
c) Normal axial tomogram of a).

Chapter 3 Maxillofacial Trauma

The radiological examination of the facial bones after trauma should be approached with three objectives in mind:
1. The accurate anatomical delineation of any fractures involving the facial bones.
2. An estimation of the severity of these fractures.
3. A determination of the portions of the facial structures and the skull which are intact. One looks for the most inferior portions of bone that can be used as the locus of stabilizing wires in reducing these fractures and stabilizing them.

General Considerations

It is helpful to have the results of the physical examination prior to obtaining the radiographic examination.

Physical and Radiographic Examinations

It is helpful to have this clinical information for two reasons:
1. The radiographic examination can be tailored to demonstrate those particular areas of the facial bones in which there is a suspicion of fracture.
For example, a depression of the malar eminence in the region of the zygomatic arch is an indication for obtaining a zygomatic arch view as well as the routine facial views, including the Caldwell, Waters, lateral, and base views. If a depressed fracture of the floor of the orbit is suspected, then the optic canal (or Rhese) view should be obtained.
2. Knowing the areas of post-traumatic contusion, laceration, tenderness or malformation of the facial bones directs special attention to these areas. If the radiographs which have been obtained do not adequately demonstrate these areas of suspected traumatic change, special views can be devised to bring out these areas.

For example, if there is tenderness of the roof of the mouth on palpation, an intraoral film should be obtained to demonstrate a possible fracture of the hard palate or the premaxilla.

Also when routine films have not demonstrated a fracture where one is strongly suspected clinically, tomograms of the suspected area of the face should be obtained before a fracture is ruled out of consideration.

Pitfalls

It is of course helpful to have the clinical information as to the suspected area of fracture. However, anyone reading post-traumatic radiographs should always keep in mind that the clinical information can be misleading.

Patients who have had trauma to the face are often in pain and the areas of injury are quite tender. These facts make it difficult to perform an accurate physical examination including adequate palpation for the purpose of revealing deformities such as a step deformity in the rim of the floor of the orbit.

The swelling and edema commonly associated with facial fractures may mask deformities of the facial structures produced by a trauma. For example, a depression of the zygomatic arch may be masked by swelling and edema of the soft tissues of the involved side of the face.

Not infrequently, the clinical suspicion of the area of the facial bones that may be fractured is incorrect. The physical examination may raise a question of a blowout fracture and yet on the radiographs it will be seen that there is no blowout fracture but rather a depressed fracture of the zygomatic arch (Fig. 3.1).

Importance of Previous Trauma

A knowledge of a history of previous trauma is important. There is no way to assess the age of a facial fracture by purely radiographic means. Old facial fractures may have the same appearance as fresh fractures.

The people who tend to have falls and blows, such as chronic alcoholics or elderly persons who have problems with stability, will often have multiple traumatic episodes. In such persons, a fracture demonstrated on the radiographs of the face may be unrelated to the current trauma and may have been produced by a previous traumatic incident.

In such circumstances a patient could present with ecchymosis of one eye and the radiographs could show a blowout fracture of the other eye. The ecchymosis is caused by the current trauma; the blowout fracture was produced in some previous traumatic incident and is completely unrelated to the present traumatic incident.

Or a woman who has been beaten up by her husband may be subject to many beatings and the most recent beating may not be the cause of an apparent fracture on the radiographs. For example such a patient may have a blowout fracture from a recent beating and a depressed fracture of the zygomatic arch from a previous beating. Thus, the zygomatic arch fracture may not be fresh and not amenable to reduction.

There may be a tendency at such times to presume that the zygomatic films are mismarked left for right and the temptation may be to try to elevate a perfectly normal zygomatic arch.

The point is that if there has been no history of recent trauma to the area of the fracture, it should never be presumed that a radiographically demonstrated fracture is actually a new fracture (Fig. 3.2).

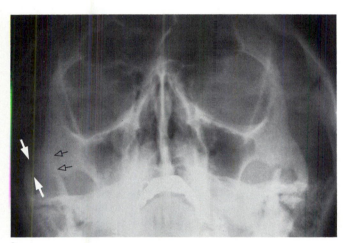

a

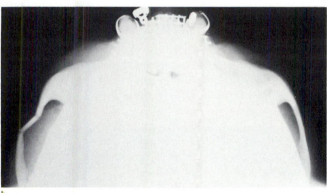

b

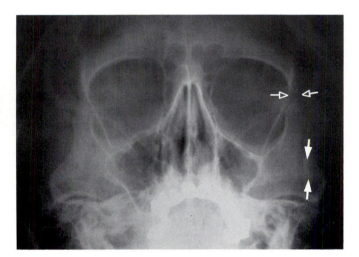

Fig. 3.1
a) Waters view showing depression of the right zygomatic arch of a patient suspected of having a blowout fracture of the floor of the orbit. The three manifestations of a depressed zygomatic arch as seen on the Waters view are demonstrated. They are (1) an oval shaped radiodensity (hollow arrows), (2) a radiolucent line crossing, but confined to, the zygomatic arch (solid arrows), and (3) a change of the normal smooth contour of the zygomatic arch to a more angulated configuration (compare the configuration of the right zygomatic arch to the left zygomatic arch).
b) Zygomatic arch view of the same patient seen in a) showing a depressed fracture of the zygomatic arch unsuspected clinically.

Fig. 3.2   Waters view of a patient who had had an unreduced trimalar fracture 2 years previously. There is separation of the left frontozygomatic suture (hollow arrows) and an oval shaped radiodensity in the zygomatic arch (solid arrows). These fractures are known to be 2 years old. However, radiographically, they cannot be differentiated from recent fractures, emphasizing the necessity of an accurate history in determining the age of facial fractures.

Categories of Fracture

Fractures of the face can be broken down into categories such as zygomatic arch fractures, maxillary sinus fractures, blowout fractures, trimalar fractures, LeFort fractures, ethmoid sinus fractures, frontal sinus fractures, and sphenoid sinus fractures.

Zygomatic Arch Fractures

On viewing routine films of the sinuses after trauma, the Waters view should be carefully evaluated for evidence of a depressed fracture of the zygomatic arch because it is often not clinically apparent that a zygomatic arch fracture is present and special zygomatic arch views are not routinely obtained. The only routine view that consistently shows the zygomatic arches is the Waters view.

Change of Contour

On the Waters view, the inferior aspect of the zygomatic arch should form a smooth curve with the lateral border of the maxillary sinus down to the maxillary alveolar ridge (Fig. 3.3).
If there is a depressed fracture of the zygomatic arch, the smooth curve will not appear the same on both sides.
A depressed fracture of the zygomatic arch may produce

two other findings in the image of the zygomatic arch as seen on the Waters view:
1. A linear lucency crossing the zygomatic arch and confined to it.
2. An oval density in the zygomatic arch.

Linear Lucency

When a linear lucency extends beyond the zygomatic arch, it is obviously not a fracture of the zygomatic arch but rather a lucency within the calvarium superimposed upon the zygomatic arch. Generally such a confusing linear lucency is a vascular marking in the temporal calvarial area superimposed on the zygomatic arch.

Oval Density

The other finding that may be seen with a depressed fracture of the zygomatic arch is an oval density. The oval density is formed by the depression in the zygomatic arch. Normally the zygomatic arch is a smooth curve. When there is a depressed fracture the smooth curve is interrupted. The bone is angulated in such a way that more bone is presented to the central beam. Thus, there is greater absorption of the beam in the area of the depression. This increased absorption produces a density of an oval shape (Fig. 3.4).

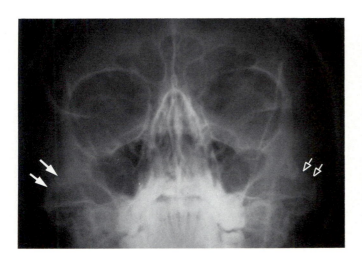

Fig. 3.**3** Waters view showing left zygomatic arch fracture manifested by a change in contour of the zygomatic arch. Compare the contour of the left zygomatic arch (hollow arrows) to that of the right zygomatic arch (solid arrows).

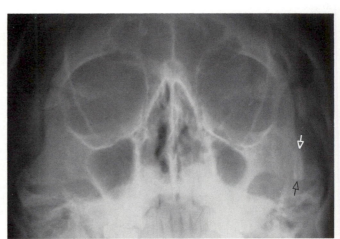

a

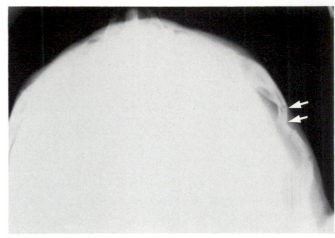

b

Fig. 3.**4** ▶
a) Waters view showing depressed fracture of the left zygomatic arch manifested by an oval shaped radiodensity (hollow arrows).
b) Zygomatic arch view of the left zygomatic arch showing the depressed fracture seen in a). The depressed fragment between the solid arrows presents more bone to the x-ray beam producing a greater absorption of x-rays when the Waters view is obtained, and thus results in the oval density seen on the Waters view.

Zygomatic Arch View

When one sees any of these findings on a Waters view – a change in the contour of the zygomatic arch, a linear lucency confined to, and crossing the zygomatic arch, or an oval-shaped radiodensity in the region of the zygomatic arch – one should then obtain special zygomatic arch views.

The zygomatic arch view is obtained by extending the head as in the base view, but then tilting the head towards the contralateral shoulder in such a way as to throw out the involved zygomatic arch.

Maxillary Sinus (Antrum) Fractures

Secondary radiographic evidence of a fracture of the maxillary sinus are three:
1. Post-traumatic air fluid level
2. Complete opacification of the maxillary sinus
3. "Bright lines"

Air Fluid Level

A post-traumatic air fluid level in the maxillary sinus indicates the presence of a fracture of the sinus whether the fracture is demonstrated radiographically or not. However, the absence of an air fluid level does not rule out a maxillary sinus fracture.

For example, a fracture which does not interrupt the mucosa but rather strips the mucosa from the underlying bone, will present as a soft tissue mass in the maxilla. The soft tissue mass is produced by submucosal hematoma.

Opacification

Quite often apparent opacification of the maxillary sinus after trauma as seen on the Waters view is due not to a clouding of the sinus but rather to soft tissue swelling of the cheek. Therefore, to evaluate opacification of the maxillary sinus one should look on the base view as well as on the Waters view.

If the opacification as seen on the Waters view is truly due to intrasinus clouding, the involved sinus will also appear opacified on the base view. However, if the clouding seen on the Waters view is due to soft tissue swelling, then the involved sinus will be clear on the base view.

Swelling in the soft tissues of the cheek produces a swollen soft tissue density superior to the palpable margin of the orbit on the Waters view. The swollen soft tissues of the cheek will produce a haziness of the ipsilateral maxillary sinus which should not be confused with intrasinus opacification. However, the presence of soft tissue swelling does not rule out the possibility that there is in addition intrasinus opacification. The appearance of the maxillary sinus on the base view can be helpful in differentiating these two causes of opacification of the maxillary sinus.

"Bright Lines"

Bright white lines superimposed upon the maxillary sinus on the Waters view which do not correspond to a cortical margin of an anatomical structure are another indication of a fracture involving the maxillary sinus.

These white lines represent fractures of the thin walls of the maxillary sinus with rotation of the fragments. Such lines can be seen on the Waters film (Fig. 3.5) and more rarely on the Caldwell view or on the lateral view.

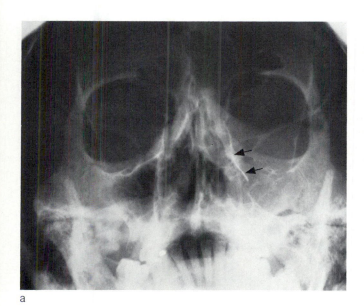

a

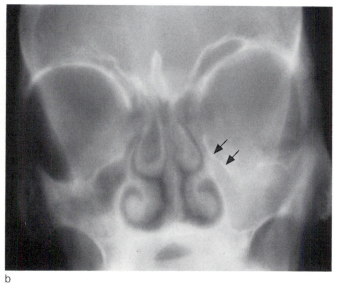

b

Fig. 3.5
a) Waters view demonstrating a "trap door" fracture of the floor and medial walls of the left orbit producing a "bright white line" (solid arrows). The whiteness is produced by rotation of the frag-

ment of bone which increases the absorption of the x-ray beam.
b) Coronal tomogram of the same patient demonstrating the fracture fragment (solid arrows) in the floor and medial wall of the left orbit which was seen as a "bright white line" on the Waters view.

Superior Orbital Fissure

A linear lucency which is often seen superimposed on the maxilla is the superior orbital fissure. This normal structure should not be confused with a fracture. To avoid this mistake of confusing the superior orbital fissure for a fracture, care should be used in interpreting as a fracture any radiolucency extending from medial to lateral as the radiolucency goes from inferior to superior, especially when you see such a radiolucency on both sides.

Blowout Fractures

A blowout fracture can also be called an isolated depressed fracture of the floor of the orbit.

Generation of Blowout Fracture

The term "blowout" fracture of the orbit originated with the original description of this type of fracture. It was postulated that a blow to the orbit put pressure on the globe, increasing the hydrostatic pressure within the orbit, and the effect of this increased intraorbital pressure is to produce a depressed fracture of the floor of the orbit.

However, if tomograms are obtained in the lateral projections of all orbits with a depressed fracture of the orbit floor, it is often evident that there is also a fracture of the

anterior wall of the maxillary sinus. There is no way that an increase in intraorbital hydrostatic pressure could produce a fracture of the anterior wall of the maxillary sinus in addition to a depressed fracture of the floor of the orbit.

It is more likely that blowout fractures are produced by the relief of the stress of trauma to the facial bones and if the force is sufficient, then the stress is relieved not only by a depressed fracture of the floor of the orbit (blowout fracture), but also in addition, a fracture of the anterior wall of maxillary sinus. Fractures of the anterior wall of the maxillary sinus are often not seen on routine radiographs and therefore are overlooked unless lateral tomograms are obtained.

Radiographic Findings

The radiographic findings of the blowout fracture are:
1. A separation of the rim of the orbit from the floor of the orbit as seen on the Waters view (Fig. 3.6).
2. Polypoid mass in the superior portion of the maxillary sinus associated with fragments of bone (Fig. 3.7).

The floor of the orbit is represented in the Waters view by two lines:
1. A superior line, the palpable margin of the orbit.
2. A more inferior line, the floor of the orbit more posterior.

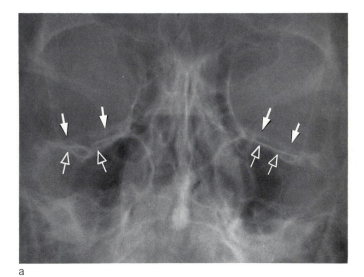

a

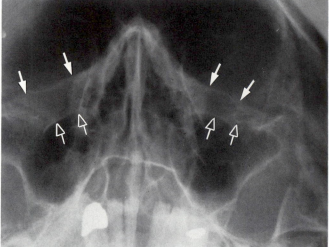

b

Fig. 3.6
a) Waters view of a patient with a right blowout fracture of the floor of the orbit showing separation of the lines, on the affected sides, representing the palpable margin of the orbit (solid arrows) and the floor of the orbit (hollow arrows). Compare the distance between the same two lines on the normal left side.

b) Same case as a). More extended Waters view. The distance between the palpable margin of the orbit (solid arrows) and the floor of the orbit (hollow arrows) is greater on the more extended Waters view on both sides but the distance between these two lines on the affected right side is still greater than on the normal left side.

By definition a blowout fracture is an isolated depressed fracture of the floor of the orbit without affecting the palpable margin of the orbit. Thus the relationship between these two areas will be changed in the presence of a blowout fracture.

Since the superior line representing the palpable margin of the orbit is not affected by the fracture, and the more inferior line representing the floor of the orbit is depressed, then these two lines must separate.

Normally these two lines, produced by the palpable margin of the orbit and the floor of the orbit more posterior, are parallel and the same distance apart on both sides on the same Waters view.

However, the distance between these two lines will increase as the head is more extended when taking the Waters view. The line representing the rim of the orbit and the line representing the floor of the orbit more posterior will be further apart on the more extended Waters view.

On any given Waters view the distance between the two lines, that is the line representing the palpable parts of the orbit and the more inferior line representing the floor of the orbit should be the same distance on each side, and if there is a blowout fracture, the distance between these two lines will be increased on the affected side.

Another sign of a blowout fracture is a polypoid mass in the superior portion of the maxillary sinus appearing to hang down from the floor of the orbit. A post-traumatic finding of a polypoid mass in the maxillary sinus is particularly significant if there are fragments of bone associated with such a polyp (Fig. 3.8).

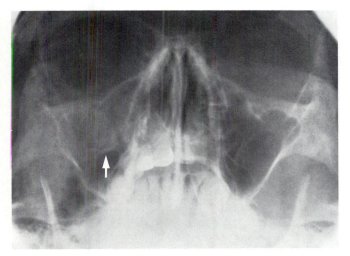

Fig. 3.7 Waters view of a right blowout fracture manifested by opacification of the superior portion of the maxillary sinus produced by a mass of prolapsed orbital tissue. There is a fragment of bone associated with the polypoid mass (solid arrow).

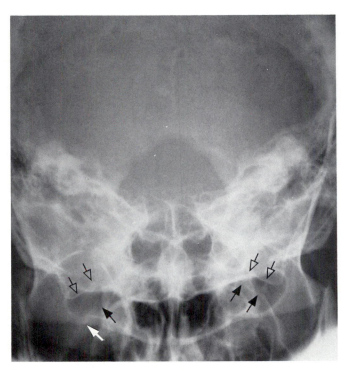

Fig. 3.9 Towne view demonstrating a fracture of the posterior portion of the floor of the orbit. The most posterior portion of the floor of the orbit forms the medial margin of the inferior orbital fissure. The inferior orbital fissure can be seen only on the Towne view. The inferior orbital fissure on the Towne view lies between the infratemporal tubercle of the greater wing of the sphenoid (hollow arrows) and the most posterior extent of the floor of the orbit (solid arrows). Note that the right inferior orbital fissure is widened and that the most posterior portion of the floor of the orbit is fuzzy and indistinct. Both of these findings are a result of the fracture of the posterior portion of the floor of the orbit.

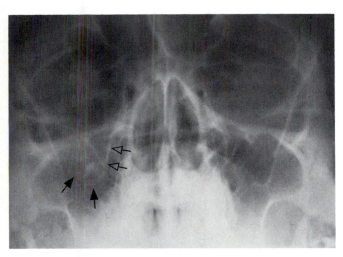

Fig. 3.8 Waters view demonstrating a blowout fracture of the floor of the right orbit manifested by a polypoid mass in the superior portion of the right maxillary sinus (solid arrows). There is also an abnormal "bright white line" (hollow arrows).

Fractures of the Posterior Portion of the Floor of the Orbit

Fractures of the posterior portion of the floor of the orbit will not be visualized on the Waters view. They can however be seen on the Towne view (Fig. 3.9).

Depression of the posterior portion of the floor of the orbit can be deduced from the Caldwell view because the posterior portion of the floor of the orbit which is usually seen on the Caldwell view will not be demonstrated if there is a depression of that portion.

Usually the posterior portion of the medial wall of the orbit as seen on the Caldwell view can be traced inferolaterally to the posterior portion of the floor of the orbit. However, if this portion of the floor of the orbit is depressed, the juncture of the posterior portion of the floor of the orbit with the medial wall of the orbit will no longer be visible. It should be pointed out that the posterior portion of the floor of the orbit will not be seen on either orbit if the Caldwell view is extended. However, if it is seen on one side it should be seen on both, and if it is not, it is abnormal.

Tomography

Most blowout fractures can be seen on routine films. However, if it is desirable to show the exact extent of the fracture, and the depth of the depression of the floor of the orbit into the maxillary sinus, tomograms will be necessary. Tomograms should be obtained in the coronal and lateral projection every 5 mm.

If tomograms are obtained and a floor fracture demonstrated, the extent of the fracture and the amount of depression of the fracture should be recorded using accessible anatomical landmarks, such as the rim of the orbit and the infraorbital canal. In this way, the size and location of the fracture, as seen on the tomograms, can be used as useful reference points at surgery.

The anterior-posterior distance should be measured on the lateral tomograms. This distance should be measured using the distance from the anterior rim of the orbit to the anterior edge of the fracture. The width should be measured on the coronal tomograms using the infraorbital canal to determine the location of the fracture (Fig. 3.10).

It is often helpful to use a diagram to outline the exact extent of the fracture as seen on the tomograms. The diagram can then become part of the patient's chart and be available at the time of surgery. Since the number of images obtained in tomography of the orbit are so great that it makes it difficult to view them all in the operating room, a diagram summarizing the tomographic findings may be helpful at surgery.

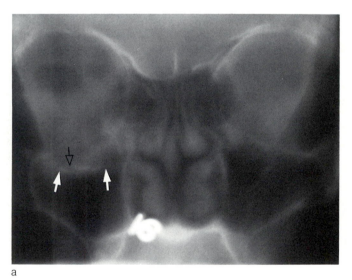

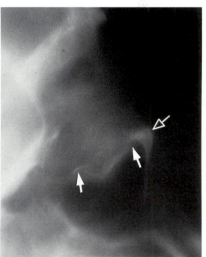

a

b

Fig. 3.**10**

a) Coronal tomogram showing a blowout fracture of the floor of the orbit (solid arrows). The position of the margins of the fracture fragment should be related to the position of the infraorbital canal (hollow arrow) in reporting the fracture so that the surgeon will have a better idea of the position of the area of the fracture.

b) Lateral tomogram showing the extent of the blowout fracture (solid arrow) seen in a). The position of this fracture should be related to the distance of the fracture from the infraorbital rim (hollow arrow).

Trimalar Fracture

A trimalar fracture is a unilateral facial fracture in which the malar eminence is mobile and is generally displaced inferiorly and medially (Fig. 3.11).

Anatomy

A trimalar fracture is really a quadripod fracture, consisting of fractures of the zygomatic arch, the lateral wall of the orbit, the inferior rim of the orbit and the lateral wall of the maxillary sinus. It is the fracture of the lateral wall of the maxillary sinus that is usually forgotten in speaking of a trimalar fracture.

All four of these fractures are connected one with the other. That is, the fracture between the lateral wall of the orbit and the rim of the orbit are connected across the floor and lateral wall of the orbit. The fracture of the lateral wall of the maxillary sinus is connected with the fracture of the floor of the orbit and across the anterior wall of the maxillary sinus. It is only by being thus connected that the fragment can be free to rotate inferiorly and medially.

Radiographic Representation

The classic radiographic representation of a trimalar fracture is:
1. Separation or diastasis of the frontozygomatic suture.
2. A radiodense line parallel to the linea innominata, indicating a rotation of a fragment in the lateral wall of the orbit.
3. A step defect in the palpable margin of the orbit.
4. A depressed fracture in the floor of the orbit.
5. An angulation of the lateral wall of the maxillary sinus (Fig. 3.12).

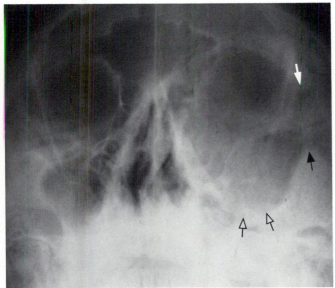

a

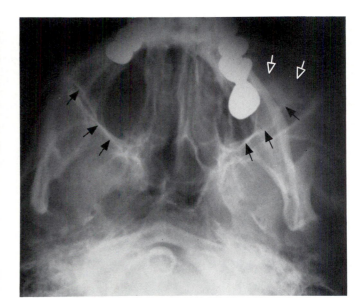

Fig. 3.**12** Base view showing posterior displacement of the left malar eminence (hollow arrows) secondary to a trimalar fracture. Compare the appearance of the lateral wall of the left maxillary sinus to the lateral wall of the right maxillary sinus (solid arrows). The anterior portion of the lateral wall of the left maxillary sinus is compressed, fuzzy and indistinct.

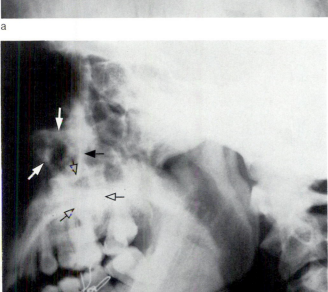

b

◀Fig. 3.**11**
a) Waters view showing a markedly depressed left trimalar fracture. There is marked distraction of the margins of the frontozygomatic suture (solid arrows) and downward displacement of the rim of the orbit (hollow arrows).
b) Lateral view demonstrating the position of the triangle formed by the right malar eminence in its normal position (solid arrows) and the position of the depressed left malar eminence (hollow arrows).

Waters View

The fracture of the lateral wall of the maxillary sinus which is always present when there is a trimalar fracture is usually not represented by a frank diastasis of the lateral wall of the maxillary sinus, but rather an angulation of the wall, resembling the "green stick" fractures that occur in the long bones of children.

When angulation of the lateral wall of the maxillary sinus is present, the usual smooth curve which incorporates the inferior border of the zygomatic arch and the lateral wall of the maxillary sinus, is no longer smooth but has a sharp angulation. The point of this angulation is the point of the fracture.

Lateral View

At times the depression of the malar eminence can be so great that the depression is obvious on the lateral view (Fig. 3.11 b). The malar eminence is seen on the lateral view as a triangle superimposed on the anterosuperior portion of the maxillary sinus. The apex of the triangle is pointed downward. The base forms the floor of the orbit. On a perfectly straight lateral view of the skull the two triangles representing the malar eminence on both sides should be completely superimposed so that one sees only one triangle. In the presence of a severe depression of one malar eminence, the two triangles will no longer be superimposed, and two triangles will be seen on a straight lateral view.

Base View

The base view will demonstrate posterior displacement of the malar eminence. The malar eminence on the affected side will be displaced posteriorly so that the frontal bone which is generally obscured by the superimposed malar eminence is seen free and clear (Fig. 3.12).

In addition, on the base view the anterior portion of the S-line representing the lateral wall of the maxillary sinus, and the anterior portion of the line representing the lateral wall of the orbit, are fuzzy and indistinct. In the presence of a trimalar fracture, the anterior portions of these lines are no longer tangent to the beam, and therefore do not present a clear cortical line on the film (Fig. 3.13).

LeFort Fractures

There are three types of LeFort fractures. All three types have the following characteristics in common:
1. They are all bilateral.
2. They extend through the pterygopalatine fossae and the pterygoid plates.
3. Some portion of the face is mobile.

Mobility of the Face

The mobility of a portion of the face may not immediately be apparent clinically, because the patients are in pain and will not tolerate palpation or movement of the fragments. But the mobility of the fragment becomes obvious under anesthesia.

Pterygopalatine Fossa

The extension of a LeFort fracture through the pterygopalatine fossae and pterygoid plates can be appreciated on a routine lateral view.

On the routine lateral view the pterygopalatine fossa makes a V-shaped lucency, immediately posterior to the maxillary sinus, the anterior wall of the pterygopalatine fossa being the posterior wall of the maxillary sinus. If there is a fracture with diastasis extending through the pterygopalatine fossa, the cortical margins of this V-shaped lucency are no longer straight lines, but rather interrupted and angulated.

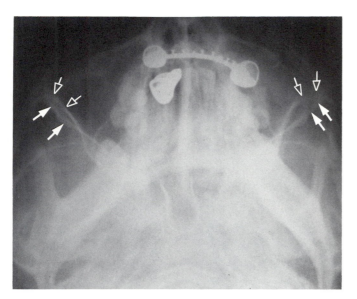

Fig. 3.**13**   Base view showing a left trimalar fracture. The anterior portions of both the lateral wall of the orbit (solid arrows) and the lateral wall of the maxillary sinus (hollow arrows) are fuzzy and indistinct due to the fracture. Then compare the same lines on the right side.

Bilateral vs. Unilateral Fracture

It should be pointed out that a unilateral fracture through the pterygopalatine fossa will also be visualized on the lateral view (Fig. 3.14). On the lateral view it is difficult to ascertain whether the fracture through the pterygopalatine fossa is bilateral or unilateral. Therefore, the demonstration of fractures through the pterygopalatine fossa on the lateral view does not necessarily confirm the presence of a LeFort fracture, which by definition is bilateral.

It may be possible to differentiate a unilateral fracture from a bilateral fracture seen in the case of a LeFort fracture. If the fracture is only unilateral, there will be one normal V-shaped lucency with intact cortical margins demonstrated on the lateral view whereas with a true LeFort type fracture with fractures going through both pterygopalatine fossae, all of the cortical lines of the radiolucent V-shaped lucencies of both pterygopalatine fossae will be interrupted (Fig. 3.15).

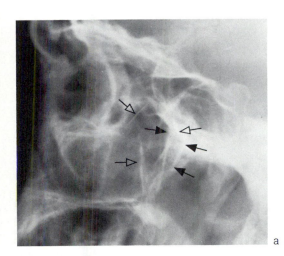

a

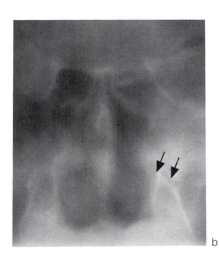

b

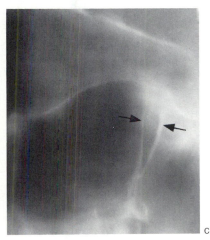

c

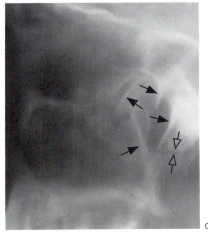

d

Fig. 3.14
a) Lateral view in a patient who has had a unilateral pterygopalatine fossa fracture with one intact pterygopalatine fossa (solid arrows) and the other pterygopalatine fossa showing diastasis of its walls (hollow arrows).
b) Coronal tomogram through the pterygoid plates showing fracture through the base of the left pterygoids (solid arrows).

c) Lateral tomogram through the normal pterygopalatine fossa (solid arrows).
d) Lateral tomogram through the fractured pterygopalatine fossa with diastasis of the anterior and posterior walls of the pterygopalatine fossa (solid arrows) and extension of the fracture posteriorly through the pterygoid plates (hollow arrows).

Associated Nasopharyngeal Soft Tissue Mass

Often there is a large soft tissue mass in the nasopharynx visualized in the lateral view in patients with LeFort fractures or for that matter any form of severe facial fracture. This nasopharyngeal soft tissue mass is produced by submucosal hematoma. Most of these patients have been lying supine for some time before the films are obtained, and during this time there has been enough dissection of blood posteriorly to demonstrate a mass in the nasopharynx. This mass is of no clinical significance, but it should not be confused with any more significant abnormality. It is merely a submucosal hematoma.

Types of LeFort Fracture

If all the types of LeFort fracture have in common bilateral fractures through the pterygopalatine fossae and pterygoid plates, how do they differ? They differ in the

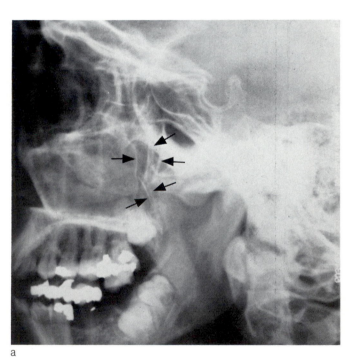

a

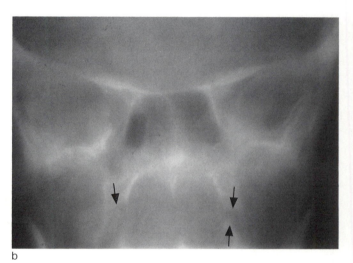

b

Fig. 3.**15**
a) Lateral view of a patient with a LeFort fracture and bilateral pterygopalatine fossa fractures. There is no normal pterygopalatine fossa seen on the lateral view. (Compare with Fig. 3.14a).

All the lines forming the pterygopalatine fossae are interrupted (solid arrows).
b) Coronal tomogram through the pterygoid plates shows fractures of both pterygoid processes (solid arrows).

level of the face through which they pass. Therefore the portion of the face which is mobile is different for each type of LeFort fracture.

LeFort I Fracture

The LeFort Type I fracture is a transverse maxillary fracture. It goes transversely (or horizontally) through the maxilla bilaterally above the level of the teeth. The fracture fragment contains the maxillary alveolar process and this process is mobile after a LeFort I fracture.

A LeFort I fracture is manifest on the Waters view (Fig. 3.16) by obvious fracture of the lateral wall of the maxillary sinuses, but the fractures of the medial wall of the maxillary sinuses are uniformly invisible on routine films. Often there is a displacement of the maxillary alveolar ridge to one side or other and if there is such a displacement it should be noted.

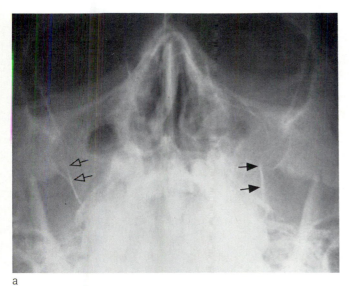

a

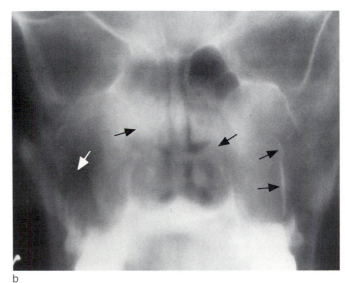

b

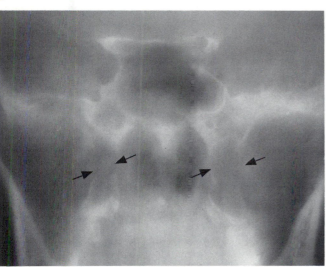

c

Fig. 3.**16**
a) Waters view, LeFort fracture I. There is an obvious fracture of the lateral wall of the left maxillary sinus with a "bright line" (solid arrows) and also a "bright line" involving the lateral wall of the right maxillary sinus (hollow arrows).
b) Coronal tomogram through the maxillary sinuses showing fractures of the lateral walls and medial walls of both maxillary sinuses (solid arrows).
c) Coronal tomogram through the pterygoid plates showing bilateral pterygoid fractures (solid arrows) confirming that this represents a LeFort I fracture.

LeFort II Fracture

The LeFort II fracture is a pyramidal fracture of the midline structures of the face. The fracture extends through the lateral wall of the maxillary sinuses, through the rims of the orbits, up to the base of the nose. The plane of the fracture extends posteroinferiorly down through pterygopalatine fossae and pterygoid plates. The result is that the middle pyramid of the face is mobile. For this reason the LeFort II fracture is also referred to as a pyramidal fracture.

In the presence of a LeFort II fracture the following fractures are demonstrated on the Waters view:
1. Fracture of the lateral wall of both maxillary sinuses.
2. Fracture through the rim of the orbit bilaterally.
3. Fracture through the base of the nose.

Generally both maxillary sinuses are opacified. As with all LeFort fractures, the pterygopalatine fossae are disrupted on the lateral view and the pterygoid plates are fractured bilaterally on coronal tomograms.

LeFort III Fracture

A LeFort III fracture is also called craniofacial dysjunction. The fracture extends across the lateral wall of the orbits and across the base of the nose. The plane of the fracture then extends posteroinferiorly through the pterygopalatine fossae and pterygoid plates, so that the entire face is mobile and separate from the skull.

Classification of Fractures

The LeFort classification of bilateral facial fractures is a convenient shorthand classification, a rough classification of facial fractures. However, nature usually does not follow classical definitions, and it is probably better to confine diagnosis to the actual fracture lines that exist. For example, a bilateral fracture of the facial bones may extend from the lateral wall of the maxillary sinus through the rim of the orbit, across the base of the nose, and through the lateral wall of the orbit with the plane of the fracture extending posteroinferiorly through the pterygopalatine fossa and pterygoid plates. Such a fracture would be a LeFort II type fracture on the side through which the fracture goes to the rim of the orbit, and LeFort III type fracture on the side through which it goes through the lateral wall of the orbit. Such a fracture would be a combination of a LeFort II and a LeFort III fracture (Fig. 3.17).

Though the LeFort classification of facial fractures is a good first approximation to describing these fractures clinically, this classification is only a first approximation and not good enough for evaluation of post-traumatic radiographs. An evaluation of post-traumatic radiographs should deal with the actual fracture lines and displacements that are present without recourse to somewhat artificial classifications. Rather the radiological evaluation should be rigorously anatomic.

Ethmoid Sinus Fractures

The radiographic signs of fracture of the medial wall of the orbit (which is the lamina papyracea) involving the ethmoid sinuses are:
1. Clouding of the ethmoid sinuses.
2. Orbital emphysema.
3. Rarely a demonstrable fracture of the lamina papyracea.

Clouding of the Ethmoid Sinuses

Clouding of the ethmoid sinuses is invariably seen in the presence of a fracture of the ethmoid sinuses.

If the fracture is in the anterior portion of the medial wall of the orbit (which is the same as the lateral plate of the ethmoids, the lamina papyracea), the clouding of the ethmoid sinuses will not be seen on the Caldwell view, but only on the Waters view.

If the fracture is more posterior, then the opacification of the ethmoid sinuses will be seen on the Caldwell view.

Orbital Emphysema

Fractures of the medial wall of the orbit into the ethmoid sinuses are common. In my consecutive series of 49 cases of fractures of the orbit, 24 (49%) had fractures of the lamina papyracea; 5 of these 24 cases had isolated fractures of the lamina papyracea of the ethmoid.

The presence of orbital emphysema almost invariably indicates a fracture of the lamina papyracea and ethmoid sinuses. In 24 cases of orbital emphysema, only 1 was due to an isolated fracture of the floor of the orbit into the maxillary sinus (or blowout fracture).

All the rest of the cases of orbital emphysema had either an isolated ethmoid sinus fracture or an ethmoid sinus fracture in association with a depressed fracture of the floor of the orbit. In all of these cases tomograms were

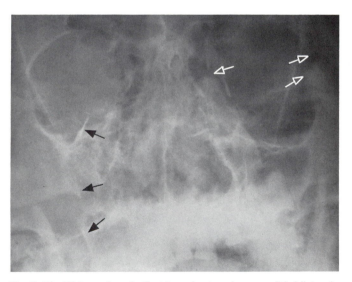

Fig. 3.17 Waters view, LeFort type fracture because it is bilateral. The fracture is like a LeFort II on the right since the fracture goes through the lateral wall of the right maxillary sinus and the floor of the right orbit (solid arrows). However, it is like a LeFort III on the left, with the fracture going across the base of the nose through the medial wall of the right orbit and diastasis of the frontozygomatic suture (hollow arrows).

obtained to confirm the presence of an ethmoid sinus fracture.

Very often a fracture of the ethmoids is not apparent on routine films and it will only be apparent on tomograms. Occasionally the actual fracture can be seen on routine films without the necessity of obtaining tomograms. Usually however, one must depend upon secondary findings to make the diagnosis of an ethmoid sinus fracture, that is, clouding of the involved ipsilateral ethmoid sinuses and orbital emphysema.

Entrapment of the Medial Rectus Muscle

Orbital emphysema is not a significant symptom and is self-limited. Occasionally a fracture of the medial wall of the orbit will produce entrapment of the medial rectus muscle which is significant.

The clinical symptoms in such a case would be diplopia on lateral gaze and enophthalmos on lateral gaze. The patient develops enophthalmos because the entrapped medial rectus muscle retracts on the eyeball when the patient tries to gaze in the lateral direction. When the patient presents with such symptoms, tomograms of the ethmoid sinuses and the orbits are mandatory.

Frontal Sinus Fractures

Direct trauma to the frontal sinus usually produces a depressed fracture of the anterior wall of the frontal sinus. Sometimes it is difficult to see the actual depres-sion of the fracture on a lateral view but it will always be demonstrated on the Caldwell view or the Waters view by an area of increased density superimposed on the frontal sinus (Fig. 3.18).

Radiographic Signs

The signs of a fracture of the frontal sinus is a radiodensity superimposed on the frontal sinus by the depressed fragment, and usually an air fluid level representing blood in the frontal sinus. Occasionally the frontal sinus will be completely filled with blood and will be completely opacified and thus not show an air fluid level.

When there is a fracture of the frontal sinus, it is important to obtain lateral tomograms to rule out a fracture of the posterior wall of the frontal sinus.

A fracture of the frontal sinus can serve as the avenue of meningitis and/or the locus of a cerebrospinal fluid leak producing cerebrospinal fluid rhinorrhea (Fig. 3.19).

Sphenoid Sinus Fractures

Sphenoid sinus fractures are seen best on the lateral view and the Caldwell view. The fracture can be seen involving the planum sphenoidale (Fig. 3.20), the sella turcica (Fig. 3.21), or the basisphenoid.

In addition to the actual demonstration of a fracture, there is the secondary evidence of a post-traumatic sphenoid sinus air fluid level.

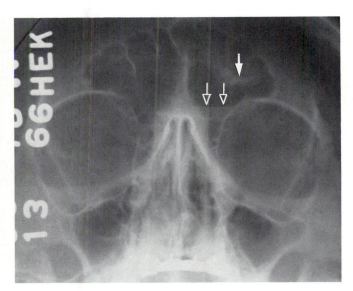

Fig. 3.18   Waters view showing a fracture of the anterior wall of the frontal sinus manifested by a linear radiodensity representing a rotated fragment of the anterior wall of the frontal sinus (solid arrow) and an air-blood level (hollow arrows).

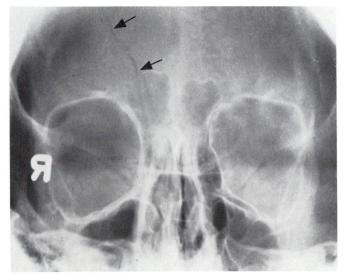

Fig. 3.19   Caldwell view in a patient with posttraumatic rhinorrhea through the right frontal sinus. There is a fracture of the right frontal bone (solid arrows) extending into the right frontal sinus.

Air Fluid Level

Fractures involving the sphenoid sinus may demonstrate an air fluid level in the sphenoid sinus. However, a post-traumatic air fluid level suggesting the presence of blood in the sphenoid sinus is not necessarily indicative of a fracture of the sphenoid sinus. The blood may have drained posteriorly from a more anterior injury, such as in the nasal fossa or the ethmoids, into the sphenoid sinus. But the sphenoid sinus itself could actually be intact.

Bilateral Lateral Rectus Paralysis

Fractures through the sella turcica or the basisphenoid have a unique clinical presentation. After such fractures, there may be the development of bilateral lateral rectus paralysis, two to three days after the trauma. Such a development is strongly suggestive of the presence of a fracture through the body of the sphenoid or the basi-sphenoid.

It is postulated that the mechanism of the lateral rectus paralysis is due to bilateral cavernous sinus hemorrhage, producing pressure on the sixth cranial nerve bilaterally and thus bilateral sixth nerve (lateral rectus) paralysis.

Loss of Vision

Fractures of the sphenoid sinus in the planum sphenoidale may involve the optic canal and the optic nerve. Whenever there is a post-traumatic loss of vision, a fracture of the optic canal should be suspected.

Sometimes such fractures of the optic canal cannot be visualized on routine optic canal views and require optic canal tomograms in order to visualize the fracture (Fig. 3.22).

Optic canal tomograms are obtained in the same manner as is the routine optic canal view, that is the head is rotated 40 degrees to the contralateral side and the head is extended 20 degrees in order to place the axis of the optic canal parallel to the beam. Then tomograms are obtained at every millimeter of the length of the optic canals.

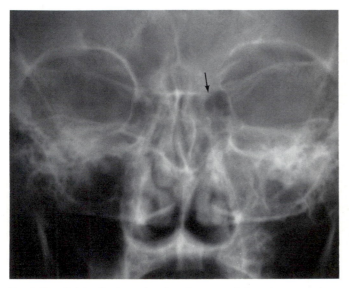

Fig. 3.20 Caldwell view showing fracture of the planum sphenoidale (solid arrow) in a patient with posttraumatic blindness in the left eye.

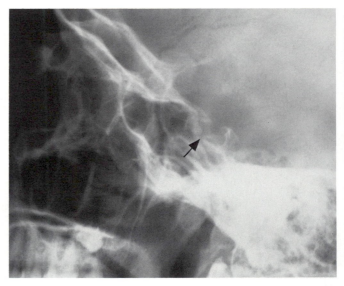

Fig. 3.21 Lateral view in a patient with posttraumatic bilateral sixth nerve palsies, showing a fracture through the floor of the sella turcica (solid arrow). The bilateral sixth nerve palsies were due to bilateral hemorrhage into the cavernous sinuses with resultant bilateral compression of the sixth nerve in the cavernous sinuses.

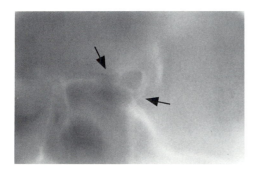

◄ Fig. 3.22 An optic canal tomogram obtained perpendicular to the axis of the optic canal in a patient who had posttraumatic blindness in the left eye. It demonstrates a fracture through the left optic canal (solid arrows).

Chapter 4 Inflammatory Disease of the Paranasal Sinuses

Radiographic Diagnosis of Sinusitis

The radiographic diagnosis of sinusitis is generally based on opacification of the paranasal sinuses. However, all apparent opacifications or clouding of the area of the paranasal sinuses are not necessarily reflections of sinus disease but may come about from other causes.

Spurious Opacification of the Maxillary Sinus

Any unilateral increase in the prominence of the soft tissues of the cheek will cause an apparent opacification of the ipsilateral maxillary sinus.

Trauma

For example, after trauma in which there is edema and swelling of the soft tissues of the cheek, the ipsilateral maxillary sinus will appear opacified.

Maxillary Sinus Hypoplasia

Another cause for an increase in density of the maxillary sinus is hypoplasia of the maxillary sinus. When there is a hypoplastic maxillary sinus, there is of course less air

content in the smaller sinus. Since one is reading decreased air content when one is reading opacification – that is, the less air the more opacified the sinus – a hypoplastic sinus which contains less air will appear opacified but may not actually be diseased.

In the presence of a hypoplastic maxillary sinus:
1. The lateral wall of the maxillary sinus will be bowed medially.
2. The lateral wall of the nasal fossa (which is the medial wall of the maxillary sinus) will be bowed laterally.
3. The floor of the orbit (which is the roof of the maxillary sinus) will appear depressed, producing an increase in the distance between the palpable margin of the floor of the orbit and the floor of the orbit more posterior, as seen on the Waters view.

Thus the inward bowing of all the walls of the maxillary sinus – the lateral wall, the medial wall, and the roof – produces a very small air cavity and thus an apparent opacification of the maxillary sinus.

Unilateral and Bilateral Hypoplasia

Hypoplasia of the maxillary sinus may be unilateral (Fig. 4.1) or bilateral (Fig. 4.2).

It should be noted that the increase in distance between

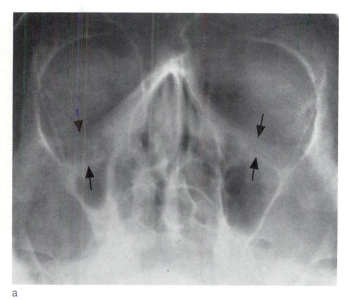

a

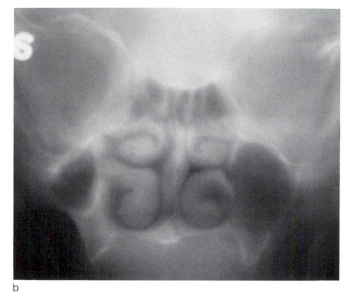

b

Fig. 4.1
a) Waters view showing hypoplasia of the right maxillary sinus. The lateral wall of the nasal fossa (which is the medial wall of the maxillary sinus) is bowed laterally. The distance between the palpable margin of the orbit and the floor of the orbit on the right is increased over the same distance on the left (solid arrows).

b) Coronal tomogram. The floor of the right orbit is lower than the floor of the left orbit. The lateral wall of the nasal fossa is displaced laterally. The right maxillary sinus is hypoplastic.

the palpable margin of the orbit and the floor of the orbit more posterior as seen on the Waters view which is present with a hypoplastic maxillary sinus (Fig. 4.1a) is also the finding that is expected on the Waters view when there is a blowout (or depressed) fracture of the orbit floor. Therefore care must be used in the diagnosis of a blowout fracture in the presence of a hypoplastic maxillary sinus.

On the base view, the maxillary sinus is small and confined to the anterior portion of the maxilla and posterior to this small air cavity is solid bone extending back to the region of the pterygoid process.

If drainage of the maxillary sinus is planned, care should be taken to note the presence of the solid bone since it would be impossible to drain a hypoplastic sinus in the usual fashion.

Spurious Opacification of the Frontal Sinus

Asymmetry

It is common for the frontal sinuses to be asymmetric in size. Naturally, since the lucency of the sinuses is only the reflection of the air content of that sinus, the smaller frontal sinus will appear more opaque than does the larger sinus.

Thick Anterior Wall

Another common cause for an apparent opacification of the frontal sinuses is a thick anterior wall.

If the anterior wall of one frontal sinus is thicker than the other, the sinus with the thicker anterior wall will appear opacified.

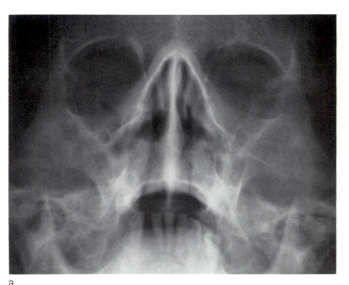

a

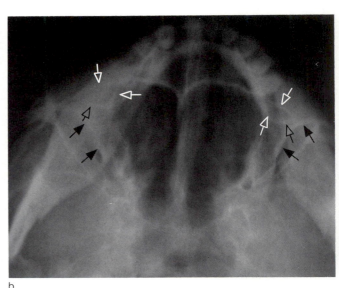

b

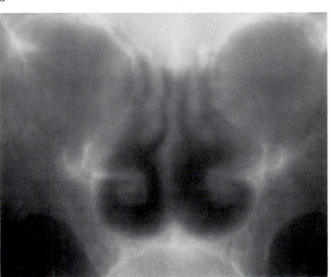

c

Fig. 4.2
a) Waters view showing bilateral maxillary sinus hypoplasia. The maxillary sinuses appear opacified bilaterally. The lateral wall of the nasal fossa cannot be seen on either side due to the lateral bowing of the lateral wall of the nasal fossa. This appearance could simulate bone destruction by a tumor. The distance between the palpable margin of the orbit and the floor of the orbit is greater than usual bilaterally.
b) Base view. Bilateral maxillary hypoplasia. There is marked lateral bowing of the lateral wall of the nasal fossa and also marked bilateral medial bowing of the lateral wall of the maxilla (solid arrows). The maxillary sinuses are represented by small triangles anteriorly (hollow arrows).
c) Coronal tomogram of bilateral maxillary hypoplasia confirms the fact that the maxillae are solid bone bilaterally except for a tiny air cavity immediately beneath the orbit.

One way to guard against misinterpreting this spurious opacification of the frontal sinus caused by a thick anterior wall is to compare the appearance of opacification on the Caldwell view and the Waters view.

Since the Waters view is a more angled view, the head is more extended, and the beam does not go through the anterior wall of the frontal sinus as perpendicularly as it does on the Caldwell view. Thus, the effect of a thick anterior wall on the image of the frontal sinus is not as great on the Waters as on the Caldwell.

Often a frontal sinus with a thick anterior wall which appears opacified on the Caldwell view will not appear so on the Waters view.

The anterior wall of the frontal sinus can be examined on the lateral view. If the anterior wall of the frontal sinus is of the same thickness, only one line will be seen on the lateral view produced by the inner surface of the anterior wall of the frontal sinuses.

On the lateral view, if the anterior wall of one frontal sinus is thicker than the other, there will be two lines produced by the inner surface of the anterior wall of the frontal sinuses. A thick anterior wall of the frontal sinus accounts for a spurious opacification of the frontal sinus as seen on the Caldwell view.

Spurious Opacification of the Ethmoid Sinus

The ethmoid sinuses are best seen on the Caldwell view. On the Caldwell view, the sphenoid sinuses are superimposed on the ethmoid sinuses. If there is opacification of one sphenoid sinus or if one sphenoid sinus is hypoplastic, the opacification produced by the sphenoid sinus will cloud the area of the ipsilateral ethmoid sinuses, thus giving a spurious appearance of opacification of the ethmoid sinuses, when in actual fact the abnormality is in the sphenoid sinuses.

Use of the Lateral View in Diagnosing Opacification

It is difficult to diagnose opacification of the paranasal sinuses on the lateral view because of superimposition of the paranasal sinuses, one on the other.

Unilateral Opacification

If there is one clear maxillary sinus and one opacified maxillary sinus, generally the area of the maxillary sinuses will appear clear on the lateral view, because of the effect of the one unaffected sinus.

Bilateral Opacification

However, if the area of the sinus – such as the frontal sinus or the maxillary sinus or the sphenoid sinus – appears opacified on the lateral view, this is an indication that there is bilateral sinus opacification.

For example, on the Caldwell view, it is often difficult to be sure whether there is bilateral opacification of the frontal sinus or whether there are normal frontal sinuses which are narrow and therefore appear opaque. This differentiation can be made on the lateral view. If there is bilateral frontal sinus opacification due to intrasinus disease on the Caldwell view, then the area of the frontal sinuses on the lateral view should appear opacified and not have the appearance of air. If the frontal sinuses appear clear on the lateral view, then the frontal sinuses are normal, the apparent bilateral opacification which was seen on the Caldwell being due to bilaterally narrow frontal sinuses.

Unilateral Opacification of the Sphenoid Sinus

The sphenoid sinuses are visualized on the lateral view but the two sphenoid sinuses are superimposed on one another and often opacification of one sinus is impossible to diagnose on the lateral view. Unilateral sphenoid sinus opacification can only be seen on the base view.

Only on the base view can we see the sphenoid sinuses as separate structures.

Evaluation of the Ethmoid Sinus

Degree of Opacity

The area of the ethmoid sinus, the ethmoid air cells, should be scrutinized carefully for any suggestion of opacity. The effect of opacification of the ethmoid air cells may be somewhat vitiated by the presence of a superimposed aerated sphenoid sinus, and therefore any slight difference in opacification of the ethmoid air cells as seen on the Caldwell view should be interpreted as abnormal.

A slight degree of opacity of the ethmoid air cells on the Caldwell view may be in fact completely and densely opacified on tomograms of the ethmoid sinus.

Nonrotated View

Opacification of the ethmoid air cells should be evaluated only on a nonrotated view. On a rotated view, the ethmoid air cells on the ipsilateral side of the rotation will appear opacified relative to the other side. This apparent opacification on a rotated view comes about due to the nose which is superimposed on the ipsilateral ethmoid air cells if the head is rotated.

Anterior and Posterior Ethmoid Air Cells

Since there are 10 to 14 ethmoid air cells normally and each of them has its own individual ostium, there may be opacification of a selected group of ethmoid air cells. Thus there may be opacification of the posterior ethmoid air cells without opacification of the anterior ethmoid air cells or vice versa.

Generally if there is opacification evident in the ethmoid region on the Caldwell view this indicates at least opacification of the posterior ethmoid air cells, if not both the anterior and the posterior ethmoid air cells.

Opacification of the anterior ethmoid air cells only will usually not produce evident opacification in the ethmoid region on the Caldwell view. Opacification of the anterior ethmoid air cells will produce clouding in the region of the ethmoids on the Waters view.

Acute and Chronic Sinusitis

Air Fluid Level

The presence of an air fluid level in a paranasal sinus indicates an acute sinusitis.

One must be first sure that there is actually an air fluid level. For example, a very edematous thickened mucosa can be so fluid laden that it assumes an air fluid level configuration in the upright position.

The only way this can be differentiated from a true air fluid level is to examine the sinus in another position. For example, an apparent air fluid level configuration due to thickened edematous mucosa on the Waters view will not produce an air fluid level on the base view when both of these views are taken in the upright position. However, true fluid within the sinus will assume an air fluid level configuration both on the Waters view and on the base view (Fig. 4.3).

One should keep in mind that patients who have recently had a washing out of the sinus may have enough of the irrigation fluid remaining in the maxillary sinus to produce an air fluid level.

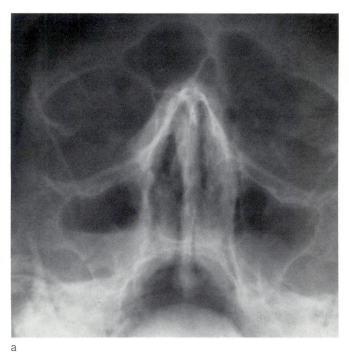

a

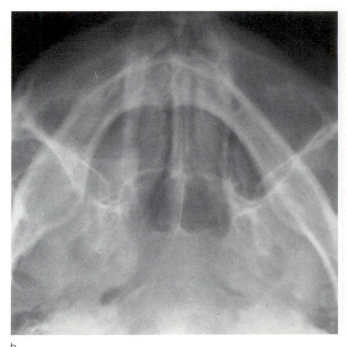

b

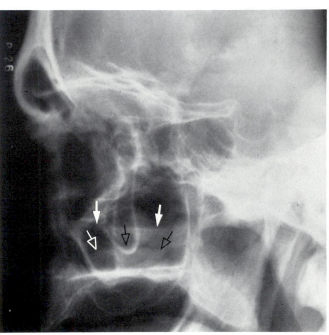

c

Fig. 4.**3**

a) Waters view in a patient with right acute sinusitis showing an air fluid level in the right maxillary sinus. Incidentally noted is a retention cyst in the left maxillary sinus.

b) Base view confirms that the apparent air fluid level seen on the Waters view is actually a fluid level because an air-fluid level is also seen on the base view. If the air-fluid level were not seen on the base view, then one would have to presume that what was seen on the Waters view was not actually an air-fluid level.

c) Lateral view. In the lateral view both the air-fluid level (solid arrows) and the dome-shaped retention cyst in the maxillary sinus (hollow arrows) can be seen superimposed one on the other. This is a typical appearance of a retention cyst: a dome-shaped homogeneous mass where the remaining portion of the sinus mucosa appears normal.

Sclerotic Wall

Thickened sclerotic sinus walls indicate a chronic inflammatory process. In the frontal sinus this periostitic reaction to the presence of chronic inflammation is reflected as a zone of sclerosis surrounding the margins of the frontal sinus.

In the maxillary sinus, chronic inflammatory periostitic reaction produces thick sclerotic walls, especially evident in the lateral wall of the maxillary sinus.

Inflammatory Masses of the Paranasal Sinuses

The inflammatory masses of the paranasal sinuses consist of:
1. nonsecretory cysts,
2. retention cysts, and
3. polyps.

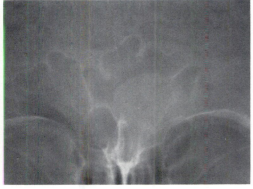

◀ Fig. 4.**4**   Caldwell view of a frontal sinus retention cyst. The mass has the typical appearance of a retention cyst: a perfectly smoothly marginated dome-shaped mass of homogeneous density.

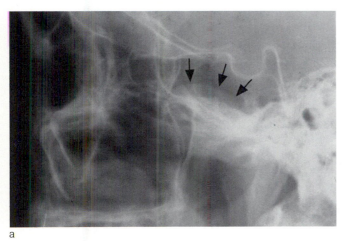

a

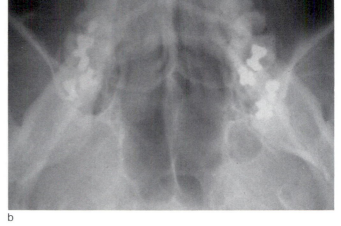

b

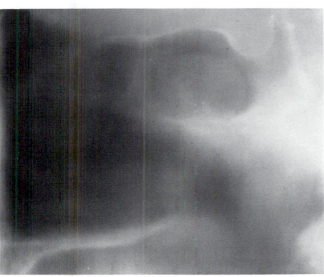

c

Fig. 4.**5**
a) Lateral view of a patient with a sphenoid sinus retention cyst. A dome-shaped mass is seen arising from the floor of the sphenoid sinus (solid arrows).
b) Base view demonstrating the retention cyst to be in the left sphenoid sinus.
c) The lateral tomogram shows the sphenoid sinus retention cyst more clearly. One can also see that the entire margin of the retention cyst is completely smooth and round.

Nonsecretory Cyst

Nonsecretory cysts arise in the maxillary sinus and are merely a collection of submucosal fluid in the inferior portion of the maxillary sinus. They produce a homogeneous dome-shaped mass with completely smooth borders in the inferior portion of the maxillary sinus.

Retention Cyst

Retention cysts are the result of obstruction of a minor seromucinous gland in the sinus mucosa. The most common location for retention cysts is also the inferior portion of the maxillary sinus but they may also be seen in other areas of the maxillary sinus, the frontal sinus (Fig. 4.4), and the sphenoid sinus (Fig. 4.5).

The radiographic appearance of a retention cyst is similar to that of a nonsecretory cyst – a smoothly marginated dome-shaped mass of homogeneous density. A retention cyst may have a thin calcific border similar in appearance to an eggshell (Fig. 4.6).

In the presence of a retention cyst, the mucoperiosteal membrane of the sinus containing the cyst is otherwise normal. In the presence of a thickened mucoperiosteal membrane, a mass in the sinus is usually produced by an inflammatory polyp.

Retention cysts are filled with a clear fluid. Therefore on transillumination in a maxillary sinus containing a retention cyst, there will be no diminution in transillumination.

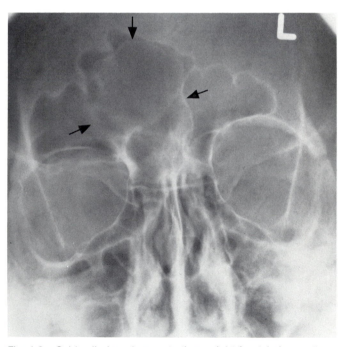

Fig. 4.6 Caldwell view demonstrating a right frontal sinus retention cyst which has an eggshell calcified border (solid arrows). Occasionally retention cysts do manifest a very thin calcified border, such as in this case.

The walls of a retention cyst are one cell thick. They are easily punctured, and the small amount of fluid in these cysts may be overlooked in the irrigation fluids used during surgery. Thus it is not uncommon for such cysts to be removed at surgery without the surgeon even being aware that they were present.

It should be kept in mind that retention cysts do not cause bone destruction, do not cause bone displacement, and do not cause symptoms. If there is bone displacement or bone destruction in association with a mass in the maxillary sinus, the mass is not a retention cyst but either a neoplasm or some form of bone destroying inflammatory condition.

If there are symptoms in the same sinus which contains a retention cyst, then either the mass is not truly a retention cyst or the patient has another condition producing the symptoms other than this mass, because the retention cyst does not cause symptoms.

A retention cyst does not cause bone destruction or bone displacement because the secretory pressure of the minor seromucinous gland is insufficient to destroy bone. However, retention cysts may become large enough to completely fill the sinus.

When a retention cyst completely fills the sinus, the resulting opacification produced by a retention cyst cannot be differentiated from an opacification produced by sinusitis.

Polyp

Inflammatory polyps also may produce isolated masses in the sinuses. However, polyps in the sinuses are usually associated with generalized thickening of the entire mucosal membrane with the polypoid mass being simply an accentuation of this thickening which is affecting the entire membrane.

Unlike retention cysts or nonsecretory cysts, inflammatory polyps can cause bone displacement and can cause bone destruction.

Often with severe nasal polyposis producing bone destruction, it is difficult to differentiate this condition radiographically from a benign or malignant tumor.

Polyps in the maxillary sinus can produce displacement or destruction of the lateral or medial wall of the maxillary sinus (Fig. 4.7).

Polyps in the ethmoid sinuses can destroy the medial wall of the orbit and even cause unilateral proptosis.

It should be kept in mind that children who present with a mucocele or severe nasal polyposis should be investigated for cystic fibrosis. The incidence of cystic fibrosis is much higher in these children than in the general population.

Choanal Polyp

A particular type of inflammatory polyp is the choanal polyp. The choanal polyp is so named because it presents at the posterior nares in the nasal choanae.

Actually these polyps have their origin in the region of the ostium of the maxillary sinus and the edematous

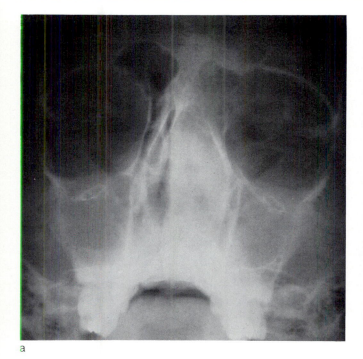

a

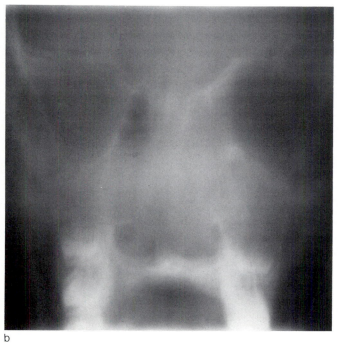

b

Fig. 4.7

a) Waters view demonstrating opacification of the left frontal and ethmoid sinuses, bilateral maxillary sinus opacification, complete opacification of the left nasal fossa and destruction of the medial wall of the orbit by inflammatory nasal polyposis. Simple inflammatory nasal polyposis can produce a radiographic appearance

which is apparently very ominous but in actual fact is due to this benign non-neoplastic condition.

b) Coronal tomogram confirms the bone destruction, not only of the medial wall of the left orbit, but also bilateral bone destruction involving the maxillary sinuses.

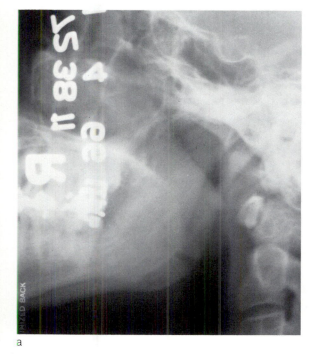

a

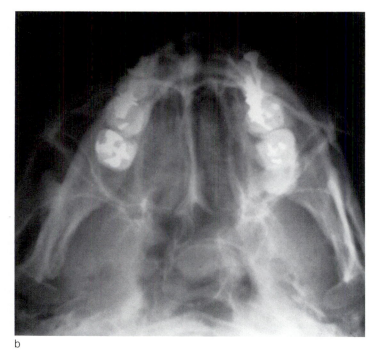

b

Fig. 4.8

a) Lateral view showing a large mass in the nasopharynx completely free of the posterior wall of the nasopharynx, smoothly marginated and extending into the oropharynx. The fact that this mass does not arise from the posterior wall of the nasopharynx confirms that it is coming from anteriorly in the region of the nasal

fossa. It has the typical appearance of a choanal polyp which arises in the maxillary sinus, enlarges, and stretches out by gravity like a teardrop until it hangs by a long stalk from the ostium of the maxillary sinus.

b) Base view demonstrates the choanal polyp superimposed upon the left sphenoid sinus.

polypoid mucosa continues to enlarge and by gravity extends downward to form a large tear-shaped mass which may occupy the nasal fossa and the nasopharynx (Fig. 4.8). Just by gravity this edematous mucosa stretches out like a teardrop until it hangs by a long stalk from the ostium of the maxillary sinus backward and downward into the nasopharynx.

Mucocele

A complication of chronic sinusitis is the formation of a mucocele.

A paranasal sinus mucocele is nothing but a blocked sinus which continues to secrete against an obstructed blocked ostium. It is a destructive expanding lesion consisting of the entire sinus with the wall of the cyst consisting of the mucosal lining of the sinus. The destruction is produced by the secretory pressure of this entire mucosal lining of the cyst.

An infected mucocele is called a pyocele.

Frontal Sinus Mucocele

The cardinal findings of a mucocele of the frontal sinus are:

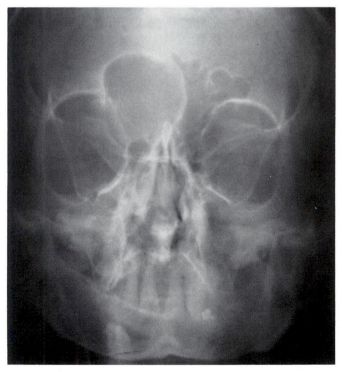

Fig. 4.9 Caldwell view of a patient with a right frontal sinus mucocele. This case shows the 3 cardinal signs of a frontal mucocele: (1) the normal scalloped border of the frontal sinus is smooth, the sinus has lost its usual scalloped margin, (2) the margin of the affected right frontal sinus is sclerotic, and (3) there is curvilinear downward displacement of the superomedial border of the right orbit. Compare the appearance of the right frontal sinus to that of the left frontal sinus.

1. The normal scalloped border of the frontal sinus becomes smoothed out to an even line.
2. There is generally a diffused zone of sclerosis external to this smoothed out border.
3. There is bone destruction or bone displacement involving the superomedial border of the orbit adjacent to the involved frontal sinus.

Most commonly patients presenting with a frontal sinus mucocele complain of a painless mass in the superomedial corner of the orbit.

Frontal sinus mucoceles are one of the most common causes of unilateral proptosis. Because of their distinct appearance, frontal sinus mucoceles are generally easy to diagnose radiographically (Fig. 4.9). Frontal sinus mucoceles may lead to intracranial complications due either to destruction or displacement of the posterior wall of the frontal sinus.

Destruction of the posterior wall of the frontal sinus puts the sac of the mucocele in direct contact with the dura. Marked posterior displacement of the posterior wall of the frontal sinus into the anterior cranial fossa acts as an intracranial mass. If it becomes extensive enough, it may even cause tentorial herniation due to the increased intracranial pressure produced by this mass.

Ethmoid Sinus Mucocele

Ethmoid sinus mucoceles may be more difficult to diagnose radiographically than frontal mucoceles. There may be a mucocele in one ethmoid air cell and the other 12 to 14 ethmoid air cells on the ipsilateral side may remain unaffected and obscure the presence of the ethmoid mucocele. The ethmoid air cells, or sinuses, are much smaller individually than is the frontal sinus, so when an ethmoid air cell develops a mucocele or when an ethmoid air cell gets blocked, it is only a small portion of the entire ethmoid labyrinth that is affected.

The radiographic findings are a round homogenous radiodensity in the ethmoid region.

Later with expansion the ethmoid sinus mucocele may cause lateral displacement of the lamina papyracea. This is the most definitive radiographic finding of an ethmoid sinus mucocele: lateral displacement or destruction of the medial wall of the orbit (Fig. 4.10).

An ethmoid sinus mucocele may also cause destruction and lateral displacement of the superomedial wall of the orbit or displacement downward of the ethmomaxillary plate Fig. 4.11).

Sphenoid Sinus Mucocele

Sphenoid sinus mucoceles are very unusual. When they occur, they generally balloon out all the walls of the sphenoid sinus.

The floor of the sella turcica may be destroyed by a sphenoid sinus mucocele (Fig. 4.12).

Maxillary Sinus Mucocele

Mucoceles of the maxillary sinus are very very rare and when they occur are difficult to differentiate from neoplastic disease or granulomatous sinusitis causing bone destruction.

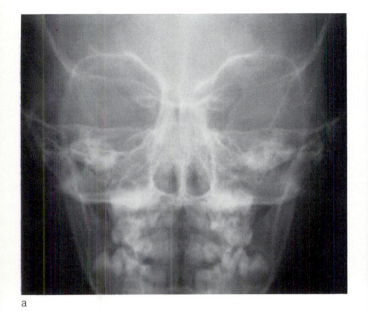

a

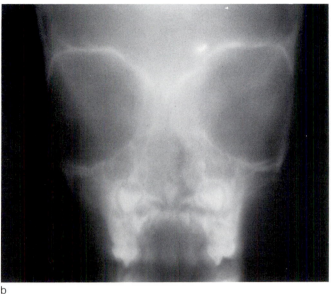

b

Fig. 4.**10**
a) Caldwell view of a 2 year old child with an ethmoid mucocele who has left exophthalmos. There is complete opacification of the maxillary sinuses and ethmoids bilaterally with destruction of the medial wall of the orbit.

b) Coronal tomogram. On subsequent testing this child was found to have cystic fibrosis. The incidence of cystic fibrosis is much higher in children with mucoceles or severe nasal polyposis.

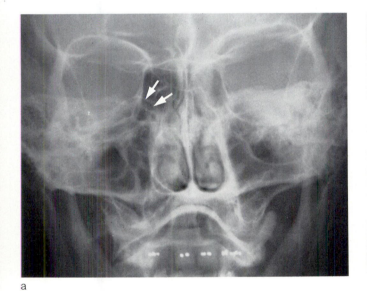

a

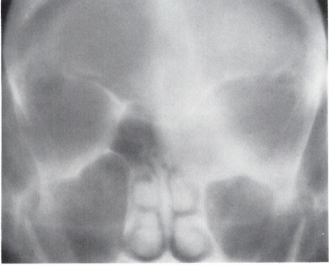

b

Fig. 4.**11**
a) Caldwell in a patient with an ethmoid mucocele who has left exophthalmos. There is opacification in the left ethmoid region. The right ethmomaxillary plate is seen (solid arrows); the left is not.

b) Coronal tomogram. The medial wall of the left orbit is destroyed. The left ethmomaxillary plate is not destroyed but rather displaced inferiorly. Displacement of the ethmomaxillary plate is another manifestation of an ethmoid mucocele as is displacement or destruction of the medial wall of the orbit.

Other Complications of Sinusitis

Orbital Cellulitis

Ethmoid sinusitis may produce orbital cellulitis. In any patient with orbital cellulitis, tomograms of the paranasal sinuses should be obtained to rule out the presence of an ethmoid sinusitis.

Tomograms are necessary in such cases because ethmoid sinusitis can often be overlooked on routine views and only by means of tomograms can one be sure that there is not opacification of the ethmoid air cells.

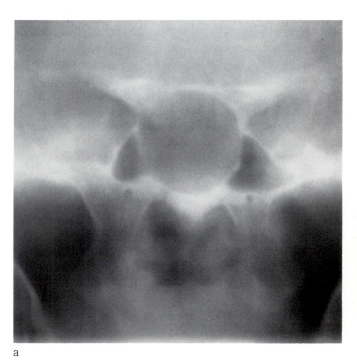

a

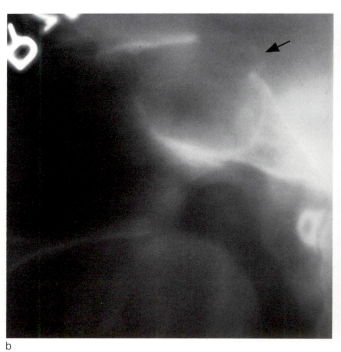

b

Fig. 4.12
a) Coronal tomogram in a patient with sphenoid mucocele and a history of years of retroorbital headaches. There is curvilinear displacement of all the walls of the sphenoid sinus.
b) Lateral tomogram through the sella turcica. Except for the dorsum sellae the sella turcica is completely destroyed. The sphenoid

sinus is expanded in a curvilinear fashion with upward displacement of the planum sphenoidale. The upward displacement of the planum sphenoidale confirms that this is a lesion arising from within the sphenoid sinus. The curvilinear expansion of the sphenoid sinus suggests that this is a benign lesion.

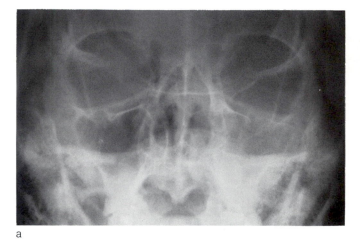

a

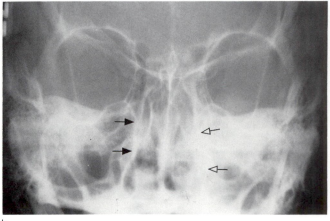

b

Fig. 4.13
a) Waters view of a patient with diabetic ketosis and mucormycosis shows opacification of the left maxillary sinus.

b) Caldwell view demonstrates that the lateral wall of the right nasal fossa is intact (solid arrows), but the lateral wall of the left nasal fossa is destroyed (hollow arrows).

Brain Abscess

A rare complication from a frontal sinusitis is the complication of brain abscess.

The only radiographic evidence of a brain abscess is when there is air in the abscess. In such a case, there will be an air fluid level in the region of the abscess. Of course a brain abscess can be diagnosed by means of computerized tomography even in the absence of air in the abscessed cavity.

Granulomatous Sinusitides

In the absence of a mucocele, routine sinusitis either allergic or bacterial, does not cause bone destruction. However, granulomatous sinusitides do cause bone destruction. They cannot be differentiated radiographically from neoplasms causing bone destruction.

Fungous Diseases

These granulomatous sinusitides should include the fungous diseases such as mucormycosis (Fig. 4.13), aspergillosis, and histoplasmosis.

Although these lesions cannot be differentiated from neoplasms radiographically, the radiographic evidence of bone destruction in a lesion where the histology shows only inflammatory reaction should make us aware of explanations for the bone destruction other than neoplasms – for example, fungi.

Any time the histological report of a biopsy of a paranasal sinus that has radiographic evidence of bone destruction shows only inflammatory reaction, one should be aware of the possibility of a fungous infection and ask for special stains for the fungi.

Rhinoscleroma

Another granulomatous sinusitis is rhinoscleroma, a chronic granulomatous affection of the respiratory tract which is believed to be caused by Klebsiella rhinoscleromatis.

It may affect the nose, the larynx, the pharynx, the nasopharynx, or the trachea. It may be characterized by bone destruction.

The patient presents with nasal obstruction and a watery discharge. Examination of the larynx and trachea may show granulomatous masses within these structures (Fig. 4.14).

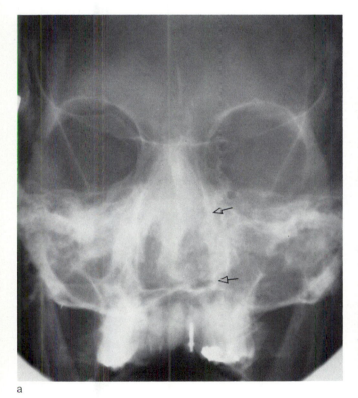

a

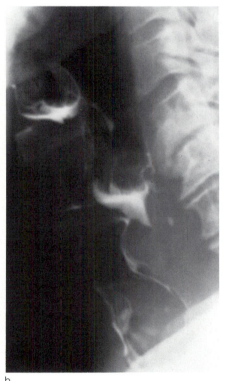

b

Fig. 4.**14**
a) Caldwell view of a patient with a 10 year history of rhinoscleroma shows opacification of the maxillary and ethmoid sinuses bilaterally and destruction of the lateral wall of the left nasal fossa (hollow arrows).

b) Lateral view of a laryngogram demonstrating two masses in the cervical trachea, one off the posterior wall, the other off the anterior wall of the trachea. Rhinoscleroma is a granulomatous disease involving the sinuses and the respiratory tract producing bone destruction of the sinuses and granulomata in the tracheobronchial tree.

Wegener's Granulomatosis

Wegener's granulomatosis also causes an opacification of the sinuses with bone destruction (Fig. 4.15).

Other Granulomatous Sinusitides

Other conditions which produce opacification of the paranasal sinuses and bone destruction include:
Syphilis (Fig. 4.16)
Tuberculosis
Sarcoid.

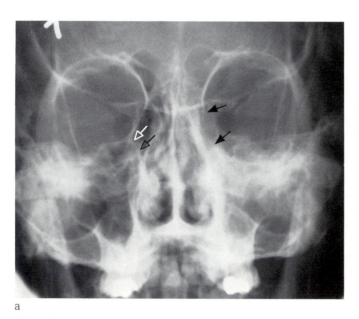

a

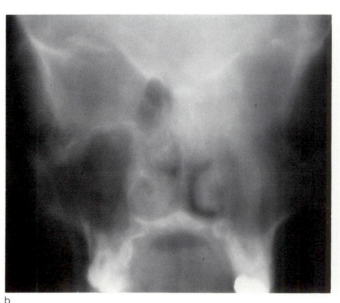

b

Fig. 4.**15**
a) Caldwell view of a patient with Wegener's granulomatosis and opacification of the left frontal, ethmoid and maxillary sinuses. There is bone destruction involving the medial wall of the left orbit (solid arrows) and the left ethmomaxillary plate. The right eth-momaxillary plate is intact (hollow arrows).

b) Coronal tomogram of the paranasal sinuses confirms the destruction of the medial wall of the left orbit and the left ethmomaxillary plate.

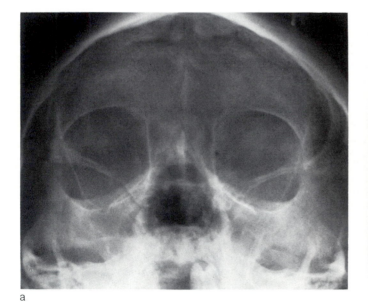

a

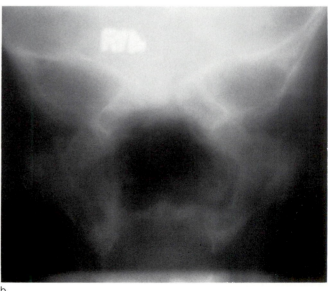

b

Fig. 4.**16**
a) Waters view of a patient with syphilis demonstrates bilateral maxillary sinus clouding, destruction of the lateral wall of the nasal fossa bilaterally, the nasal septum and the nasal turbinates.

b) Coronal tomogram confirms the destruction of all the midline structures of the face.

Chapter 5   Tumors of the Nasal Fossa and Paranasal Sinuses

The radiographic manifestation of sinus disease is clouding or opacification of the sinus and the differential between the opacification of a sinus produced by a usual type of sinusitis — bacterial, viral or allergic sinusitis — and a tumor is the presence of bone destruction. Therefore in the presence of an opacified sinus one should examine the sinus walls carefully for evidence of bone destruction and if necessary obtain tomograms to confirm or deny the presence of bone destruction.

If bone destruction is present, the lesion must be biopsied. The usual conservative therapy for inflammatory sinus disease such as antibiotics, antihistamine and/or vasoconstrictors is not adequate. Therefore the determination of the presence or absence of bone destruction is the most important information to be gained from the radiographic examination of the paranasal sinuses. The differential diagnosis of such bone destruction is not nearly so important as the simple absence or presence of bone destruction.

Where will bone destruction be manifest? The answer to this question depends on the specific sinus or sinuses which are opacified.

In the presence of an opacified maxillary sinus one should examine the lateral and medial walls of the maxillary sinus, the ethmomaxillary plate, the floor of the orbit, both anterior and posterior, and the maxillary alveolar process.

When there are clouded ethmoid sinuses, one should look carefully at the lamina papyracea, both the anterior and posterior portions, and at the ethmomaxillary plate. Frontal sinus bone destruction usually involves the adjacent medial portion of the roof of the orbit, or perhaps the margins of the frontal sinus.

Many of these sinus tumors are quite silent.

Therefore as an aid to early diagnosis, the radiographic examination is extremely important.

Maxillary Sinus Destruction

In the presence of maxillary sinus opacification, a careful examination of the walls of the maxillary sinus for evidence of bone destruction should be conducted. If there is the slightest indication or suggestion of bone destruction, tomograms of the paranasal sinuses are mandatory. If the tomograms confirm the presence of bone destruction, a biopsy of the lesion is indicated to make the final diagnosis. If bone destruction is seen, the specific diagnosis is not as important as the decision to obtain a biopsy.

Destruction of the Lateral Wall of the Maxillary Sinus

Destruction of the lateral wall of the maxillary sinus is best seen on the Waters film. On the Waters film the inferior surface of the zygomatic arch and the lateral wall of the maxillary sinus makes a smooth curve down to the alveolar process of the maxilla (Fig. 1.2). When there is bone destruction involving the lateral wall of the maxillary sinus, this curve will be interrupted.

At times, however, destruction of the lateral wall of the maxillary sinus will be manifest on the Waters view not as an interrupted line, but rather the bone destruction will produce a change in contour of the curve produced by the lateral wall of the maxillary sinus.

For example, destruction of the lateral wall of the maxillary sinus may change the contour so that it is no longer a curve but rather a straight line. The reason for the change in contour of this curve in the presence of bone destruction is due to the fact that part of the lateral wall of the maxillary sinus is destroyed. That portion of the lateral wall of the maxillary sinus which is tangential to the x-ray beam produces the contour seen on the radiograph. Destruction of a portion of the lateral wall of the maxillary sinus leaves behind a different portion of the sinus wall tangential to the x-ray beam than is normally seen. This accounts for the difference in the radiographic appearance on the Waters view between a normal lateral wall of the maxillary sinus and one in which the bone has been partially destroyed.

Destruction of the lateral wall of the maxillary sinus may also be seen on the base view. Normally on the base view, the lateral wall of the maxillary sinus is seen as an S-shaped line extending from the zygomatic arch anterolaterally to the pterygoid region posteromedially (Fig. 1.3).

Destruction of the Medial Wall of the Maxillary Sinus

Usually, destruction of the lateral wall of the maxillary sinus is visualized easily but it can be much more difficult to visualize bone destruction involving the medial wall of the maxillary sinus (which is the lateral wall of the nasal fossa).

The reason for this difficulty is the fact that the medial wall of the maxillary sinus is a more or less vertical plate of bone measuring about 5 cm in length. Therefore there can be considerable bone destruction and there will still be enough bone remaining to produce an image.

Bone destruction involving the medial wall of the maxillary sinus does not produce a hole or frank destruction but rather a difference between the two sides. This difference is manifest by the side in which there is bone destruction being thinner and less distinct than the normal side.

This sort of vaguely suspicious finding in association with an opacified maxillary sinus indicates the need for tomograms of the paranasal sinuses to rule out bone destruction and the need for biopsy.

Bone destruction of the medial wall of the maxillary sinus is seen best on the Caldwell view (Fig. 5.1). and the Waters view.

It should be emphasized that what one is looking for is a slight decrease in the visibility of the medial wall of the maxillary sinus, not its complete absence.

Destruction of the posterior portion of the medial wall of the maxillary sinus will not be visualized on the Waters view because posterior facial structures are not seen on the Waters view. Everything seen on the Waters view is anterior. So if we have the combination of a normal appearing medial wall of the maxillary sinus on the Waters view and a Caldwell view showing an abnormal indistinctness of the medial wall of the maxillary sinus, we know that the bone destruction, if present, involves the posterior portion of the maxillary sinus.

Conversely, if we have a Waters view more clearly revealing the differences between the two medial walls of the maxillary sinuses than the Caldwell view does, then we know that the bone destruction is in the anterior portion of the medial wall of the maxillary sinus. The Waters view can reveal nothing about the posterior portion of the medial wall of the maxillary sinus. Therefore if the Waters view does reveal differences between the medial walls of the maxillary sinuses more clearly than the Caldwell view, this must mean that we are seeing differences in the anterior portion of the medial wall of the two maxillary sinuses.

On the Caldwell view the medial wall of the maxillary sinus will normally be represented by a clear bright white line from top to bottom. But if we compare the two sides, where there is bone destruction involving the medial wall of the maxillary sinus, this line will be smudged, unclear and indistinct. The two sides will look different and this is what bone destruction of the medial wall of the maxillary sinus looks like – not a clear punched out hole like one would see with bone destruction in a long bone, but a difference in texture, a difference in density.

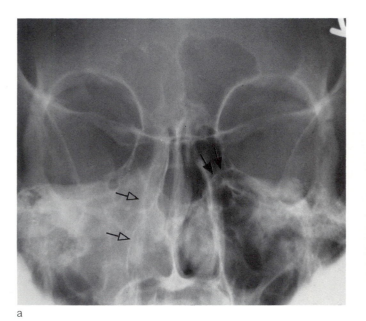

a

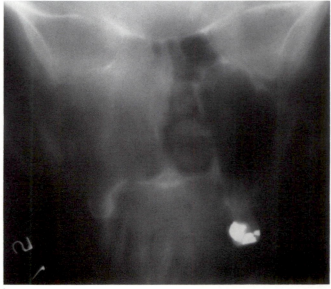

b

Fig. 5.**1**
a) Caldwell view of a patient with squamous cell carcinoma of the right paranasal sinuses who presented with nasal obstruction. The right frontal, ethmoid, and maxillary sinuses are opacified. The right ethmomaxillary plate is not seen. The left ethmomaxillary plate (solid arrows) is intact. The lateral wall of the right nasal fossa is thinner and much less distinct (hollow arrows) than is the lateral

wall of the left nasal fossa. This difference in texture and density of the lateral wall of the nasal fossa as seen on the Caldwell view or the Waters view is the earliest radiographic evidence of bone destruction involving these structures.
b) Coronal tomogram confirms the destruction of the medial wall of the right maxillary sinus and the right ethmomaxillary plate.

Destruction of the Ethmomaxillary Plate

Very often destruction of the medial wall of the maxillary sinus will be accompanied by destruction of the ethmomaxillary plate, an extension of the tumor into the ethmoid region.

The ethmomaxillary plate is a thin curvilinear plate of bone separating the ethmoid sinuses from the maxillary sinus. It is best visualized on the Caldwell view (Fig. 1.1). Any bone destroying process involving the superior portion of the maxillary sinus or the ethmoid sinuses will often destroy this plate first.

Therefore in any case of opacified ethmoid sinuses or an opacified maxillary sinus, the ethmomaxillary plate should be looked for and if it cannot be seen on the Caldwell view, tomograms should be obtained.

The ethmomaxillary plate is usually not seen well on the Waters view.

Destruction of the Roof of the Maxillary Sinus

The anterior portion of the roof of the maxillary sinus is seen on the Waters view and the Caldwell view. Therefore destruction of the anterior portion of the roof of the maxillary sinus should be looked for on these two views. On the Waters view two lines represent the floor of the orbit (which is the roof of the maxillary sinus):

The more superior line is the palpable margin of the floor of the orbit. The palpable margin of the orbit should be approximately the same width in both sides. If it is much thinner or indistinct or irregular on one side in association with an opacified sinus, destruction of this most anterior portion of the roof of the maxillary sinus should be suspected and tomograms obtained (Fig. 5.2).

The more inferior line representing the floor of the orbit as seen on the Waters view is a very delicate line. In the presence of opacification of the maxillary sinus, this line is often not visible even though it is actually present and not destroyed, because it is so delicate that the superimposition of an opacified sinus makes it disappear. Therefore the nonvisualization of the more inferior line representing the floor of the orbit and the presence of an opacified maxillary sinus should not be interpreted as bone destruction.

However, by tracing the anterior portion of the medial wall of the orbit as seen on the Waters view (Fig. 1.2) inferolaterally to where it should join the floor of the orbit, obvious bone destruction may be appreciated.

Bone destruction involving the anterior portion of the roof of the maxillary sinus may also be seen on the Caldwell view. However, to appreciate this bone destruction as seen on the Caldwell view, a careful search is necessary. The way to conduct this search is to trace the anterior portion of the medial wall of the orbit inferolaterally to where it joins the anterior portion of the floor of the orbit. By following this meticulous method of looking for bone destruction, destruction in this area might be appreciated which might be otherwise overlooked.

One should keep in mind that the medial wall of the orbit (which is the lateral wall of the ethmoid sinuses, the lamina papyracea) is represented on the Caldwell view by two lines:

1. A more lateral oblique line,
2. a more medial vertical line.

The medial vertical line is the anterior portion of the lamina papyracea. This is the line which should be traced downward to try to envisage the presence of bone de-

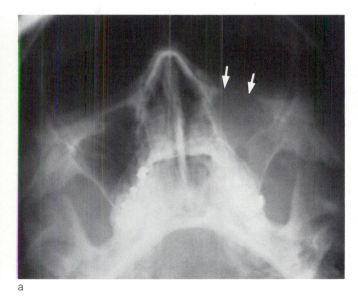

a

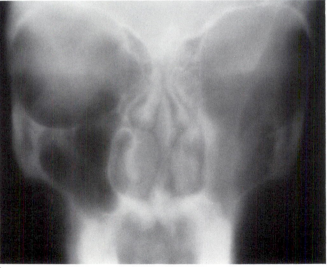

b

Fig. 5.**2**
a) Waters view of a patient with numbness in the left cheek and a malignant giant cell tumor of the left maxillary sinus. The left maxillary sinus is opacified. The inferior rim of the left orbit (solid arrows) is much thinner and less distinct than is the inferior rim of the right orbit. Generally the inferior rim of the orbit as seen on the

Waters view will have the same thickness bilaterally. If it appears thinner on the side where there is an opacified maxillary sinus, this is suspicious for bone destruction involving the anterior portion of the floor of the orbit.
b) Coronal tomogram confirms the destruction of the floor of the left orbit.

struction involving the anterior portion of the roof of the maxillary sinus.

The Caldwell may be used for analyzing the condition of the posterior portion as well as the anterior portion of the roof of the maxillary sinus. The lateral oblique line which represents the posterior portion of the lamina papyracea merges smoothly inferolaterally with the posterior portion of the roof of the maxillary sinus (Fig. 1.1). If the Caldwell view is obtained with the head extended, then the posterior portion of the roof of the maxillary sinus will not be seen on either side. However, if it is seen on one side, it should be seen on both. The unilateral absence of the image of the posterior portion of the roof of the maxillary sinus indicates bone destruction in this area (Fig. 5.3).

The posterior portion of the roof of the maxillary sinus is

also seen on the Towne view. The Towne view is usually not thought of as a sinus view. However, this portion of the maxillary sinus can be seen well on the Towne view (Fig. 5.4).

If the Towne view is not positioned correctly, the posterior portion of the roof of the maxillary sinus will not be seen on either side. But if the Towne view is positioned correctly, the posterior portion of the roof of the maxillary sinus should be seen on both sides if the posterior portion of the roof of the maxillary sinus is intact bilaterally.

If the posterior portion of the roof of the maxillary sinus is seen on one side and not on the other, in association with an opacified maxillary sinus, this means that there is bone destruction in this region (Fig. 5.5).

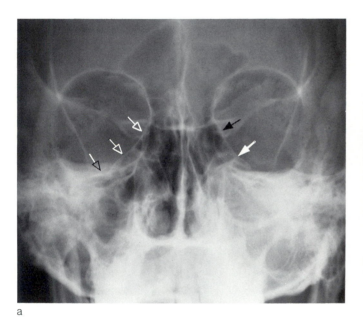

a

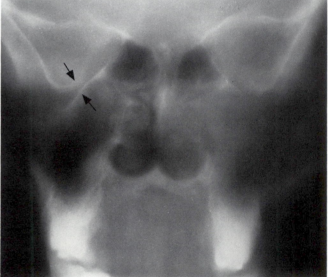

b

Fig. 5.**3**

a) Caldwell view of a patient with pain in the left cheek. The patient had leiomyosarcoma. The posterior portion of the floor of the orbit on the left which should be a continuation of the posterior portion of the medial wall of the orbit (solid arrows) is not seen. The posterior portion of the floor of the orbit as a continuation of the posterior portion of the medial wall of the orbit (hollow arrows) is seen on the right. This finding suggests destruction of the pos-

terior portion of the floor of the orbit which is the same as the roof of the maxillary sinus.

b) Coronal tomogram confirming destruction of the posterior portion of the floor of the left orbit and destruction in the region of the left inferior orbital fissure. Compare the appearance of the left inferior orbital fissure to that of the right inferior orbital fissure (solid arrows).

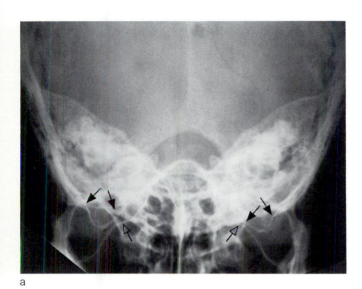

a

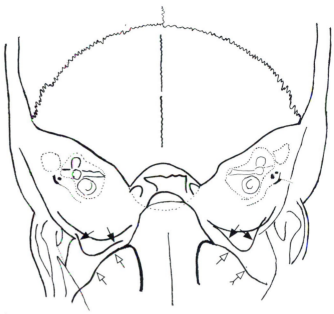

b

Fig. 5.4
a) Normal Towne view. The Towne view is the best view for demonstrating the posterior portion of the floor of the orbit and the inferior orbital fissure. The inferior orbital fissure lies between the infratemporal tubercle of the greater wing of the sphenoid (solid

arrows) and the most posterior portion of the floor of the orbit which is the roof of the maxillary sinus (hollow arrows).
b) Line drawing of Towne view.

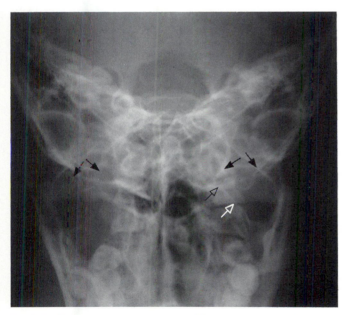

Fig. 5.5 Towne view of a patient with swelling and pain in the right cheek who had squamous cell carcinoma of the maxillary sinus. The infratemporal tubercle is seen bilaterally (solid arrows). The posterior portion of the floor of the left orbit is seen (hollow arrows), but the posterior portion of the floor of the right orbit is destroyed.

Destruction of the Maxillary Alveolar Ridge

Bone destruction involving the maxillary alveolar ridge can be seen both on the Caldwell view (Fig. 5.6) and on the Waters view (Fig. 5.7).

Bone destruction involving the maxillary alveolar ridge is most obvious when the patient is edentulous.

But even when the teeth are present, careful search can sometimes elicit the presence of bone destruction which might be otherwise overlooked. This careful search is done by tracing the lateral wall of the maxillary sinus downward on both the Waters view and the Caldwell view to include the alveolar ridge. If this is done, an interruption in the bony wall of the lateral wall of the maxillary sinus as it approaches the maxillary alveolar ridge may be appreciated.

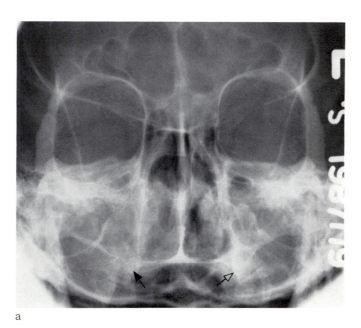

a

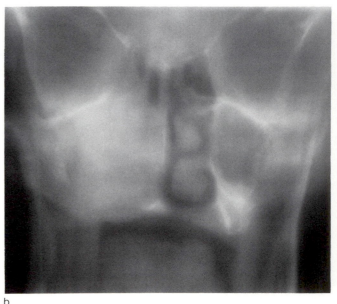

b

Fig. 5.6
a) Caldwell view of a patient with a right maxillary sinus opacified by squamous cell carcinoma. The right alveolar ridge is destroyed by the cancer (solid arrow). The left alveolar ridge (hollow arrow) is intact. There is also destruction of the lateral and medial walls of the maxillary sinus. Destruction of the lateral wall of the maxillary sinus is reflected by the changing contour of the lateral wall rather than complete absence.
b) Coronal tomogram confirming the destruction of the alveolar ridge and the medial and lateral walls of the maxillary sinus.

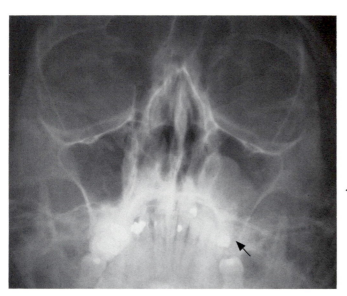

◀ Fig. 5.7 Waters view of a patient with left maxillary cylindroma. There is a slightly lobulated mass in the inferior portion of the left maxillary sinus and destruction of the outer margin of the left alveolar ridge (solid arrow). This mass in the left maxillary sinus might be confused with a retention cyst except for 2 findings: (1) the lobulated margin. Retention cysts always have a smooth dome-shaped margin. (2) The bone destruction. Retention cysts never produce bone destruction.

Summary

In summary, radiographic evidence of a tumor in the maxillary sinus is bone destruction associated with opacification of the sinus or the presence of a mass in the sinus.

Bone destruction involving the maxillary sinus should be searched for in the following areas on the appropriate views:

1. The lateral wall as seen on the Waters view and base view.
2. The anterior portion of the medial wall as seen on the Waters view.
3. The posterior portion of the medial wall as seen on the Caldwell view.
4. The ethmomaxillary plate as seen on the Caldwell view.
5. The anterior portion of the roof of the maxillary sinus as seen on the Caldwell and Waters views.
6. The posterior portion of the roof of the maxillary sinus as seen on the Caldwell and Towne views.
7. The maxillary alveolar ridge as seen on the Caldwell and Waters views.

Ethmoid Sinus Destruction

In the presence of opacification of the ethmoid sinuses, one should look for destruction of the ethmomaxillary plate and of the lamina papyracea (the medial wall of the orbit) (Fig. 5.8).

Destruction of the Posterior Portion of the Lamina Papyracea

The posterior portion of the lamina papyracea is best seen on the Caldwell view. The anterior portion is best seen on the Waters view.

Destruction of the posterior portion of the lamina papyracea is quite often obvious. Occasionally however the manifestation of bone destruction involving the posterior portion of the lamina papyracea can be similar to the presentation of destruction of the medial wall of the maxillary sinus, that is, rather than frank destruction or absence of the line, the line is fuzzier and more indistinct on the side of the opacified ethmoid sinuses than it is on the normal side.

When there is opacification of the ethmoid sinuses and a slight difference in the visualization of the posterior portion of the lamina papyracea as seen on the Caldwell view, this is an indication to obtain tomograms of the paranasal sinuses.

Destruction of the Anterior Portion of the Lamina Papyracea

Destruction of the anterior portion of the lamina papyracea in the presence of opacification of the ethmoid sinuses is virtually impossible to visualize on the Caldwell view. The anterior portion of the lamina papyracea is often not seen on the Caldwell view normally. Therefore no significance can be attached to the absence of this

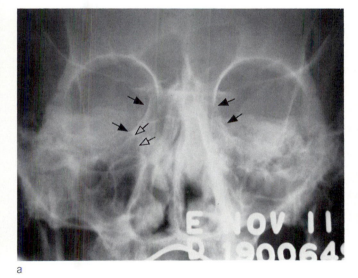

a

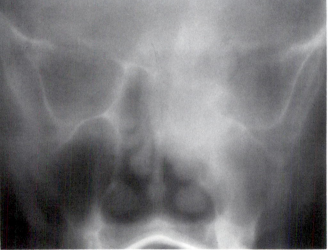

b

Fig. 5.8

a) Caldwell view of a patient with reticulum cell sarcoma of the ethmoid sinuses. The left ethmoid region is opacified as is the left maxillary sinus. The posterior portion of the lamina papyracea (solid arrows) on the left is indistinct. The left ethomaxillary plate is not seen; the right ethmomaxillary plate is intact (hollow arrows).

b) Coronal tomogram through the posterior portion of the ethmoid sinuses confirms the destruction of the posterior portion of the lamina papyracea on the left and the ethmomaxillary plate with opacification of the left maxillary sinus and ethmoid sinuses.

line even in the presence of opacification of the ethmoid sinuses.

The anterior portion of the lamina papyracea is well seen on every Waters view, so in the presence of opacification of the ethmoid air cells, this region of the medial wall of the orbit should be carefully scrutinized on the Waters view.

The anterior portion of the lamina papyracea should appear the same on both sides in the Waters view. If they do not appear the same on both sides, the presence of bone destruction is suggested in the anterior portion of the lamina papyracea (Fig. 5.9).

Summary

In summary, opacification of the ethmoid sinuses associated with bone destruction suggests the presence of tumor and indicates the necessity of obtaining tomograms of the paranasal sinuses.

Bone destruction should be looked for:

1. In the posterior portion of the lamina papyracea on the Caldwell view,
2. in the anterior portion of the lamina papyracea on the Waters view, and
3. in the ethmomaxillary plate on the Caldwell view.

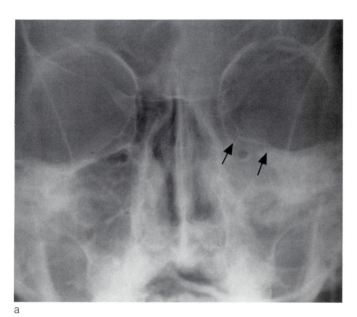

a

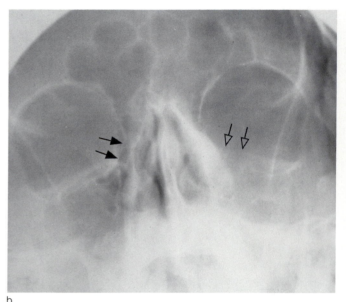

b

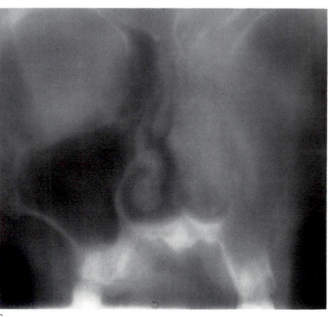

c

Fig. 5.**9**

a) Caldwell view of a patient with squamous cell carcinoma of the left ethmoids and maxillary sinus. There is opacification of the left frontal, ethmoid and maxillary sinuses. Both the posterior and the anterior portion of the lamina papyracea appear intact bilaterally. The only area that is suspicious for bone destruction is the anterior portion of the floor of the orbit where it joins the anterior portion of the lamina papyracea (solid arrows).

b) Waters view. There is destruction of the anterior portion of the left lamina papyracea. The anterior portion of the right lamina papyracea is intact (solid arrows). There is also thinning of the medial portion of the inferior rim of the orbit on the left (hollow arrows).

c) Coronal tomogram shows opacification of the left nasal fossa and maxillary and ethmoid sinuses and confirms destruction of the anterior portion of the left lamina papyracea. The anterior portion of the floor of the left orbit and the lateral wall of the left nasal fossa are also destroyed. This case shows the need for carefully examining the Waters view for destruction of the anterior portion of the lamina papyracea. Otherwise such destruction might be overlooked.

Frontal Sinus Destruction

Bone destruction involving the frontal sinus usually affects the adjacent superomedial border of the rim of the orbit as seen on the Caldwell view. This area of the rim of the orbit should only be evaluated on the Caldwell view (Fig. 5.10). On the Waters view because of the angulation of the beam, this portion of the orbit wall is never visualized well.

Usually such bone destruction of the rim of the orbit adjacent to the frontal sinus is quite obvious. The only difficulty comes in the differential diagnosis from a frontal mucocele.

Generally a tumor destroying the party wall between the orbit and the frontal sinus will not affect the entire frontal sinus, whereas a mucocele destroying the superomedial border of the orbit will also expand the entire frontal sinus. Bone destruction of this area due to tumor will leave the scalloped margin of the frontal sinus intact.

Sphenoid Sinus Destruction

Bone destruction involving the sphenoid sinuses can be difficult to visualize on routine views. Therefore whenever there is opacification of the sphenoid sinus, tomograms are probably indicated.

Occasionally bone destruction involving the sphenoid sinuses can be appreciated on the routine views. The roof of the sphenoid sinus formed by the planum sphenoidale and the sella turcica can be seen on the lateral view.

Bone destruction of the posterior wall of the sphenoid sinus can also be seen on the lateral view.

In the presence of an opacified sphenoid sinus, the base view should be carefully examined. The cortical margins of both sphenoid sinuses should be traced from the most lateral portion of the midline. In the presence of an opacified sphenoid sinus, the absence of a portion of this corticated margin is suggestive of bone destruction (Fig. 5.11).

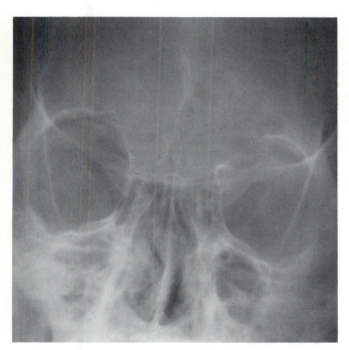

Fig. 5.10   Caldwell view of a patient with left frontal sinus carcinoma. Both frontal sinuses are opacified as are the left ethmoid sinuses. The superomedial border of the left orbit is destroyed. This area of destruction in the orbit can also be seen with a mucocele. However the scalloped border of the frontal sinus which is still demonstrated here would be smoothed out if the orbit destruction were caused by a mucocele.

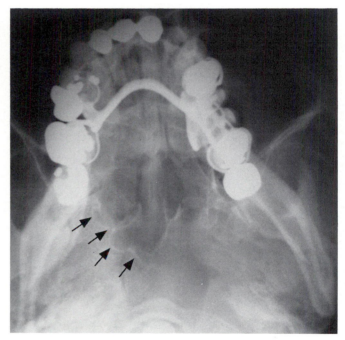

Fig. 5.11   Base view of a patient with squamous cell carcinoma of the sphenoid sinus. The cortex of the right sphenoid sinus is seen (solid arrows). The cortex of the left sphenoid sinus is destroyed.

Differential Diagnosis of Bone Destruction

The presence of bone destruction in association with a mass or opacification of a paranasal sinus is an indication for biopsy to make the conclusive diagnosis.

The differential diagnosis of bone destruction of the paranasal sinuses must include all neoplasms as well as granulomatous sinusitides. The granulomatous sinusitides include all fungi such as aspergillosis and mucormycosis. The granulomatous sinusitides also include nonspecific granulomatous disease such as Wegener's granulomatosis, sarcoidosis, and rhinoscleroma, as well as tuberculosis and syphilis.

All the above entities will destroy bone in the paranasal sinuses and all the above entities require a biopsy to make the diagnosis.

If there is curvilinear displacement of bone, this indicates that the lesion or tumor if not benign is at least slow growing and would suggest a more benign lesion such as an odontogenic cyst, a mucocele, or a slow growing tumor such as an ameloblastoma (Fig. 5.12).

The presence of a tooth suggests that the bone destroying lesion is dental in origin and a follicular cyst (Fig. 5.13). Multiple dentigerous cysts in children should suggest the diagnosis of the basal cell nevus syndrome characterized by multiple dentigerous cysts, skeletal anomalies and eventually the development of basal cell nevi and carcinoma of the skin (Fig. 5.14).

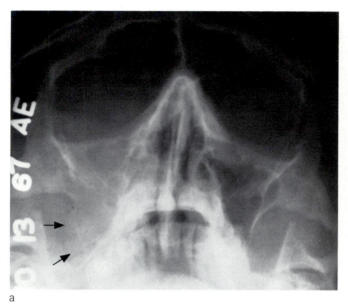

a

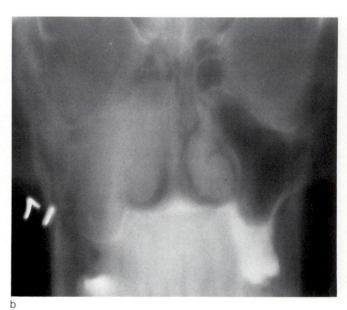

b

Fig. 5.**12**
a) Waters view of a patient with a right maxillary ameloblastoma. The right maxillary sinus is opacified and there is curvilinear displacement with thinning of the lateral wall of the right maxillary sinus (solid arrows). Curvilinear displacement of the bone indicates slow growth and probable benignity.

b) Coronal tomogram confirms a curvilinear displacement of the lateral wall of the opacified right maxillary sinus and destruction of the medial wall of the right maxillary sinus.

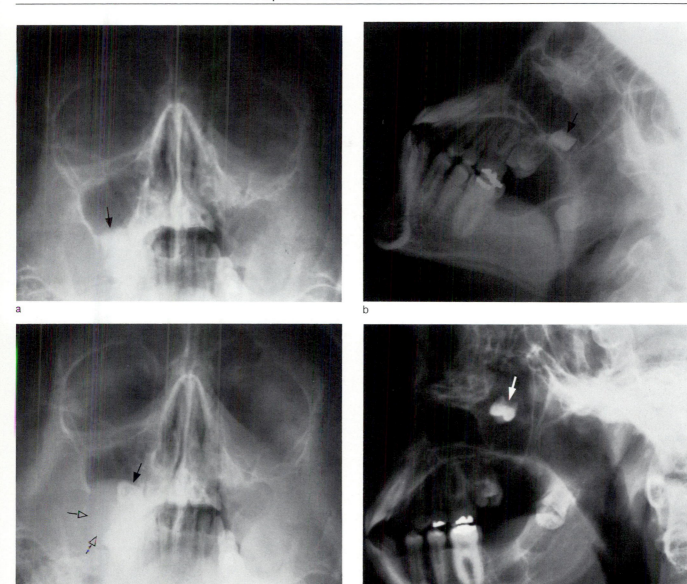

a

b

c

d

Fig. 5.**13**

a) Waters view and b) lateral view. The uninterrupted right third molar (solid arrow) is in a normal position in the alveolar process. The patient had had a previous left maxillectomy.

c) Waters view and d) Lateral view of the same patient 18 months later than a) and b). The right third molar is now displaced superiorly and medially (solid arrow). There is a mass in the inferior portion of the right maxillary sinus with a curvilinear lateral displacement of the lateral wall of the right maxillary sinus (hollow arrows). This illustration shows the natural evolution and development of a dentigerous cyst. In a period of 18 months this 15 year old male developed a dentigerous cyst which displaced the involved tooth superiorly and medially as such cysts usually do.

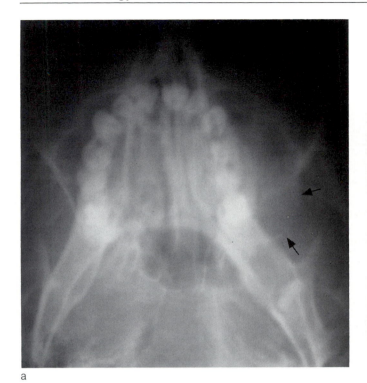

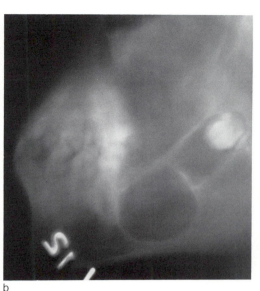

a

b

Fig. 5.**14**
a) Waters view of a patient with basal cell nevus syndrome illustrates a mass in the left maxillary sinus and curvilinear displacement of the lateral wall of the left maxillary sinus (solid arrows). This is a primordial cyst, a dentigerous cyst which does not contain a tooth.

b) Lateral tomogram demonstrating two dentigerous cysts in the body of the left mandible; the anterior one, a primordial cyst without a tooth; the posterior one, the more usual one, a dentigerous cyst containing a tooth.

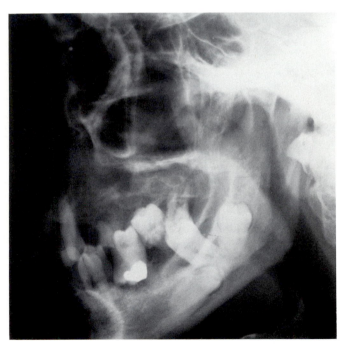

Fig. 5.**15** Lateral view of a patient with a squamous cell carcinoma showing destruction of the premaxilla. The maxillary incisor teeth appear to be floating with no bony support at all due to the destruction of the premaxilla.

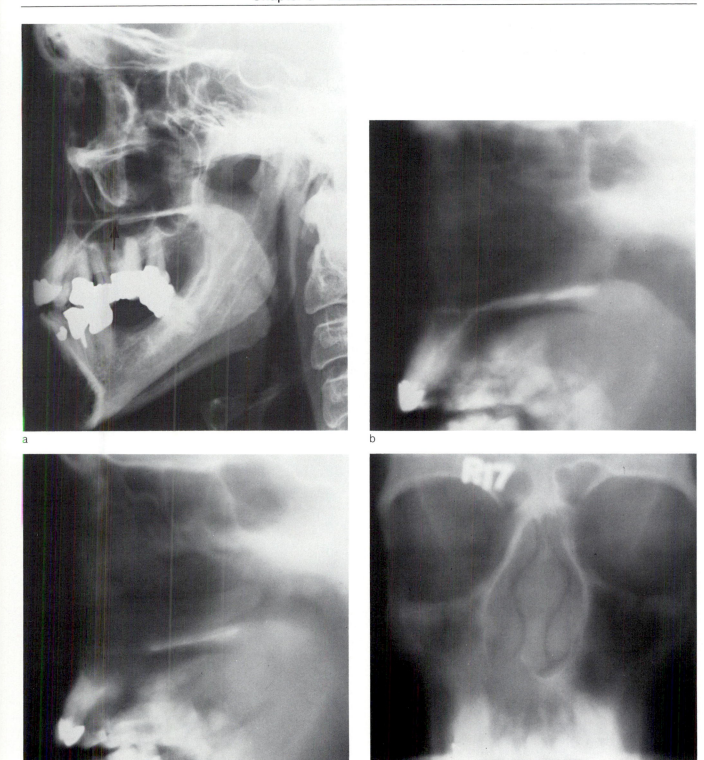

Fig. 5.**16**

a) Lateral view of a patient with a right maxillary cylindroma. In order for the image of the hard palate on the lateral view to disappear, more than half of the width of the hard palate must be destroyed. However, destruction of less than half of the width of the hard palate will produce a change in its appearance, such as in this case where there is destruction on the right side of the premaxilla. There is an abrupt change in the thickness of the hard palate (solid arrow).

b) Lateral tomogram of the left side of the hard palate. The premaxilla is intact.

c) Lateral tomogram of the right side of the hard palate. The premaxilla is destroyed.

d) Coronal tomogram shows destruction of the right side of the hard palate.

Destruction of the Hard Palate

The hard palate is another area in which the facial bones associated with the paranasal sinuses may also show bone destruction in the presence of a tumor. The hard palate should extend from the pterygopalatine fossa posteriorly to the premaxilla anteriorly as seen on the lateral view.

The posterior portion of the hard palate is generally seen as a single corticated line because of the thinness of the bone in the posterior portion. Anteriorly there are two cortical margins produced by the superior and inferior surface of the premaxilla which is the anterior thicker portion of the hard palate. If the two cortical lines anteriorly are missing, there is erosion of the premaxilla (Figs. 5.15 and 5.16).

If the thin corticated line of the hard palate does not extend posteriorly as far as the pterygopalatine fossa, then the posterior portion of the hard palate is destroyed (Fig. 5.17).

Alveolar Recesses

When both portions of the hard palate are missing, both the posterior portion and the anterior portion, then none of the hard palate will be visualized on the lateral view but what will be visualized is the inferior or alveolar recesses of the maxillary sinus.

Since these alveolar recesses are scalloped, the irregular scalloped form of the alveolar recesses may give an impression of abnormality in the absence of the hard palate. They are not usually visualized on the lateral view, since the hard palate is usually superimposed on the alveolar recesses. Thus the absence of the hard palate makes them visible and since this visibility is unusual, it could be misinterpreted as abnormal. The abnormality is not in the alveolar recesses of the maxillary sinus but rather the abnormality lies in the absence of the hard palate (Fig. 5.18).

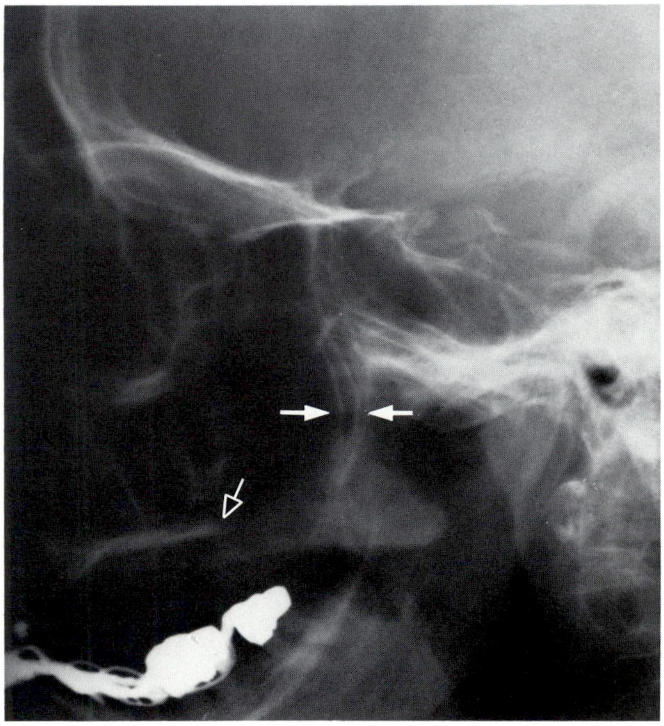

Fig. 5.**17**
Lateral view of a patient with a plasmacytoma of the hard palate. The posterior portion of the hard palate is destroyed. Normally, the image of the hard palate would extend posteriorly as far as the pterygopalatine fossa (solid arrows). In this instance, the most posterior edge of the hard palate (hollow arrow) is anterior to the pterygopalatine fossa.

Carcinoma of the Nasopharynx

Carcinoma of the nasopharynx should be suspected any time there is a mass visualized in the nasopharynx on the lateral view in an adult.

Often such a mass turns out to be nothing more than lymphoid hyperplasia or adenoidal hyperplasia such as seen in children, even though it appears in the adult. But whenever there is a mass in the nasopharynx associated with sclerosis of the base of the skull in the region of the sphenoid sinuses and the pterygoid plates, a mass in the nasopharynx is much more ominous.

The association of a nasopharyngeal mass with sclerosis of the adjacent bone of the base of the skull should pro-duce an assiduous search by biopsy for nasopharyngeal carcinoma.

Nasopharyngeal carcinomas are often difficult to find by biopsy. One negative biopsy is not sufficient to rule out carcinoma if radiographically there is a mass in the nasopharynx and sclerosis of the base of the skull (Fig. 5.19). In the presence of a nasopharyngeal mass and sclerosis, repeated biopsies are indicated.

The demonstration of sclerosis of the base of the skull is so important that tomograms are probably indicated in every adult who has a mass in the nasopharynx and a search should be made for sclerosis of the bony walls of the nasopharynx which might be overlooked on routine views.

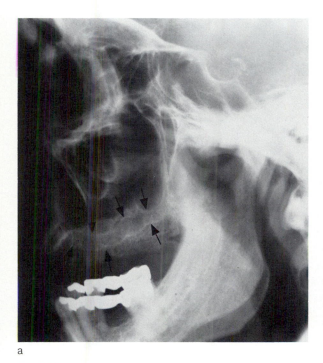
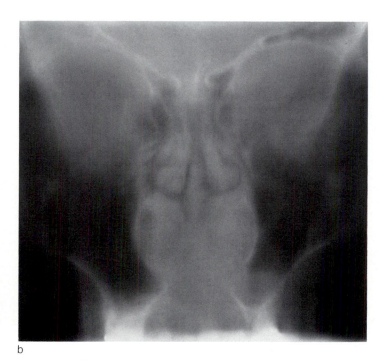

a   b

Fig. 5.**18**

a) Lateral view of a patient with a reticulum cell sarcoma of the hard palate. The hard palate is completely destroyed. There is no visualization of any of the hard palate, either the posterior portion or the premaxilla. The absence of the hard palate makes it possible to visualize the contour of the normal borders of the alveolar recesses of the maxillary sinuses (solid arrows) which are nor-mally obscured by the intact hard palate.

b) Coronal tomogram showing the destruction of the hard palate and a mass in the inferior portion of the nasal fossa.

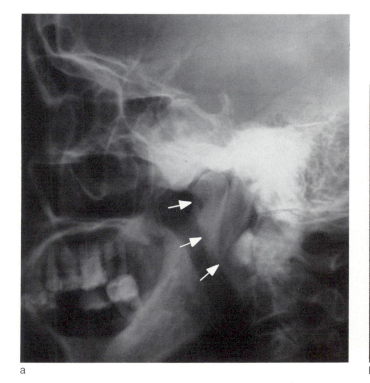

a

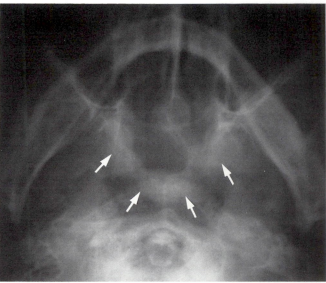

b

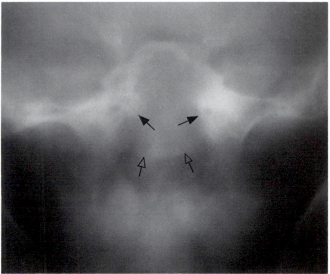

c

Fig. 5.**19**
a) Lateral view of a patient with squamous cell carcinoma of the nasopharynx. There is a mass in the nasopharynx (solid arrows).
b) Base view. There is a zone of sclerosis surrounding the sphenoid sinuses (solid arrows).
c) Coronal tomogram confirming the presence of the sclerosis surrounding the sphenoid sinuses (solid arrows), the destruction of the floor of the sphenoid sinuses, complete opacification of the sphenoid sinuses and a mass in the nasopharynx (hollow arrows).

Acknowledgment

Figures 1.1, 1.2, 1.3 and 1.4 are reprinted from my article *Radiographic Analysis of the Skull* by Potter GD, Gold RP, Medical Radiography and Photography, 51: 2–15, 1975, by permission of the publisher.

Figures 2.1, 2.2, 2.3, 2.4, 2.5, 2.6, 2.7, 2.8, 2.9, 2.10, 2.11, 2.12, 2.13, 2.14, 2.15, 2.16 and 2.17 are reprinted from my book, *Sectional Anatomy and Tomography of the Head,* by Potter GD, Grune and Stratton, New York City, 1971, by permission of the publisher.

References

1. Adkins WY, Cassone PD, Putney FJ: Solitary frontal sinus fracture. Laryngoscope 89: 1099, 1979
2. Crikelair GF, Rein JM, Potter GD, Cosman B: A critical look at the blowout fracture. Plast Reconstr Surg 49: 374, 1972.
3. Dodd GD, Jing B: Radiology of the nose, paranasal sinuses and nasopharynx. Williams & Wilkins, Baltimore 1977
4. Dolan KD, Hayden J Jr: Maxillary "pseudofracture" line. Radiology 107: 321, 1973
5. Dolan KD, Jacoby CG: Facial fractures. Semin Roentgenol. 13: 37, 1978
6. Gregory JA, Turner PT, Reynolds AF: A complication of nasogastric intubation: Intracranial penetration. J Trauma 18: 823, 1978
7. Knowles, DM, Jakobiec FA, Potter GD, Jones IS: The diagnosis and treatment of rhabdomyosarcoma of the orbit. In: Ocular and Adnexal Tumors, ed. by Jakobiec FA. Aesculapius Publishing Company, Birmingham 1978
8. LeFort R: Etude expérimentale sur les fractures de la machoire superieure. Rev Chir 23: 208, 1901
9. Merrell RA Jr, Yanigasawa E: Radiographic anatomy of the paranasal sinuses I. Waters view. Arch Otolaryngol 87: 184. 1968
10. Nakamura T, Gross CW: Facial fractures: An analysis of 5 years of experience. Arch Otolaryngol 97: 288, 1973
11. Potter GD: Maxillary sinus. In: Disorders of the Head and Neck (Second Series) Syllabus, ed. by Rogers, Meschan, Potter, Weinberg and Wilson. American College of Radiology, Chicago 1977
12. Potter GD: Radiographic and differential diagnosis of sinus disease. Appl Radiol 5: 57, 1976
13. Potter GD: Tomography of the head. CRC Critical Reviews in Clinical Radiology and Nuclear Medicine 6: 282, 1975
14. Potter GD: The hard palate. Am J Roentgenol 118: 415, 1973
15. Potter GD: Tomography of the orbit. Radiol Clin North Am 10: 21, 1972
16. Potter GD: The radiological examination of the orbit. CRC Critical Reviews in Radiological Sciences 2: 145, 1971
17. Potter GD: Sectional anatomy and tomography of the head. Grune & Stratton, New York 1971
18. Potter GD: Sclerosis of the base of the skull as a manifestation of nasopharyngeal carcinoma. Radiology 94: 35, 1970
19. Potter GD: The pterygopalatine fossa and canal. Am J Roentgenol 107: 520, 1969
20. Potter GD: Tomography of the optic canal. Am J Roentgenol 106: 530, 1969
21. Potter GD, McClennan BL: Malignant giant cell tumor of the sphenoid bone and its differential diagnosis. Cancer 25: 167, 1970
22. Potter GD, Trokel SL: The optic canal. In: Radiology of the skull and brain. Vol. I, ed by Newton RH, Potts DG, Mosby, St. Louis 1971
23. Smith B, Regan WF Jr: Blowout fractures of the orbit: mechanism and correction of inferior orbital floor fracture. Am J Ophthalmol 44: 733, 1957
24. Trokel SL, Potter GD: Radiographic diagnosis of fracture of the medial wall of the orbit. Am J Ophthalmol 67: 772, 1969
25. Turvey TA: Midfacial fracture: a retrospective analysis of 593 cases. J Oral Surg 35: 887, 1977
26. Valvassori GE, Hord GE: Traumatic sinus disease. Sem Roentgenol 3: 160, 1968
27. Yanigasawa E, Smith HW, Thaler S: Radiographic anatomy of the paranasal sinuses II. Lateral view. Arch Otolaryngol 87: 96, 1968
28. Zizmor J, Noyek AM: Cysts, benign tumors and malignant tumors of the paranasal sinuses. Otolaryngol Clin North Am 6: 487, 1973
29. Zizmor J, Noyek AM: Fractures of the paranasal sinuses. Otolaryngol Clin North Am 6: 473, 1973

Part III

Computed Tomography

Barbara L. Carter

Chapter 1 Introduction

Radiographic imaging in otorhinolaryngology has become considerably more sophisticated during the past few years. The most recent advance, computed tomography (CT) provides clear definition and differentiation of soft tissue structures as well as sharp bone detail. Radiographic film has been replaced by a series of detectors linked to a computer which, by solving thousands of equations instantaneously, reconstructs an image in a transverse plane (35) equivalent to an anatomical section. The computer is much more sensitive than film in the detection of areas of varying photon absorption by different soft tissue structures. CT is therefore particularly useful for the depiction of anatomical detail of soft tissues and in the measurement of the relative absorption coefficients of abnormal areas. This information provides an accurate assessment of the total extent of disease, in the soft tissue identification of fatty tumors, cystic structures, necrotic areas, abscess cavities, and recent hemorrhage (46). Areas previously inaccessible to radiographic study, such as the infratemporal fossa and soft tissues of the neck, can now be accurately evaluated. CT is particularly important in determining the presence of any intra-orbital or intracranial extension of tumors or infection.

Part III is devoted to a study of the application of CT to the various diseases encountered in the radiology of otorhinolaryngology (2, 7, 9, 10, 12, 13, 26, 28, 55, 56, 63, 67). Particular emphasis has been placed on the role of this new tool as complementary to or a replacement for other imaging modalities.

CT makes the following unique contributions:

1) demarcating the entire extent of tumor;
2) differentiating solid from cystic lesions;
3) identifying recent hematoma or abscess;
4) depicting the presence of minute calcification and of fat or necrosis within a tumor;
5) demonstrating the vascularity of a tumor (with intravenous contrast enhancement);
6) identifying intra-orbital or intracranial extension of tumor;
7) assisting in the precise localization of a lesion for biopsy;
8) assisting in decision making for primary therapy, i.e. surgery, radiotherapy, or chemotherapy;
9) demonstrating the best surgical approach;
10) assisting in planning radiotherapy portal (14, 36, 44) and calculating dose to tumor and to adjacent tissue;
11) following patients for the detection of recurrent tumor or metastases; and
12) following patients to determine the effectiveness of radiotherapy or chemotherapy.

Following a discussion of the methodology, the normal CT anatomy and the various diseases amenable to CT diagnosis will be presented. The format will be similar to that of the other parts of the book to include congenital anomalies, functional disorders, trauma, infection, and tumors. The anatomical areas to be covered in this section are the orbit, skull base, infratemporal fossa, nasopharynx, nasal cavity, sinuses, and oropharynx. CT of the petrous bone, salivary gland, and larynx have been included in other sections. All of the CT images are shown without contrast enhancement and in the transverse plane unless otherwise stated.

Method

Tomographic Plane

Images are obtained in the transverse plane at 8 mm–10 mm increments with the patient in a supine position. Angulation of the gantry is predetermined for each examination as with conventional tomography. The optic nerve and optic canal for example, are best visualized with the gantry angled minus 10 degrees to Reid's base line. The clivus and intracranial structures are studied with the gantry angled plus 20 degrees to Reid's base line. Particular attention must be paid to the precise positioning of the patient to attain maximum symmetry between the two sides.

Coronal tomograms (25) are performed by angling the gantry and hyperextending the head with the patient in a supine or prone position (Fig. 1.1). If the gantry is fixed in an upright position, coronals may be obtained by hyperextending the head and tilting the tabletop to such a degree that the gantry is at right angles to Reid's base line. The degree of angulation varies with the degree of hyperextension and should be modified to decrease artifacts caused by dental fillings, caps, clips, etc. The quality of the examination is dependent upon patient cooperation, i.e. keeping the same degree of hyperextension and refraining from moving, swallowing, and chewing.

An alternative method for doing direct sagittal (48) and coronal tomograms is to reconstruct a computer image from the data obtained in the transverse plane at 2 mm intervals (43). Many serial tomograms in close proximity may be needed to provide sufficient data input to the computer to reconstruct images of good quality. Because the additional scans result in greater patient exposure, reconstructed data should be limited to the immediate area of interest. Reconstructed images from the same data base may be obtained in varying degrees of obliquity in addition to the coronal and sagittal planes, all from the same data base, if appropriate software is available.

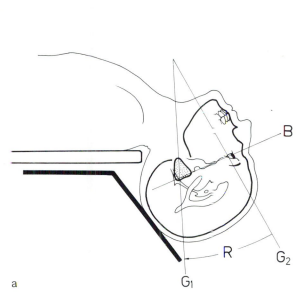

a

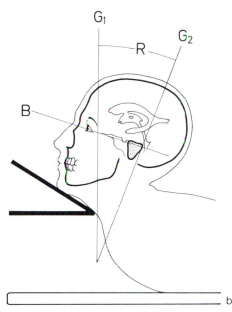

b

Fig. 1.1   Diagram of position for coronal scan. The patient is in a supine (a) or prone (b) position with the head hyperextended. The gantry (G) is angled (R) to obtain a scan 90 degrees to Reid's baseline (B).

Contrast Material

Contrast enhancement is occasionally used to detect vascular tumors and to differentiate normal neck vessels from an abnormal mass. The enhancement is accomplished either by scanning during a rapid drip infusion or by a bolus injection of iodinated contrast material through a 19-gauge needle positioned in a peripheral vein (8). With scan times of two minutes or more, rapid infusion is preferred to bolus injection because it provides a high blood level of contrast material over a longer period of time (24), allowing visualization of blood vessels on several sequential images. With bolus injection, a higher peak concentration is obtained in the blood pool and in the extra cellular fluid, but for a shorter time interval. With the rapid scan times (1–5 seconds) of the newest CT scanners, the bolus technique is preferable for showing normal vessels and vascular tumors. Repeated scans of the same area during the arterial, capillary, venous and subsequent phases often help to characterize the type of lesion present.

For improved CT visualization of the subarachnoid space, particularly in the cerebellopontine angles and basal cisterns, dilute aqueous iodinated contrast material is injected into the subarachnoid space (1, 47, 53, 55, 58). Metrizamide has been used extensively for myelography in Europe and more recently in the United States. Arachnoiditis has not been reported in over 1100 cases, but 25–57% of patients with whom Metrizamide has been used may have other complications such as headaches, occasionally severe, with nausea and vomiting. On rare occasions generalized seizures may occur. The amount of Metrizamide used for CT studies is considerably less than that required for myelography, with a concomitant reduction in morbidity.

The procedure is performed by injecting 4 ml of 170 mg of iodine per ml into the subarachnoid space via a lumbar puncture. The patient is turned supine and placed into a Trendelenburg position for approximately one minute during which the contrast material is allowed to flow into the basal cisterns and ventricles. The patient is then placed into a horizontal position minus 10 degrees and CT images are obtained. The contrast material is absorbed by the subarachnoid villi and the brain and is excreted from the body within 24 hours. 5–10 ml of air injected into the subarachnoid space with the patient in a decubitus position has also been used to good advantage for visualization of the CP angle and internal auditory canal. Other contrast agents are used for specific areas of the face, neck, and body. Dilute aqueous contrast material (3–5%) or dilute barium is given by mouth for opacification of the esophagus in order to differentiate a dilated esophagus or hiatal hernia from a tumor. Improved visualization of the salivary gland is accomplished by scanning immediately after a sialogram (13, 28), using either Ethiodol or aqueous contrast material. Barium paste is placed on the skin surface for external landmarks to localize a palpable mass or to outline portals for radiation therapy.

Technical Considerations

Equipment

Some images in this chapter were made with an Ohio Nuclear whole body scanner having a scan time of 2.5 minutes with a 256 × 256 matrix and at 120 KV and 30 MA. Each slice is nominally 12 mm thick. The more detailed images were made with a Somatome II body scanner with a scan time of 5 seconds, a 256 × 256 matrix, 125 KV and 45–75 MA. These slices are 4–8 mm thick.

The earlier CT machines use a traverse-rotate system with one to twenty detectors opposite the x-ray tube, which emits a finely collimated x-ray beam. The scan time varies with the number of detectors used. For example, three detectors per beam require a tube rotation of three degrees after each traverse whereas twenty detectors permit a twenty degree rotation after each traverse. Thus, as the total number of traverses decreases, e.g. from 60 to 8, the scan time is shortened from 2.5 minutes to 18 seconds.

Third and fourth generation scanners now employ 500–1,000 detectors. The detectors rotate opposite the tube with the "third generation" scanners and are permanently mounted in the ring with the "fourth generation". A well collimated fan beam from the tube rotating about the patient permits a scan time of 1–5 seconds. Other recent advances have added significantly to the capabilities of CT. Preliminary "scout views" are obtained by moving the patient through the gantry at 2–4 mm increments while keeping the tube and detectors stationary. This can be done in AP and/or lateral projections, permitting precise localization and angulation of the gantry for the subsequent tomographic images. Zooming capabilities permit better definition and differentiation of small areas such as portions of the spine, the middle ear cavity, internal auditory canal, etc. This is accomplished by increased sampling of data from the smaller selected area. The improved detail permits the identification of the ligamentum flavum, herniated discs, nerve roots, etc. within the spinal canal. In the middle ear it is even possible to see the muscles and ligaments attached to the ossicles and to identify the canal for the endolymphatic duct.

By using larger discs, more raw data can be stored, temporarily or even permanently, permitting greater software manipulation of the information obtained. Data may be selected from the early or later part of the 360° rotation giving serial images in rapid sequence. "Dynamic scanning" therefore makes it possible to see sequential images throughout the arterial, capillary, and venous phases. By using cardiac gating, images may be displayed that were obtained during cardiac systole or diastole resulting in improved visualization of the cardiac chambers, the myocardium, the coronary arteries and even bypass grafts. When automatic table incrementation is used, rapid images may be obtained in sequence during the peak blood level of contrast medium with a bolus injection and/or with one breath-holding. Rapid successive scans at different levels increase the potential usefulness of CT for the evaluation of vessels and tumors over relatively long segments. Recording these images during a single breath-hold eliminates the problems encountered by varied positions of anatomical structures during inspiration, expiration, swallowing, phonation, etc.

Artifacts

Motion artifacts are a major cause of degradation of the image and have been a particular problem with the prolonged scan times of earlier CT machines. The artifacts result in stellate streaks of high and low densities due to motion of sharply contrasted structures (air, bone, etc.) caused by swallowing, breathing, coughing, and other movement during scanning. High metallic densities (such as dental fillings and clips) are particularly apt to produce artifacts. Imbalance between detectors, faulty detectors, or improper alignment between the x-ray tube and the detectors will also produce a variety of artifacts. Structures that are only partially imaged may be difficult to identify, particularly with a beam collimated to 10 mm. Small structures are more accurately depicted and artifacts such as those seen between the petrous bones minimized with a beam collimation of 2 mm.

Partial Imaging

It is particularly important to recognize the phenomenon of partial imaging. If a structure such as the jugular tubercle of the occipital bone is only partially seen within the plane of the scan, it may simulate a tumor.

A cyst of low absorption is accurately imaged only if the scan is obtained through the mid portion of the cyst. If the scan is made through the edge of the cyst, which is thus partially imaged together with adjacent soft tissues of higher absorption, the resulting image will have a total absorption value equal to the amount of cyst plus the amount of soft tissue included in the scan.

Centering and Window Setting

Images from a CT scanner are visualized on a gray scale varying from black to white as with an x-ray film. Calculations by the computer to determine the relative absorption coefficients of the structures within the body are expressed as Hounsfield units (H) with water being zero H, the center of the gray scale. Air is black ($-1,000$ H), fat less black (-50 to -100 H), water gray (0 to $+10$ H), brain slightly lighter gray ($+25$ H), circulating blood ($+40$ H), hemorrhage ($+50$ to $+70$ H), calcium ($+200$ H) and bone light gray to white ($+1,000$ H). Determination of the relative absorption value by the computer is accurate within 0.5–1%.

The image as viewed in the TV monitor and subsequently photographed on film varies with the window width (total amount of gray scale included) and with the centering of the window used. Visualization of soft tissue detail requires a narrower window (100 to 500 H) and thus is a more highly contrasted image. Centering of this window is changed according to the area of interest (high of $+100$ to $+200$ H for bone, $+20$ to $+40$ H for muscle, and -20 H for fat). A wide window includes more of the gray scale (1500 to 2500 H) and thus results in a flatter image. Sharply contrasting structures such as air and bone are better seen with a wide window.

All of the data are stored on the disc and subsequently transferred to tape. Several different gradations of contrast may be obtained from the same data base by varying the window width and centering for viewing or photographing the images. The actual measurements of the absorption coefficient (expressed as Hounsfield units) is obtained by placing a cursor over the area of interest. This remains constant despite any variations in the window settings for viewing the image. Various structures, such as cysts, fatty tumors, necrosis, calcification, etc., are thus consistently characterized by these measurements.

Radiation Exposure

The dose of radiation absorbed by the patient varies with the equipment, the efficiency of photon capture by the detector system, the filtration, and the type of collimation used (4, 57). Since the entrance dose is greater than the exit dose, many units are designed so that the tube passes around the back of the head with the detectors being in front in order to minimize the exposure to the lens of the eye. If scans are obtained in close proximity or are overlapping, the absorbed dose is increased accordingly. A larger matrix with small pixel sizes requires a greater radiation dose than that used for the same signal-noise ratio used with a smaller matrix and larger pixel sizes. The spatial resolution is improved by employing a smaller pixel size (35), but at the expense of greater radiation exposure. Most units deliver 1–4 rads at the entrance and 0.5 to 1 rad at the exit portals. The usual head scan results in an exposure equivalent to a total skull series which is considerably less than an arteriogram or pneumonencephalogram.

Chapter 2   Orbit

Normal Anatomy

CT scanning has surpassed all other modalities of investigating the orbit because of its unique ability to identify normal and abnormal structures within the area (Fig. 2.1–2.4).* The lens within the globe, the exact dimensions of the globe, the orbital muscles, orbital fat within and outside of the muscle cone, the optic nerve, ophthalmic artery and branches, orbital veins and the lacrimal gland are all sharply defined (33, 34, 39, 62, 66). Dimensions of the globe should be measured through the mid-plane, identified by the lens. The degree of proptosis or enophthalmus can also be measured at this level. The patient should fix vision on an object during the scanning procedure so that the eyes are immobilized.

Although the medial and lateral rectus muscles are readily seen on the same image that includes the mid-plane of the globe, the inferior and superior recti are identified

---

* Orbit is included in this section since it is often involved by trauma, inflammatory disease, and tumors of the paranasal sinuses and nasal cavity.

---

only on sections taken at the superior and inferior aspects of the globe (transverse plane) and should be recognized as such lest they be mistaken for tumors. The levator palpebrae, immediately above the superior rectus muscle, is so close to the latter that the two muscles are usually imaged as one. The superior oblique muscle, close to the medial rectus, can usually be seen (coronal plane), whereas the inferior oblique is small and difficult to identify. All except the inferior oblique muscle originate at the apex of the orbit from a common tendon (annulus of Zinn) attached to the sphenoid bone. They insert distally on the surface of the globe (59).

The lacrimal gland, above and lateral to the globe, appears on the superior sections. The superior ophthalmic vein courses obliquely to the superior rectus muscle and can usually be identified, particularly with contrast enhancement studies. Peripheral fat is located between the muscles and the bony wall, whereas central fat is within the muscle cone behind the globe and contrasts sharply with the optic nerve throughout its course from the optic canal to the retina. The optic chiasm and its cistern are usually visible intracranially.

The sharp definition of the bony walls of the orbit is also

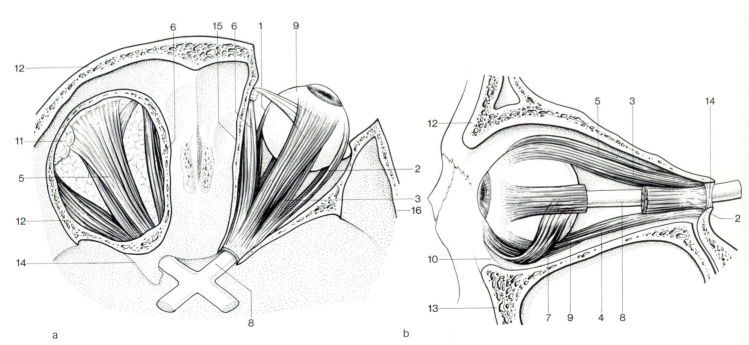

a

b

Fig. 2.1   Diagram of orbit, transverse (a) and sagittal (b) planes. The extra-ocular muscles are: medial rectus (1), lateral rectus (2), superior rectus (3), inferior rectus (4), levator palpebrae (5), superior oblique (6) and inferior oblique (7). The optic nerve (8) is surrounded by intraconal fat. The globe (9) is surrounded

anteriorly by the orbital septum (10). The lacrimal gland (11) is superior and lateral to the globe. The bony walls of the orbit, the frontal (12), maxillary (13), sphenoid (14), ethmoid (15), zygoma (16), and lacrimal bones are readily identified.

clearly seen (Fig. 2.2–2.4). Although the anatomical detail of the transverse and coronal planes is not quite comparable to the AP and lateral projections of poly-directional tomography, it is sufficient for the identification of gross changes due to tumor, infection, or trauma involving the orbit and immediately adjacent structures.

The optic canal, medial to the anterior clinoid (Fig. 2.4), and the superior orbital fissure may be identified by CT scanning but supplemental films by polydirectional tomography may be necessary for more detailed analysis of other structures such as the infraorbital canal.

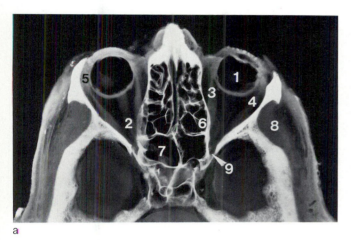

a

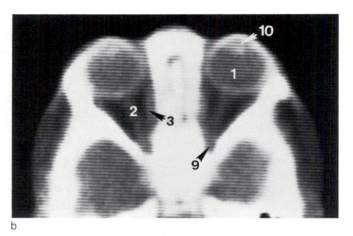

b

Fig. 2.2   Normal orbit, transverse section through a specimen (a) and transverse scan of a child (b) before enhancement showing the: globe (1), optic nerve (2), medial rectus muscle (3), lateral rectus muscle (4), lacrimal gland region (5), ethmoid (6) and

sphenoid (7) sinuses, temporalis muscle (8) in temporal fossa formed by the greater wing of the sphenoid bone. The superior orbital fissure (9) is at the apex of the orbit. The lens (10) is best seen through the mid-plane of the orbit.

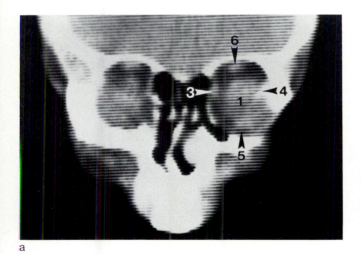

a

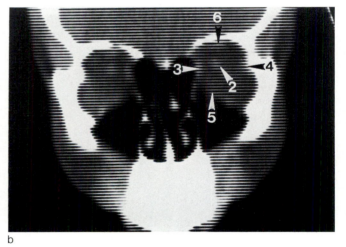

b

Fig. 2.3   Coronal tomograms of orbit; (a) is 1.5 cm anterior to (b). (a) is taken through the posterior aspect of the globe and (b) behind the globe. The globe (1), optic nerve (2), medial rectus (3),

lateral rectus (4), inferior rectus (5), and superior rectus (6) muscles are clearly seen.

Abnormal

Computed tomography is superior to all other methods of identifying intraorbital but extrabulbar structures; however, the imaging of anatomical structures and disease entities within the globe (e.g. detached retina) may be better accomplished by ultrasonography. Occasionally, both CT and ultrasound are needed to make a definitive diagnosis (29, 34, 66).

Congenital malformations, such as hypoplasia of the orbit and/or globe, are discernible by CT as is agenesis of the optic nerve. Small optic canals are indicative of hypoplasia. Hypertrophy of the extraocular muscles connotes a functional disorder, Graves' disease, which results in a muscle mass effect large enough to simulate a tumor. This is particularly evident at the apex of the orbit where the hypertrophied muscles converge to produce this mass. Occasionally, the initial diagnosis of Graves' disease in a patient presenting with proptosis is made by CT. The degree of proptosis due to hyperthyroidism, tumor, or infection is measurable by CT as is the degree of enophthalmus due to absence of fat, atrophy of the muscle cone, or deformity of the floor of the orbit.

Trauma to the orbit may be seen incidentally on CT scans obtained for the detection of intracranial hematoma in patients with severe head injury. Although a gross fracture resulting in deformity of the orbit is usually apparent on conventional radiography, this can also be seen on CT image. Fracture fragments and foreign bodies projecting into the orbit are readily identified together with any hematoma and/or subcutaneous emphysema (Fig. 2.5). Minimal deformities associated with fractures of the ethmoid, blow-out fractures into the maxillary sinus, and fractures through the optic canal, optic strut, etc., may require conventional thin section tomography for evaluation. Old post-traumatic calcifica-tions in the globe, lens, and retrobulbar area are clearly seen by CT, often as incidental findings.

Inflammatory changes caused by sinusitis, granulomata, or pseudotumor appear as a homogenous soft tissue mass of a density similar to that of the rectus muscles. The inflammatory area may have either sharply defined or irregular and poorly defined edges. A localized abscess may contain an area of lower absorption value due to the fluid content. Although Wegener's granulomatosis tends to manifest itself as a diffuse involvement of the paranasal sinuses, it is sometimes confined to the orbit (30). Pseudotumor (3, 21) is an idiopathic orbital inflammation that can be unilateral or bilateral, diffuse or multifocal, or an isolated localized mass simulating a tumor. Several follow-up scans may be needed for the confirmation of this diagnosis by documenting the response to treatment with corticosteroids. Other disease entities which should be considered in the differential diagnosis are sarcoidosis and myositis. Proptosis is often present with any of these (Fig. 2.6–2.8).

Many neoplasms involving the orbit can be clearly identified by CT (62, 66), although it is difficult to distinguish benign from malignant lesions. Different types of tumors (Table I) tend to occur within the muscle cone (intraconal), within the orbit but outside the muscle cone (extraconal), and in the wall of the orbit (extra-orbital). Vascular tumors can be identified by intravenous enhancement particularly with a bolus injection with rapid scanners and by obtaining the scans at appropriate intervals after the intravenous injection. Angiography is necessary, however, for the evaluation of other vascular pathology.

A detailed discussion of the various disease entities of the orbit is limited by the scope of this book. The reader is referred to the literature for more complete coverage of all disease entities that involve this area.

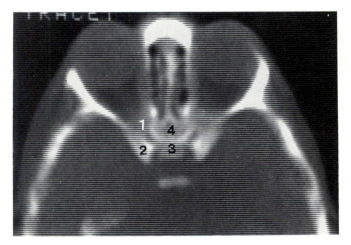

Fig. 2.4   Transverse scan through the canal for the optic nerve (1) which is medial to the anterior clinoid (2), lateral to the tuberculum sella (3) and planum sphenoidale (4); taken for bone technique.

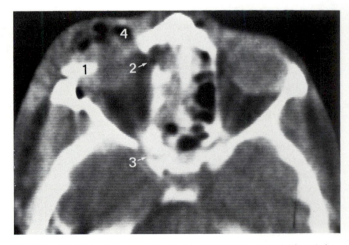

Fig. 2.5   Multiple fractures right orbit, transverse scan before infusion. A bone fragment (1) is projecting into the orbit. The lamina papyracia (2) of the ethmoid is depressed and the ethmoid sinuses are opaque. A fracture is also present across the base of the right anterior clinoid (3). Note the subcutaneous emphysema (4).

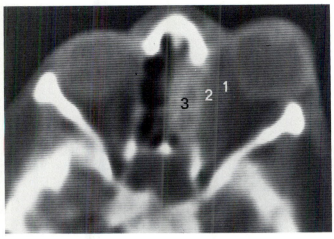

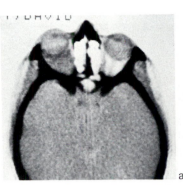
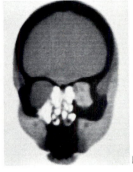

Fig. 2.6   Proptosis due to ethmoiditis in a three year old child; transverse scan before infusion. The medial rectus (1) is displaced by an inflammatory mass (2) due to ethmoiditis (3). This mass (2) also extends superior to the globe (not shown). (From: Seminars in Roentgenology, Vol. 13, 1978, Carter & Karmody-Computed Tomography of the Face & Neck).

Fig. 2.7   Wegener's granulomatosis – causing proptosis, (a) transverse and (b) coronal scans before infusion. A large soft tissue mass behind the globe is within and outside of the muscle cone. There is no bone involvement. The patient had no other manifestation of Wegener's granulomatosis.

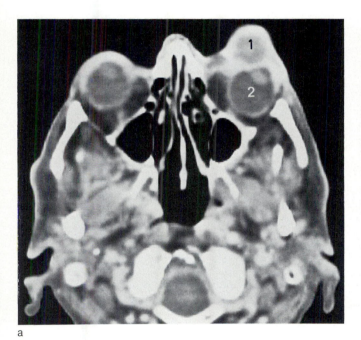

a

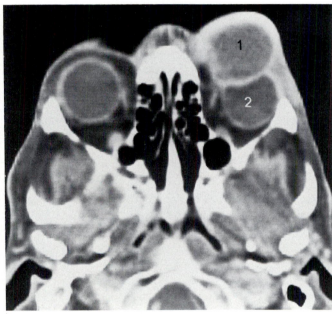

b

Fig. 2.8   Metastatic CA to orbit, transverse scans after infusion, (a) is caudad to (b). A slight bump over the eye became much larger after a fall. The resultant hematoma (1) from a metastatic lesion to the supraorbital bone displaced the globe (2) caudad, causing diplopia.

Table I   Common Orbital Tumors (Random Order)

Intraconal	Extra-orbital
Neuroma, neurofibroma of optic nerve	Benign and malignant primary tumors of ethmoid, sphenoid or maxillary sinuses. Benign and malignant primary tumors of nasal cavity. Primary bone tumors, walls of the orbit. Mucocele of frontal, ethmoid, maxillary or sphenoid sinus. Metastasis involving adjacent bone, sinuses, nasal cavity. Primary or metastatic carcinoma or sarcoma of the infratemporal fossa. Primary or metastatic tumor of the intracranial cavity. Fibrous dysplasia, Paget's disease. Histiocytosis. Lymphoma. Osteoma of adjacent sinuses.
Meningioma and glioma of optic nerve	
Venous angioma, hemangioma, lymphangioma	
Retinoblastoma	
Melanoma	
Extraconal, intraorbital	
Venous angioma, hemangioma, lymphangioma	
Lacrimal gland tumor	
Lymphoma	
Metastasis	
Rhabdomyosarcoma	

Chapter 3   Skull Base

Normal Anatomy

CT imaging of the base of the skull is almost equal in detail to conventional tomography (Fig. 3.1). The bones of the skull base are adjacent to and thus affected by tumors of the nasopharynx, nasal cavity, paranasal sinuses and infratemporal fossa (27, 45).

Computed tomography provides important information in the evaluation of patients with lesions of the skull base because of the clear soft tissue detail (described in subsequent sections), the identification of normal vascular structures, and the good definition of bone. The foramen ovale and spinosum, the spinous process of the sphenoid and styloid process of the mastoid, the carotid canal, jugular fossa, foramen magnum, clivus, petrous bone, mastoid tip, greater wing and body of the sphenoid bone and the zygomatic arch are only a few of the structures which are readily identified. The temporalis muscle, arising from the temporalis fossa, passes deep to the zygomatic arch to insert on the coronoid process of the mandible. The fascial plane passing over the surface of this muscle is often relatively dense on the CT scan and thus clearly seen overlying the muscle mass.

Abnormal

Congenital anomalies of the base of the skull are readily visualized by CT scan. An enlarged, deformed or small foramen magnum, basilar invagination, sclerosis of the bone, and defects associated with meningoceles are clearly evident. Metrizamide cisternography combined with CT defines the size of the meningocele and establishes the presence of neural elements of an encephalocele.

CT of the head is indicated post traumatically for the detection of intracranial hematoma or contusion. When there is a question of a fracture, the skull base should also be evaluated, since such fractures are often visible when the proper technique is used. This is of particular importance in the presence of a cerebrospinal fluid leak (16). As indicated above, polydirectional tomography can then be used for better definition as needed.

Reactive sclerosis or lytic defects of bone due to infections adjacent to the skull base including the infratemporal fossa are appropriately studied by CT particularly if there is a moderately large area of involvement.

Primary and metastatic tumors cause destruction and/or sclerotic reaction of the bones of the base (Fig. 3.2, 3.3), enlargement and/or destruction of the jugular fossa, hypoglossal canals, foramen ovale, etc. CT documents these bone defects and is the procedure of choice for evaluating any soft tissue extension of tumor within or outside of the skull.

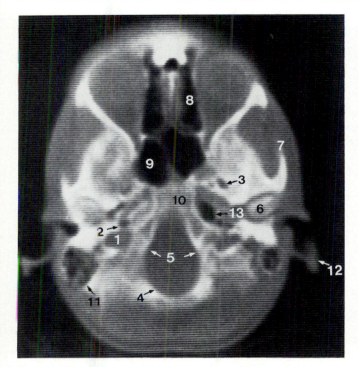

Fig. 3.1 Normal skull base, transverse scan. Image obtained for bone detail reveals the jugular fossa (1), carotid canal (2), foramen ovale (3), foramen magnum (4), hypoglossal canal (5), temporomandibular joint (6), zygomatic arch (7), ethmoid air cells (8). Also note the sphenoid sinus (9) clivus (10) mastoid tip (11) pinna of the ear (12) and pneumatized cell of the left petrous apex (13).

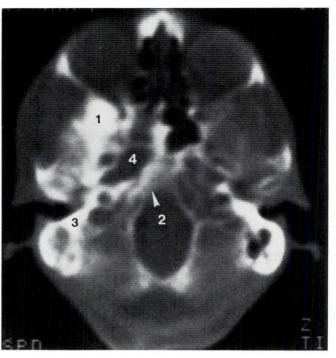

Fig. 3.2 Carcinoma nasopharynx, transverse scan before infusion. Reactive sclerosis of the sphenoid bone (1) clivus (2) and temporal bone (3) is due to carcinoma. Some bone destruction (4), petrous apex and sphenoid bone is also present. This sixty-two year old woman had been unable to oper her mouth for six months. She was found to have an ulceration of her gums which was biopsied and proved to be squamous cell carcinoma. It had been diagnosed as a primary tumor of the maxillary sinus before CT demonstrated it to be of the nasopharynx.

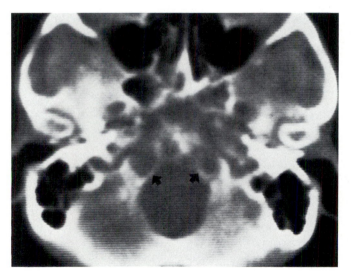

Fig. 3.3 Nasopharyngeal carcinoma, transverse scan before infusion. Destruction of the clivus back to and including the hypoglossal canals (arrows) is due to carcinoma. Ulceration of the mucosa was seen; no soft tissue mass was noted. The patient presented with dysphagia and was found to have bilateral atrophy due to involvement of both hypoglossal nerves.

Chapter 4 Infratemporal Fossa

Normal Anatomy

The boundaries and content of the infratemporal fossa (52) were inaccessible to radiographic imaging prior to the advent of CT scanning. Now it is possible to study this region in detail (Fig. 4.1–4.3).

The Boundaries of the infratemporal fossa

a) Superior: sphenoid bone, floor of the middle cranial fossa.
b) Anterior: pterygoid plates, spheno-palatine fossa, posterior wall maxillary sinus, nasal cavity.
c) Lateral: mandibular condyle, coronoid process and ramus, parotid gland.
d) Posterior: deep portion of parotid gland, posterior belly of the digastric muscle, styloid process, stylopharyngeal aponeurosis, the stylopharyngeal, stylohyoid, and styloglossus muscles.
e) Medial: clivus, nasopharynx.

The pharyngobasilar fascia is a membrane enclosing the nasopharyngeal structures and is contiguous with the pterygomandibular ligament (52). Portions of the superior pharyngeal constrictor and buccinator muscles arise from this ligament whereas the middle pharyngeal constrictor arises from the stylohyoid ligament. The stylopharyngeus muscle noted above passes from the styloid process to the thyroid cartilage whereas the stylohyoid muscle passes to the hyoid bone and the styloglossus muscle to the side of the tongue.

The contents of the infratemporal fossa

Muscles

1) Temporalis muscle insertion on the coronoid process of the mandible;
2) Lateral pterygoid muscle origin with lower and upper heads attached to the lateral border of the lateral pterygoid plate and to the greater wing of the sphenoid bone respectively; insertion on the capsule of the temporomandibular ligament and the neck of the condyle;
3) Medial pterygoid muscle (more caudad) origin from the medial surface of the lateral pterygoid plate, insertion on the ramus and angle of the mandible;
4) The superior pharyngeal constrictor origin from the medial pterygoid plate, pterygoid hamulus and the pterygomandibular ligament, interlaces with the tongue;

5) Tensor veli palatini from the greater wing of the sphenoid immediately lateral to the eustachian tube, passes anteriorly and inferiorly to join its counterpart on the palate (increase tension during swallowing);
6) Levator veli palatini origin medial to the eustachian tube and from the apex of the petrous temporal bone, decends vertically to the palatal aponeurosis (raises the soft palate during swallowing).

Vessels and Nerves

1) Mandibular division of the trigeminal nerve
The auriculotemporal nerve arises from the mandibular nerve passing to the temporo-mandibular joint, tympanic membrane of the ear and preauricular and auricular skin (source of referred otalgia from the infratemporal fossa and teeth). The lingual and inferior alveolar nerves also arise from this mandibular division as do the branches to the pterygoid muscles.
2) Otic ganglion-lesser superficial petrosal nerve to the parotid gland;
3) Chorda tympani nerve through the petro-tympanic fissure lateral to the tensor palatini, to the submandibular and sublingual glands, and to the anterior two-thirds of the tongue;
4) Internal maxillary artery and branches (deep auricular, anterior tympanic, middle meningeal, accessory meningeal, inferior alveolar);
5) Pterygoid venous plexus to the maxillary vein. The carotid sheath containing the internal carotid artery and internal jugular vein are within the retro-styloid space abutting but separated from the infratemporal fossa by the styloid "diaphragm" (an aponeurotic sheet of the pharyngobasilar fascia passing from the pharyngeal wall to the styloid process and its muscles). This space also contains the superior sympathetic ganglion of the cervical chain as well as cranial nerves 9–12.

Deep-seated pain, either in the lower jaws, the ear or the temporo-mandibular joint may be the only symptom of an abnormality of the infratemporal fossa. Infection or tumor of this area or spasm of the pterygoid muscles impedes normal motion of the mandible. Identification of the specific abnormality requires CT scanning.

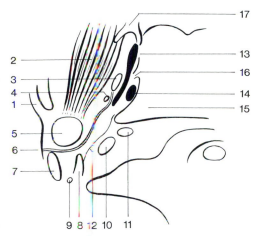

Fig. 4.**1**   Diagram of infratemporal fossa.
1) Zygomatic arch (1), lateral pterygoid m. (2), F. ovale (3), F. spinosum (4), condylar fossa (5), auriculotemporal nerve (6), external auditory canal (7), styloid process (8), stylomastoid foramen (9), internal jugular vein (10), internal carotid artery (11), styloid diaphragm (12), tensor palatini m. (13), levator palatini m. (14), fossa of Rosenmüller (15), orifice eustachian tube (16), pterygoid plates (17).

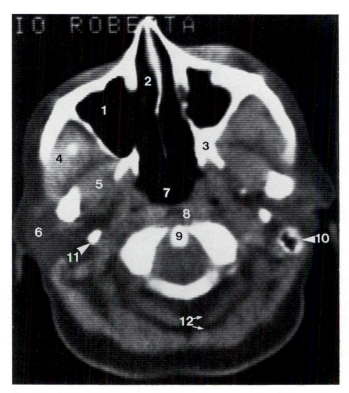

Fig. 4.**2**   Normal infratemporal fossa, transverse scan before infusion. Note the maxillary sinus (1) nasal cavity (2), pterygoid plate (3), temporalis muscle (4) around coronoid process, lateral pterygoid muscle (5), parotid gland (6), nasopharynx (7), longus capitis muscle (8), dens (9), mastoid tip (10) styloid process (11), splenius and semispinalis capitis (12). The carotid sheath containing the internal carotid artery, internal jugular vein, and cranial nerves 9–12 are medial to the styloid process.

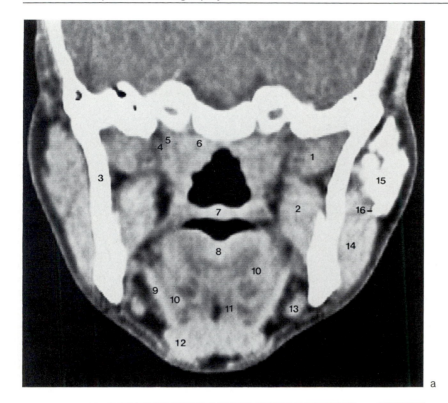

a

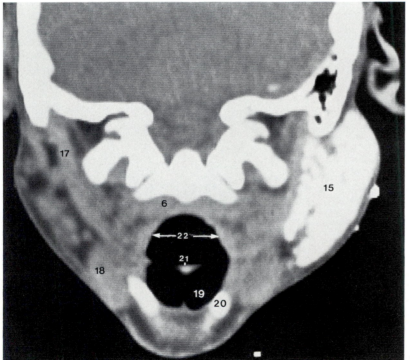

b

Fig. 4.**3**   Normal infratemporal fossa, pharynx and tongue, coronal scans after sialography (a) is anterior to (b). These show the lateral pterygoid muscle (1), medial pterygoid muscle (2), mandible (3), tensor (4), and levator palatine (5), longus capitus (6), soft palate (7), intrinsic tongue muscles-superior, longitudinal, and transverse (8), myelohyoid (9), hyoglossus, styloglossus (10), geniohyoid (11), anterior belly of digastric (12), submental a. & v. (13), masseter muscle (14), parotid (15), Stenson's duct (16), posterior belly of digastric (b 17), submandibular gland (b 18), vallecula (b 19), hyoid bone (b 20), epiglottis (b 21), pharyngeal constrictor (b 22).

Abnormal

Infection as well as both benign and malignant tumors of the infratemporal fossa are manifested by obliteration of the normal soft tissue planes and/or by a mass effect (10).

Clinical evaluation is necessary to distinguish between infection and tumor, whereas differentation between benign and malignant neoplasms often requires a biopsy, Table II lists the more common types of tumors encountered in the infratemporal fossa and in the nasopharynx.

Tumors in these areas are difficult to assess clinically. Otalgia might be the initial symptom with pain along the lower jaw indicating involvement of the mandibular nerve. Invasion of the pterygoid muscles causes trismus. Extension of tumor to the skull base may affect multiple cranial nerves. Although infection tends to be limited to the various compartments as described under the discussion of normal anatomy (see above), tumors may encroach on or invade adjacent compartments with eventual bone erosion resulting from tumor expansion.

CT is the procedure of choice for determining the total soft tissue involvement, the degree of bone destruction and the intra-orbital (Fig. 4.4–4.6) or intracranial extension. This technique also defines the precise relationship

Table II   More Common Tumors of the Infratemporal Fossa (Random Order)

Benign
  Neurilemmoma or Schwannoma
  Hemangioma and arteriovenous malformation
  Salivary gland tumor

Malignant
  Carcinoma
  Sarcoma
  Lymphoepithelioma
  Lymphoma
  Metastatic CA
  Adenoid cystic carcinoma (cylindroma)

of the tumor to adjacent structures (e.g. spine, parotid gland, etc.). Primary and metastatic tumors extend into the infratemporal fossa from adjacent structures such as the mandible, sphenoid bone, clivus, temporal bone (including the ear, external auditory canal, jugular fossa), etc. These malignant masses are most readily identified by CT with or without intravenous contrast enhancement.

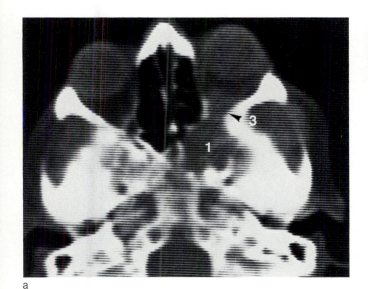

a

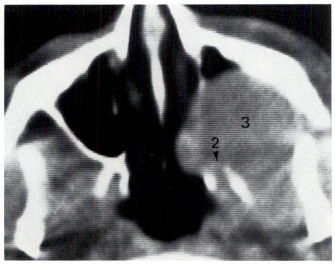

b

Fig. 4.4   Schwannoma Vth nerve, transverse scans before infusion. (a) is cephalad to (b). This patient was diagnosed as having trigeminal neuralgia and was admitted for electrocoagulation. She had been known to have an opaque sinus for years, diagnosed as

"chronic sinusitis". CT revealed destruction of sphenoid bone (1), pterygoid bone (2), and a soft tissue mass (3) of the infratemporal fossa extending into the orbit.

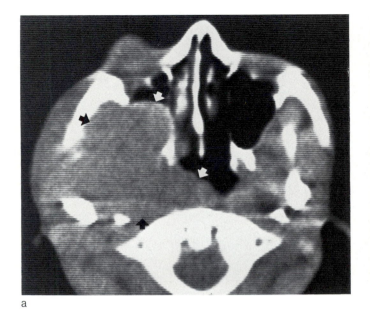

a

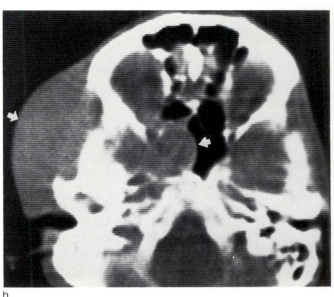

b

Fig. 4.**5** Infratemporal fossa sarcoma, transverse scan before infusion. (a is caudad to b). This twenty month old male had headache, nausea and vomiting with progressive cranial nerve signs on the right (2–7). He developed a cavernous sinus syndrome but had a negative angiogram, pneumoencephalogram and middle cranial fossa exploration. The CT scan performed post-operatively revealed a mass (arrows) arising a) from the right infratemporal fossa extending into the nasopharynx and maxillary sinus and b) into the sphenoid sinus and retro-orbital area. Soft tissue swelling laterally is post-op change. (From: Computer Assisted Tomography, Vol. 1, 1977, Hammerschlag, Wolpert & Carter-Computed Tomography of the Skull Base).

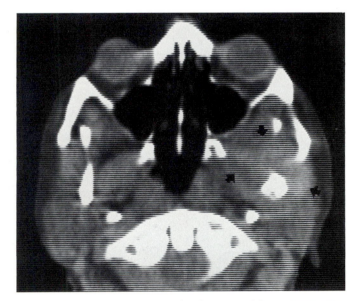

Fig. 4.**6**   Metastatic carcinoma left infratemporal fossa, transverse scan before infusion. Tumor mass (arrows) is obliterating the normal muscle planes of the left infratemporal fossa. Only irregularity of the condylar neck could be seen on plain films and conventional tomograms. This was proven to be metastatic bronchogenic carcinoma.

Chapter 5   Nasopharynx, Nasal Cavity, and Paranasal Sinuses

Normal Anatomy

The air-containing cavity of the nasopharynx is symmetrical and is adjacent to the base of the skull (unless there is residual adenoid tissue) as well as to the first and second cervical vertebrae. Parallel muscle bundles, the longus capitus and longus colli, are found between the airway and the spine (Fig. 5.1). The pharyngeal recess or fossa of Rosenmüller extends anteromedial to the internal carotid artery and internal jugular vein and reaches as far as the petrosphenoid angle, between the spine of the sphenoid and the petrous portion of the temporal bone. The anterolateral portion of this recess is bordered by the cartilaginous portion of the eustachian tube, visualized in the pharynx as the torus tubarius (7, 13). The pharyngeal opening of the eustachian tube is clearly visible anterior to the torus tubarius.

The tympanic end is seen as a thin triangular air-containing structure extending anteriorly and inferiorly from the tympanic cavity. The major portion of the eustachian tube is not air-containing and thus not normally visualized on the CT image. The average length of the tube is 37 mm (52), the medial 2/3rds being cartilaginous, the lateral 1/3rd osseous. Opening of the eustachian tube, a function of the tensor palati muscle, occurs with swallowing, yawning, and sneezing. The tensor palati originates from the lateral aspect of the pterygoid plate, the spine of the sphenoid bone and lateral aspect of the eustachian tube. It is triangular at its origin but narrows to a slender tendon which winds around the lateral surface of the pterygoid hamulus to insert on the posterior border of the hard palate and the aponeurosis of the soft palate. It fuses with the aponeurosis of the opposite side, tensing and flattening the soft palate during swallowing. The levator palati elevates the palate, passing from the medial portion of the eustachian tube and the petrous apex to the palatine aponeurosis. Pliability of the structures in the nasopharynx can be ascertained by scanning during various maneuvers such as the Valsalva and the Meuller (41).

The most cephalic portion of the maxillary sinus is visible just below the floor of the orbit and lateral to the nasal cavity. The floor of this sinus can often be seen extending inferiorly into the alveolar process of the maxilla at the level of the palate. The frontal, supra-orbital, ethmoid, and sphenoid sinuses are all clearly seen on more cephalic cuts through and just above the skull base (23, 31). The nasal cavity, septum and tubinates are visible throughout their length.

The masseter muscle, originating from the zygomatic arch, inserts on the lateral aspect of the ramus and body of the mandible. The zygomaticus muscle, originating from the zygoma, has an oblique course antero-inferiorly and can be seen below the zygomatic arch, anterolateral to the masseter muscle to its insertion at the angle of the mouth. It should not be mistaken for Stenson's duct which is close to the masseter muscle and is best seen after sialography. The buccinator muscle originates from the maxilla, inserting on the mandible, and is thus seen immediately lateral to the alveolar process of the maxilla. The orbicularis oris muscles are seen anteriorly, as is the angular or anterior facial vein.

The lymph nodes in the area are divided into the superficial and deep cervical group.

a) The superficial nodes include the occipital, the retroauricular, the parotid (imbeded within the gland), the buccal, submandibular, submental and anterior cervical as well as superficial nodes along the external jugular vein and the sternocleidomastoid muscle.

b) Deep cervical nodes are closely associated with the carotid sheath.

1. Superior – upper part of the internal jugular vein, deep to the sternocleidomastoid muscle and the jugulodigastric group in the triangle between the posterior belly of the digastric, the facial vein and the internal jugular vein.

2. Inferior deep cervical group: deep to the sternocleidomastoid muscle in the subclavian triangle related to the subclavian vessels and the brachial plexus.

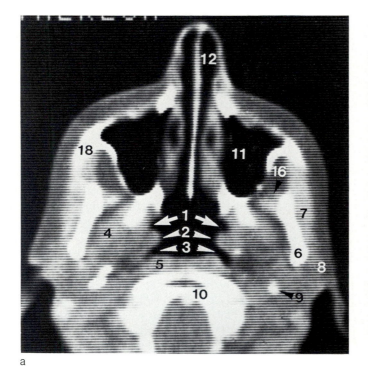

a

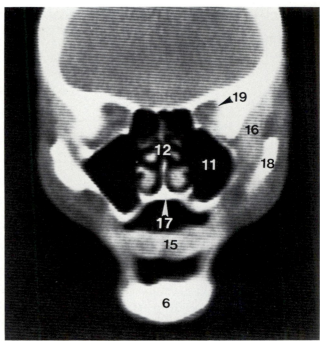

b

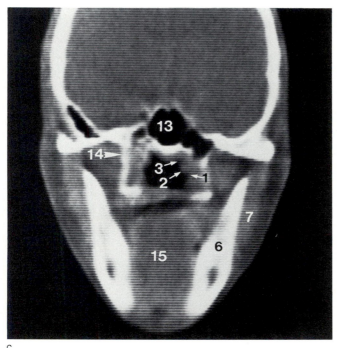

c

Fig. 5.1 Normal sinuses, nasopharynx (a) transverse scan (b) coronal scan of maxillary sinus and (c) coronal scan of sphenoid sinus and nasopharynx. Clearly seen are: orifice eustachian tube (1), torus tubarius (2), pharyngeal recess (3) medial pterygoid muscle (4), longus capitis (5), mandible (6), masseter muscle (7), parotid gland (8), styloid process (9), C-1 (10), maxillary sinus (11), nasal cavity (12), sphenoid sinus (13), pterygoid plate (14), tongue (15), temporalis muscle (16), hard palate (17), zygoma (18) and apex of orbit with optic nerve (19).

Abnormal

Development

CT scanning provides the most complete, noninvasive technique for the diagnosis of complicated or serious disease in the nasopharynx, nasal cavity and paranasal sinuses (5, 6). Developmental anomalies such as hypoplasia, hyperplasia, and the varying degrees of pneumatization of the sinuses are clearly seen with a plain film examination and with CT (Fig. 5.2). The diagnosis of an encephalocele, however, requires sharp definition of the defect in the sphenoid, ethmoid, or frontal bone and identification of the soft tissue mass. This is all within the realm of the CT scan (Fig. 5.3). The sac and its contents as well as any associated change or deformity of the intracranial structures can be identified by Metrizamide cisternography with CT.

Soft tissue densities, such as fluid retention within a turbinate (Fig. 5.4) may simulate an encephalocele except for the lack of the bony anomaly associated with the latter. Cysts arising from embryonic cell rests (e. g. Thornwaldt cyst) appear as mid-line soft tissue masses; para-pharyngeal or retention cysts appear as mid-line or more lateral soft tissue masses. The density of the mass, or the relative absorption coefficient, varies with the protein content of the cystic fluid. Adenoid tissue appears as a solid mass and is common in young adults as well as in children.

A mass effect can be simulated by paresis or paralysis of the pharyngeal muscles (Fig. 5.5). Good clinical correlation is necessary for the identification of paralysis and/or atrophy to differentiate functional abnormalities from tumor.

Trauma

CT is effectively used for the documentation of fractures of the facial bones and sinuses (Fig. 5.6). In patients with facial injuries associated with head trauma, CT is used for the demonstration of intracranial hemtomas. As indicated earlier, inclusion of the facial area at the time of the initial head scan may save the patient from additional studies (15). Various projections (AP, lateral, base) of thin section tomography may still be required at a later date for more precise delineation of the fracture fragments associated with blow-out injuries to the orbit, tripod injuries, LeForte I, II, and III fractures, etc. Preliminary assessment of the various deformities at the time of the head scan is important in the planning for overall patient care. CT combined with Metrizamide is recommended for the detection of CSF leaks due to trauma.

Infection

Chronic inflammatory diseases often associated with sclerosis of bone, particularly in the sinuses and infratemporal fossa (Fig. 5.7). Wegener's granulomatosis and midline lethal granulomatosis are usually aggressive, causing extensive destruction. Other infectious agents may be more chronic, causing reactive sclerosis, osteomyelitis and even sequestration. Mucormycosis must be considered to be a possible causative agent, particularly in diabetics. TB, actinomycosis, sarcoidosis and many other organisms have been incriminated in infections of this area. The accompanying diffuse soft tissue change with and adjacent to the paranasal sinuses are visible on CT. This is the best method for evaluating the total extent of severe infections and any subsequent complications.

Many patients may present initially with one or more of these complications which are found incidentally to be due to an unexpected sinusitis (38). Severe complications of sinusitis include: osteomyelitis, meningitis, epidural and intracerebral abscess, cavernous sinus thrombosis, intra-orbital infection and extension of the infection to the infratemporal fossa.

Benign Tumor

Differentiation between a mucocele (Fig. 5.8) and a benign, slowly growing tumor is possible with CT. Although mucoceles occur primarily in the frontal sinuses, they may arise in any of the sinuses (Fig. 5.9) and are usually spontaneous in origin, but may develop after trauma. They tend to be less dense than adjacent soft tissue structures due to the relatively lower absorption coefficient but have been reported as equal to or of greater density than adjacent soft tissue structures. An infected mucocele (pyocele) may have a high protein content and thus appear equal to or more dense than a solid tumor mass and may have an enhancing wall.

Mucoceles and benign tumors tend to expand the area of origin by their slow growth (17, 60, 61). The gradual pressure of the enlarging soft tissue mass pushes bone before it. This displacement and/or destruction of bone is visible on the CT image as well as the conventional tomograms. Mucoceles may extend into the orbit from the frontal and ethmoid sinuses or intracranially from the sphenoid sinus (49).

Intravenous contrast infusion is indicated for the identification of vascular tumors such as angiofibromas (18, 65), which do enhance. Although benign, they destroy bone, invade the sinuses (Fig. 5.10), and sometimes extend into the intracranial cavity via the neural foramina, carotid canal, etc. The latter circumstance may be discernible only by CT, as is also the case with other vascular tumors arising from the paranasal sinuses, nasal cavity, nasopharynx and infratemporal fossa such as Schwannoma, paraganglioma, etc. Benign avascular tumors such as reparative granuloma, papilloma (40), adenoma, fibroma, etc., should also be considered in the differential diagnosis (Table III).

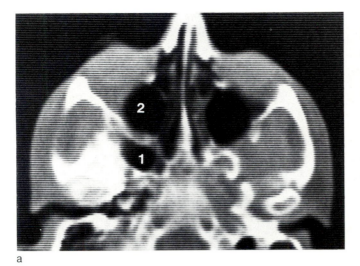

a

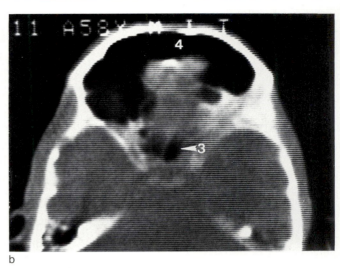

b

Fig. 5.2 Variation of normal, transverse scans before infusion. a) Lateral recess of sphenoid sinus (1) posterior to the maxillary sinus (2) near the floor of the orbit. b) Large supraorbital cells.

Pneumatization of the tuberculum sella (3) and large frontal sinuses (4) with supraorbital extension.

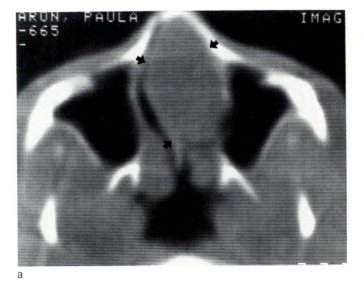

a

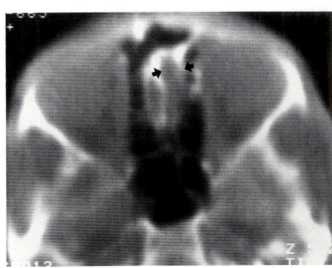

b

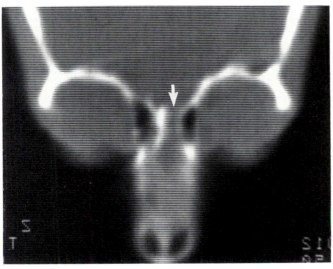

c

Fig. 5.3 Encephalocele through left cribiform plate a) transverse scan through nasal cavity, b) transverse scan through cribiform plate, c) coronal scan, all before infusion. A large soft tissue mass (arrows) left nasal cavity (a) is associated with a defect in the cribiform plate (arrows) seen in (b) transverse and (c) coronal plane. Relative absorption value is 21 H.

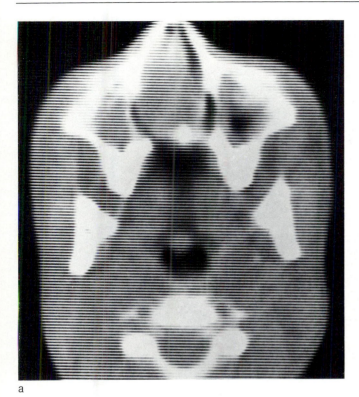

a

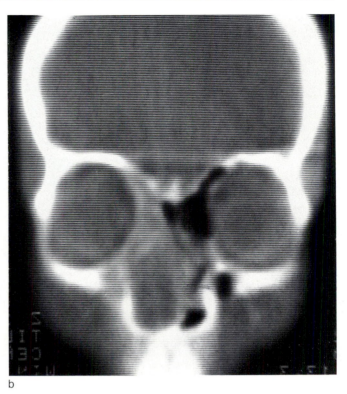

b

Fig. 5.4 Fluid filled turbinate occluding nasal cavity, (a) transverse and (b) coronal scan before infusion, simulating an encephalocele. Ethmoid bone is intact and olfactory portion of nasal cavity is clear. Relative absorption value of soft tissue mass is 7 H. Right ethmoid air cells are opaque (b).

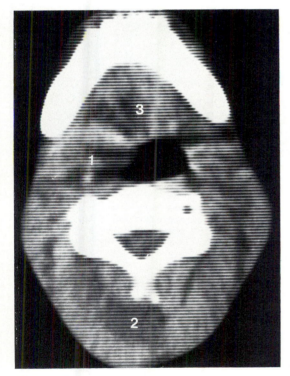

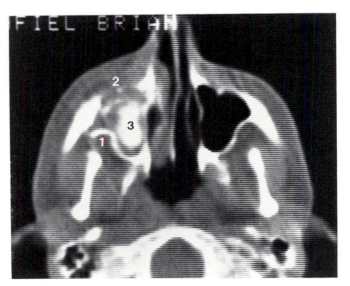

Fig. 5.5 Paresis right oropharynx and infection neck, posteriorly, transverse scan before infusion. A pseudomass is simulated by paresis of the right oropharynx (1) in a patient with mastoiditis. Infection between the deep and superficial neck muscles (2) occurred via the sigmoid sinus and mastoid emissary vein. Artifacts over tongue (3) are due to motion. (From: Seminars in Roentgenology, Vol. 13, 1978, Carter & Karmody-Computed Tomography of the Face & Neck).

Fig. 5.6 Fracture and calcified hematoma right maxillary sinus, transverse scan before infusion. Fractures are present lateral (1) and anterior (2) walls. Increased density within the sinus is attributed to calcified hematoma (3). Relative absorption value is 473 H.

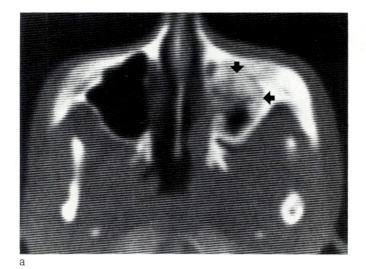

a

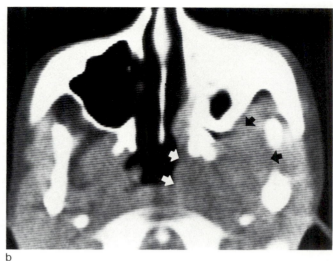

b

Fig. 5.**7** Chronic sinusitis, transverse scan before infusion, a) bone technique, b) soft tissue technique, (a) Extensive reactive sclerosis (arrows) of the left maxillary sinus and (b) diffuse inflam-matory reaction (arrows) of the infratemporal fossa and nasopharynx is present in a patient with leukemia of the sinus and superimposed pseudomonas infection.

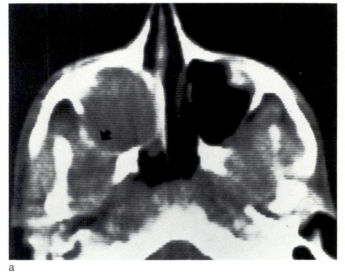

a

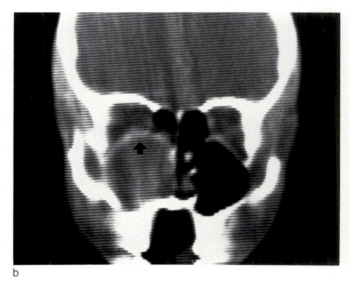

b

Fig. 5.**8** Mucocele maxillary sinus a) transverse and b) coronal scans after infusion. Expansion of the sinus is evident in the transverse (a) and coronal (b) planes. Admitting diagnosis was tumor of the maxillary sinus. Patient had had swelling of the right cheek for one month, a "clogged feeling" of the right nostril and a history of nose bleeds. The right intraocular pressure was found to be elevated. An avascular, slowly expanding cystic mass was found by CT. (From: Seminars in Roentgenology, Vol. 13, 1978, Carter & Karmody-Computed Tomography of the Face & Neck).

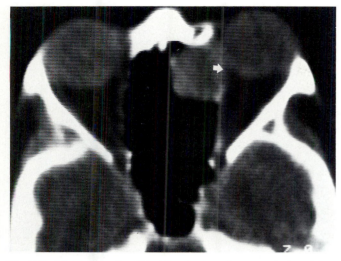

Fig. 5.9   Mucocele ethmoid sinus, transverse scan before infusion. There is erosion of the medial wall of the orbit (arrow) displacing the medial rectus muscle and the globe.

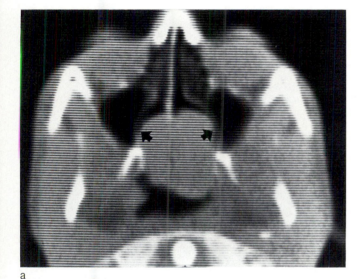

a

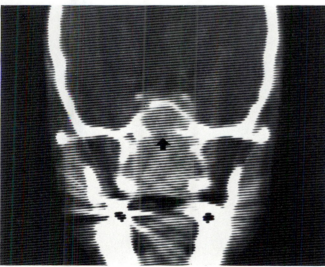

b

Table III   More Common Tumors of the Nasopharynx, Nasal Cavity, and Paranasal Sinuses (Random Order)

Benign
Encephalocele, glioma
Dermoid, Teratoma
Hamartoma
Thornwaldt cyst (notocord remnant)
Inclusion cyst
Mucous retention cyst
Branchial cleft cyst
Nasoalveolar cyst
Antral Choanal polyp
Inverted papilloma
Benign adenoma
Angiofibroma
Hemangioma
Arteriovenous fistulae
Lymphangioma
Histiocytosis
Neurogenic tumor (neurofibroma, neurilemmoma)
Salivary gland tumor (Warthins, oncocytoma)
Fibroma, desmoid tumor
Lipoma
Chondroma
Osteoma
Reparative granuloma
Dentigerous cyst
Odontoma
Ameloblastoma
Rhinolith

Malignant
Carcinoma (epidermoid, adenocarcinoma, anaplastic)
Sarcoma (melanoma, neurosarcoma, rhabdomyosarcoma, spindle cell sarcoma, fibrosarcoma, etc.)
Malignant histiocytoma
Hemangiopericytoma
Esthesioneuroblastoma
Malignant tumor of salivary gland origin
Lymphoma
Plasmacytoma
Metastatic carcinoma
Chordoma

Extension of tumors from intracranial cavity to nasopharynx
Craniopharyngioma
Chromophobe adenoma
Meningioma
Neurinoma, paraganglioma from jugular fossa
Tumors from tympanic cavity, external auditory canal

◀ Fig. 5.10   Angiofibroma, a) transverse and b) coronal scan after infusion. The tumor, which enhances after infusion, is a) displacing the medial walls of the maxillary sinuses and b) invading the sphenoid sinus (arrow). The tumor decreased slightly in size after a course of estrogen therapy. This thirteen year old boy had had a stuffy nose for one year but no nosebleeds. Artifacts on (b) are due to dental fillings.

Malignant tumor

The major contribution of CT to the evaluation of disorders of the nasopharyngeal area, however, is in the assessment of primary and metastatic tumors (Table III) (37, 50, 68). The nasopharynx, in particular, is often difficult to assess clinically. Patients may, for example, present with such occult findings as a fluid filled middle ear cavity due to obstruction of the pharyngeal orifice of the eustachian tube (Fig. 5.11). Paresis of the tongue may be the only manifestation of an invasive nasopharyngeal tumor eroding the hypoglossal canal (Fig. 3.3). Tumors of the nasopharynx, nasal cavity and paranasal sinuses destroy bone, invade adjacent soft tissue structures (Fig. 5.12–5.15) and extend into the orbit causing proptosis, diplopia and pain. These tumors also extend intracranially resulting in varied neurological defects.

Carcinoma is the most common type of malignancy, but the final diagnosis can only be made after biopsy (Table III). The type of tumor may be characterized by its location (19, 20, 42) degree of vascularity, etc. For instance, an esthesioneuroblastoma (54) or olfactory neuroblastoma arises from the olfactory mucosa of the nasal cavity immediately below the cribiform plate. This tumor tends to extend into the ethmoid and sphenoid sinuses, the orbit and intracranial cavity. Tumors arising from adjacent areas such as neurilemmomas and paragangliomas of the jugular fossa, chromophobe adenomas, craniopharyngiomas, etc. may first become manifest in the nasopharynx (see Table III).

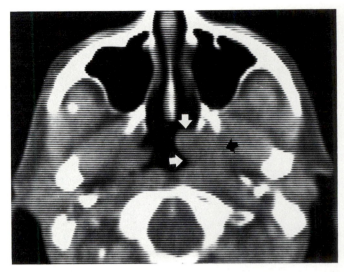

Fig. 5.**11**   Mass left nasopharynx, transverse scan before infusion. Patient presented with fluid in the left tympanic cavity, due to obstruction of the eustachian tube by a mass effect (arrows) lateral wall of the nasopharynx. This was apparently inflammatory since it resolved to normal at a later date. (From: Seminars in Roentgenology, Vol. 13, 1978, Carter & Karmody-Computed Tomography of the Face & Neck).

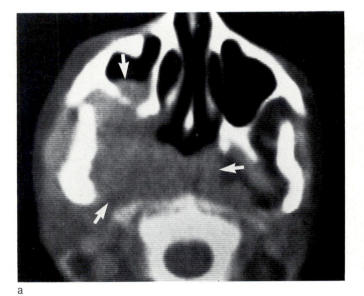

a

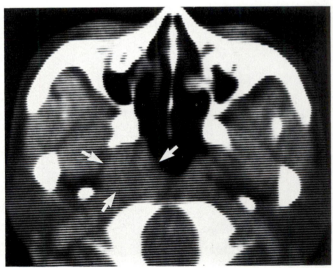

b

Fig. 5.**12**   Carcinoma nasopharynx, transverse scans before infusion. Two cases: a) large mass (arrows) involving the infratemporal fossa and extending forward to the maxillary sinus and b) smaller, more subtle tumor invading the lateral wall (arrows) and extending posteriorly. (From: Seminars in Roentgenology, Vol. 13, 1978, Carter & Karmody-Computed Tomography of the Face & Neck).

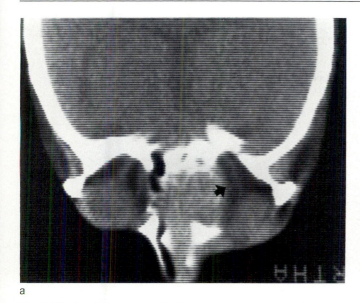

a

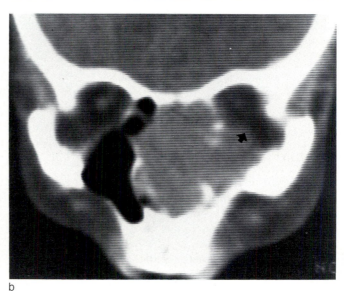

b

Fig. 5.**13**   Carcinoma nasal cavity eroding through into the orbit (arrow), causing proptosis. Transverse (a) and coronal (b) scans before infusion show (a) the tumor, the globe and optic nerve and

(b) the apex of the orbit, optic nerve and tumor extension from nasal cavity. (From: Seminars in Roentgenology, Vol. 13, 1978, Carter & Karmody-Computed Tomography of the Face & Neck).

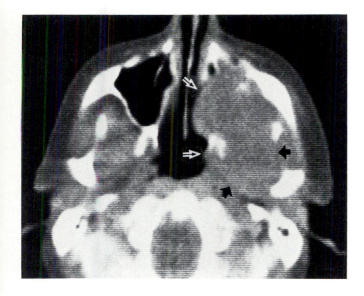

Fig. 5.**14**   Poorly differentiated histiocytic lymphoma left maxillary sinus, transverse scan before infusion. Extensive bone destruction is due to large mass (arrows) extending into the infratemporal fossa back to the styloid process and encroaching on the lateral wall of the nasopharynx. Patient had had a testicular tumor, resected in 1970, which had been called seminoma but in retrospect was considered to be a histiocytic lymphoma also. (From: Advances in Oto-Rhino-Laryngology, Vol. 24, 1978, Carter, Hammerschlag & Wolpert-Computerized Scanning in Otorhinolaryngology).

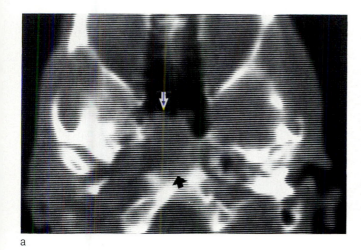

a

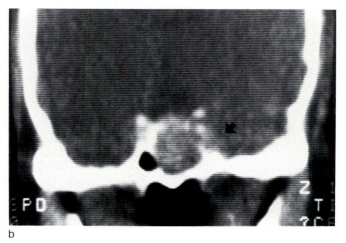

b

Fig. 5.**15**   Myeloma sphenoid sinus, a) transverse and b) coronal scans after infusion. There is destruction of the clivus (arrow) seen

with the transverse scan and extension laterally to the cavernous sinus (arrow) apparent on the coronal image.

Chapter 6   Oropharynx and Mandible

Normal Anatomy

The superior pharyngeal constrictor, levator veli palatini, and tensor veli palatini muscles originate from the skull base anterior and posterior to the orifice of the eustachian tube, partially surround the oropharynx and blend into the soft palate (Fig. 4.2, 4.3, 6.1). The medial pterygoid muscle, which inserts on the ramus of the mandible, is quite distinct. The soft and hard palates are seen, limited laterally by the alveolar process of the maxilla. The maxilla sinus, if large, may extend into the alveolar process. The facial, masseter, and pharyngeal muscles have been described in the previous section. The ramus, angle, body and symphysis of the mandible are seen at different levels. The mandibular nerve is found in a groove along the medial surface of the ramus of the mandible. The facial vein is usually seen anterior and inferior to the maxilla.

The muscles of the tongue are divided into two groups, the extrinsic and the intrinsic. The former have attachments outside the tongue and include the genioglossus, hyoglossus, styloglossus, chondroglossus, and palatoglossus. Some of these muscles can be identified on the CT scan just above the anterior belly of the digastric which inserts on the mandible near the symphysis. The genioglossus, an extrinsic muscle, is triangular in shape and arises from the inner surface of the symphysis. It spreads out in a fan-like form to the ventral surface of the tongue intermingling with the intrinsic muscles. The hyoglossus and chondroglossus are thin, quadrilateral muscles arising from the hyoid bone extending to the side of the tongue.

The styloglossus passes from the styloid process to the side of the tongue. These extrinsic muscles are separated from the intrinsic muscles by a median raphe and are often visible on the CT image.

The muscles below the tongue, forming the floor of the mouth are as follows: The myelohyoid muscle, a sling along the inferior aspect of the tongue passes from each side of the mandible to the hyoid bone, thus forming the muscular floor of of the oral cavity. The geniohyoid is a narrow muscle above the myelohyoid which passes from the symphysis of the mandible to the hyoid bone occasionally fusing with the genioglossus. The anterior belly of the digastric, immediately inferior to the myelohyoid is often seen on the transverse and coronal images as it passes from the hyoid bone to the symphysis. The stylohyoid is lateral in position, passing from the styloid process to the hyoid bone. In summary, the muscles of the tongue are divided into an intrinsic and extrinsic group as follows:

Intrinsic:
    Superior longitudinal
    Inferior longitudinal
    Transverse
    Vertical

Extrinsic:
    Genioglossus
    Hyoglossus
    Styloglossus
    Chondroglossus
    Palatoglossus

Beneath the tongue, along the floor of the mouth are found:
    Geniohyoid
    Myelohyoid
    Anterior belly of the digastric
    Stylohyoid

The aperture, communicating the mouth with the pharynx (the isthmus faucium) is bounded by the palate, the glossopalatine arch and the dorsum of the tongue. The glossopalatine arch is formed by the glossopalatinus muscle anteriorly and by the pharyngopalatinus posteriorly.

Abnormal

Congenital anomalies, developmental variations, infection, trauma, and tumor in this area are usually adequately evaluated by clinical examination, plain films and a barium swallow. However, CT occasionally provides additional important information. Limitations of space restrict adequate discussion and illustration of the various congenital anomalies, cysts, benign and malignant tumors that occur in the oropharynx, mandible and neck. The reader is referred to the literature (2, 52), for a more comprehensive review of this area.

Cystic lesions, infections, abscess cavities, hematomas and certain benign tumors may be specifically identified and localized by CT. Branchial cleft cysts often occur from a line extending from the skin in the lower neck through the carotid bifurcation to the upper tonsillar fossa. These lesions often present with signs and symptoms of acute inflammation, usually originate from the second branchial cleft or groove, and should be differentiated from a cystic hygroma, a multiloculated fluid containing structure of lymphatic origin. The latter are thin walled, irregular, lobulated and are often asymptomatic; they may become enlarged or regress over a period of time and are most commonly seen in the neck. The absorption coefficient of these and other cystic structures tends to be low (0 to 20H) but may vary depending upon the protein content. Thyroglossal duct cysts are usually midline and subcutaneous in location (2).

CT is particularly useful for the identification of lipomas and liposarcomas and for the determination of the total extent of deep-seated malignant tumors. This is especially true for lesions of the retro-molar trigone and the palatine fossa (Fig. 6.2). Since the various muscle groups of the tongue and sublingual area can now be identified, the CT scan is a valuable tool in planning the surgical approach or radiotherapy treatment.

Tumors of the mandible are usually confined to bone, but extension deep into adjacent soft tissue structures (i.e. oropharynx, infratemporal fossa) may occur (Fig. 4.6). Knowledge of the total extent of a tumor is important to the clinician in the determination of the optimum therapeutic approach.

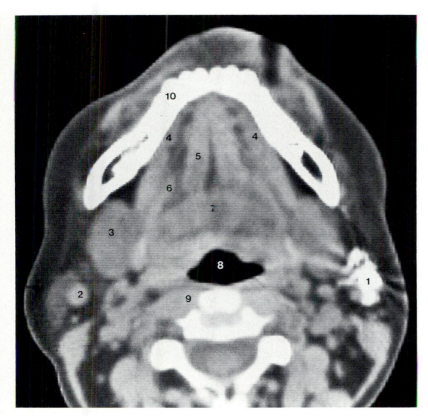

Fig. 6.1 Normal oropharynx, transverse scan after intravenous infusion and sialography. The tip of the parotid gland (1) is overlying the lateral facial vein (2) and both are posterolateral to the submandibular gland (3). The myelohyoid (4) arising from the mandible bilaterally to insert on the hyoid bone forms the muscular floor for the oral cavity. The geniohyoid (5) immediately above the medial border of the myelohyoid passes from the symphysis of the mandible down to the hyoid bone. The hyoglossus and styloglossus (6) are along the lateral border of the tongue. These extrinsic muscles interlace with the intrinsic (7) muscles of the tongue. The pharyngeal constrictors encompass the airway (8). The longus colli muscles (9) are anterior to the spine, retropharyngeal in location. The body and symphysis of the mandible (10) are clearly seen.

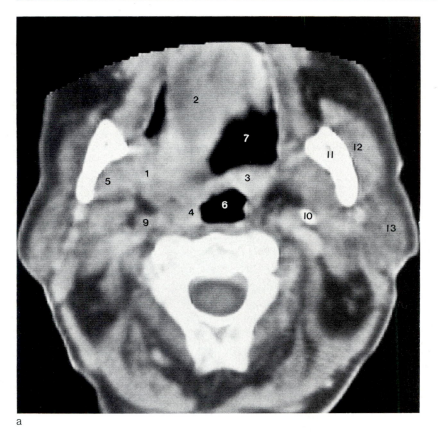

a

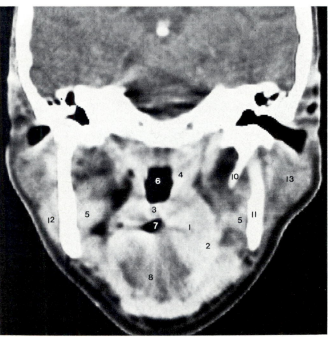

b

Fig. 6.2 Carcinoma of the palatine fossa and tongue a) transverse and b) coronal plane after intravenous infusion. The tumor (1) extends from the posterolateral aspect of the tongue (2) to the soft palate (3), the tensor and levator palatini (4), and toward the medial pterygoid (5). Air is seen in the nasopharynx (6) and oropharynx (7). The anterior and deep portions of the tongue (8) are free of tumor. The structures within the carotid sheath (9), the internal carotid A, internal jugular V, and cranial nerves 9–12, seen medial to the styloid process (10) are close to but free from the tumor. Other structures clearly seen are: ramus of mandible (11) masseter muscle (12) and the parotid (13).

Chapter 7 Conclusions

CT scanning has made major contributions to the diagnosis and treatment of various disease entities involving the skull base, sinuses, infratemporal fossa, pharynx, larynx, and neck. It is of particular value to these areas because of its unique sensitivity in the identification of various soft tissue structures and for the measurement of their relative absorption coefficients. CT also reveals the degree of involvement of bone and extension of masses through bone to the orbit and intracranial fossa.

Generally speaking, the computed tomography technique is indicated in specific problem cases:

1) Identification of congenital anomalies or developmental variations which require clarification;
2) Assessment of abscesses, hematomas, or fractures;
3) Evaluation of patients in whom a tumor is suspected;
4) As an aid in choosing and planning an appropriate mode of therapy (e. g. deciding between surgery and radiotherapy);
5) For follow-up evaluation (e. g., to determine recurrence of tumor after surgery, response to radiotherapy or response to chemotherapy);
6) Assistance in the biopsy of problem cases.

Acknowledgements

The author wishes to acknowledge with sincere appreciation the advice and recommendations of Samuel M. Wolpert, M. D., Chief of the Section of Neuroradiology and for his permission to use some of the material in this chapter. Deep gratitude is also expressed to Werner Chasin, M. D. and Collin Karmody, M. D. both of the Department of Otolaryngology, for reviewing the chapter and for their assistance in the revision and reorganization of this material. The author is also most grateful to Ms. Patricia Butler and Mrs. Eleanor Markham for their hard work and unlimited patience in retyping the manuscript with each revision and to Ms. Linda Nevins for her editorial assistance in the final writing and in the labeling of the prints. Mrs. Barbara Billings deserves a most sincere thank you for all her help in many areas in the preparation of this chapter.

References

1. Baker, RA, Hillman, BJ, McLennan, JE, et. al.: Sequelae of Metrizamide Myelography in 200 examinations. Am. J. Roentgenol. 130: 499–502, 1978
2. Batsakis, JG: Tumors of the Head and Neck-Clinical and Pathological considerations. Baltimore, Williams and Wilkins Company, 1979
3. Bernardino, ME, Zimmerman, RD, Citrin, CM, et. al.: Scleral thickening: A CT sign of orbital pseudotumor. Am. J. Roentgenol. 129: 703–706, 1977
4. Bhave, DG, Kelsey, CA, Burstein, J, et. al.: Scattered radiation doses to infants and children during EMI head scans. Radiology 124: 379–380, 1977
5. Bohman, L, Mancuso, A, Thompson, J, Hanafee, W: CT approach to benign nasopharyngeal masses. Am. J. Roentgenol. 136: 173–180, 1981
6. Burnam, JA, Benson, J, Cohen, I.: Giant cell tumor of the ethmoid sinuses: Diagnostic Dilemma. Laryngoscope 89: 1415–1424, 1979
7. Carter, BL, Moorehead, J, Wolpert, SM, et. al.: Cross sectional anatomy: computed tomography and ultrasound correlation. New York, Appleton-Century-Crofts, 1977
8. Carter, BL, Ignatow, SB: Neck and mediastinal angiography by computed tomography scan. Radiology 122: 515–516, 1977
9. Carter, BL, Hammerschlag, SB, Wolpert, SM: Computerized scanning in otorhinolaryngology. Adv. Otorhinolaryngol. 24: 21–31, 1978
10. Carter, BL, Karmody, CS: Computed tomography of the face and neck. Semin. Roentgenol. 3: 257–266, 1978
11. Carter, BL, Karmody, CS: Computerized Tomography of cancer of the head and neck. Caribbean Medical Journal, pages 17–21, Vol. 40 Nos. 3/4, 1980.
12. Carter, BL: Computed tomographic scanning in head and neck tumors. Otolaryngol. Clin. North Am. Vol. 13: 449–457, 1980
13. Carter, BL, Karmody, CS, Blickman, JR, Panders, AK: CT and sialography: Part I and II. J. of Computer Assisted Tomography Vol. 5: 42–53, 1981
14. Chernak, ES, Rodriguez-Antunez, A, Jelden, GL, et. al.: The use of computed tomography for radiation therapy treatment planning. Radiology 117: 613–614, 1975
15. Claussen, CD, Lohkamp, FW, Krastel, A: Computed tomography of trauma involving brain and facial skull (craniofacial injuries). J of Computer Assisted Tomography 1(4): 472–481, 1977
16. Drayer, BP, Wilkins, RH, Boehnke, M, et. al.: Cerebrospinal fluid rhinorrhea demonstrated by Metrizamide CT cisternography. Am. J. Roentgenol. 129: 149–151, 1977
17. Dubois, P, Schultz, JC, Perrin, RL, Dastur, KJ: Tomography in expansile lesions of the nasal and paranasal sinuses. Radiology 1925: 149–158, 1977
18. Duckert, LG, Carley, RB, Hilger, JA: Computerized axial tomography in the preoperative evaluation of an angiofibroma. Laryngoscope 88: 613–618, 1978
19. Duncan, AW, Lack, EE, Deck, MF: Radiological evaluation of paragangliomas of the head and neck. Radiology 132: 99–105, 1979
20. Elie G, Renauk-Salis, JJ, Guibert-Trainer, F, Le Truet, A, Caille, JM: CT of primary malignant tumors of the nasopharynx. Computed Tomography Vol. 4: 235–241, 1980
21. Enzmann, D, Donaldson SS, Marshall WH, et al.: Computed tomography in orbital pseudotumor (idiopathic orbital inflammation). Radiology 120: 597–610, 1976
22. Forbes, WSTC, Fawcitt, RA, Isherwood I, Webb, R, Farrington, T: Computed tomography in the diagnosis of diseases of the paranasal sinuses. Clin. Radiol. 29: 501–511, 1978
23. Forssell, A, Liliequist, B: Computed tomography of the paranasal sinuses. Adv. Otorhinolaryngol. 24: 42–50, 1978
24. Gado, MH, Phelps, ME, Coleman, RE: An extravascular component of contrast enhancement in cranial computed tomography. Part I and II. Radiology 117: 589–597, 1975
25. Hammerschlag, SB, Wolpert, SM, Carter, BL: Computed coronal tomography. Radiology 120: 219-220, 1976
26. Hammerschlag, SB, Wolpert, SM, Carter, BL: Computed tomography of the spinal canal. Radiology 121: 361–367, 1976
27. Hammerschlag, SB, Wolpert, SM, Carter, BL: Computed

tomography of the skull base. J. of Computer Assisted Tomography 1: 75–80, 1977

28. Hanafee, W.: Otolaryngology and Ophthalmology-Current Radiology, Ed. Wilson, GH, Houghton Mifflin Professional Publishers, 1979

29. Hassani, SN, Bard, RL: Real time ophthalmic ultrasonography. Radiology 127: 213–219, 1978

30. Haynes, BF, Fishman, ML, Fauci, AS, et. al.: The ocular manifestation of Wegener's granulomatosis. Am. J. Med. 63: 131–141, 1977

31. Hesselink, JR, New, PF, Davis, KR, et. al.: Computed tomography of the paransal sinuses and face. Part I an II. J. of Computed Assisted Tomography 2: 559–576, 1978

32. Hesselink, JR, Weber, AL, New, PF, Davis, KR, Roberson, GH, Taveras, JM: Evaluation of mucoceles of the paranasal sinuses with computed tomography. Radiology 133: 397–400, 1979

33. Hilal, SK, Trokel SL: Computerized tomography of the orbit using thin sections. Semin. Roentgenol. 12: 137–147, 1977

34. Hilal, SK, Trokle SL, Coleman, DJ: High resolution computerized tomography and B-scan ultrasonography of the orbits. Trans. AM. Acad. Ophthalmol. Otolaryngol. 81: 607–617, 1976

35. Hounsfield, GN: Picture quality of computed tomography. Am. J. Roentgenol. 127: 3–9, 1976

36. Jelden, GL, Chernak, ES, Rodriguez-Antunez, A, et. al.: Further progress in CT scanning and computerized radiation therapy treatment planning. Am. J. Roentgenol. 127: 179–185, 1976

37. Jing, BS, Geopfert, H, Close LG: Computerized tomography of paranasal sinus neoplasms. Laryngoscope 88: 1485–1490, 1978

38. Leopold, DA, Kellman, RA, Gould, LV: Retro-orbital hematoma and proptosis associated with chronic sinus disease. Arch. Otolaryngol. Vol. 106: 442–443, 1980

39. Lloyd, GA: The impact of CT scanning and ultrasonography on orbital diagnosis. Clin. Radiol. 28: 583–593, 1977

40. Mamose, KJ, Weber, AL, Goodman, M, MacMillan, AS, Roberson, GH: Radiological aspects of inverted papilloma. Radiology 134: 73–79, 1980

41. Mancuso, AA, Bohman, L, Hanafee, W, Maxwell D: Computed tomography of the nasopharynx: Normal and variations of Normal. Radiology 137: 113–121, 1980

42. Maniglia, AJ, Chandler, JR, Goodwin, WJ, and Parker, JC: Schwannomas of the parapharyngeal space and jugular foramen. Laryngoscope 89: 1405–1414, 1979

43. Maravilla, KR: Computer reconstructed sagittal and coronal computed tomography head scans: clinical applications. J. Computer Assisted Tomography 2: 189–198, 1978

44. Munzenrider, JR, Pilepich, M, Rene-Ferrero, JB, et. al.: Use of body scanner in radiotherapy treatment planning. CA 40: 170–179, 1977

45. Nakagawa, H, Wolf, BS: Delineation of lesions of the base of the skull by computed tomography. Radiology 124: 75–80, 1977

46. New, PF, Aronow, S: Attenuation measurements of whole blood and blood fractions in computed tomography. Radiology 121: 635–640, 1976

47. Nickel, AR, Salem, JJ: Clinical experience in North America Metrizamide. Acta. Radiol. (Suppl) (Stockh) 355: 409–416, 1977

48. Osborn, AG, Anderson, RE: Direct sagittal computed tomographic scans of the face and paranasal sinuses. Radiology 129: 81–87, 1978

49. Osborn, AG, Johnson, L, Roberts, TS: Sphenoidal mucoceles with intracranial extension. J. of Computer Assisted Tomography 3: 335–338, 1979

50. Pagani, JJ, Thompson, J, Mancuso, A, Hanafee, W: Lateral wall of olfactory fossa in determining intracranial extension of sinus carcinomas. Am. J. Roentgenol. 133: 497–501, 1979

51. Palacios, E, Valvassori, G: Computed axial tomography in otorhinolaryngology. Adv. otorhinolaryng. 24: 1–8, 1978

52. Paparella, Shumrick: Otolaryngology, basic sciences and related disciplines. Philadelphia, WB Saunders Co., 129–140, 1973

53. Rosenbaum, AE, Drayer, BP: CT cisternography with Metrizamide. Acta. Radiol. (Suppl) (Stockh) 355: 323–337, 1977

54. Rosengren, JE, Jing, BS, Wallace, S, Danziger, J: Radiographic features of olfactory neuroblastoma. Am. J. Roentgenol. 132: 945–948, 1979

55. Sackett, JF, Strother, CM, Quaglieri, CE, et. al.: Metrizamide CSF contrast medium. Radiology 123: 779–782, 1977

56. Schindler, E, Aulich, A, Wende, S: Value and limits of computerized axial tomography in ORL. Adv. Otorhinolaryngol. 24: 9–20, 1978

57. Shrivastava, PN, Lynn, SL, Ting, JY: Exposures to patient and personnel in computed axial tomography. Radiology 125: 411–415, 1977

58. Skalpe, IO: Adverse effects of water-soluble contrast media in myelography, cisternography and venticulography. Acta. Radiol. (Suppl) (Stockh) 355: 359–370, 1977

59. Sobotta, J: Atlas of human anatomy. New York, Hafner Publishing Co., 1968

60. Som, PM, Shugar, JMA: The CT classification of ethmoid mucoceles. J. of Computed Assisted Tomography Vol. 4: 199–203, 1980

61. Som, PM, Shugar, JMA: Antral mucocele: a new look. J. of Computer Assisted Tomography Vol. 4: 484–488, 1980

62. Tadmor, R, New, PF: Computed tomography of the orbit with special emphasis on coronal sections: Part I and II Normal and pathological anatomy. J. Computer Assisted Tomography 2: 24–44, 1978

63. Thawley, SE, Gado, M, Fuller, TR: Computerized tomography in the evaluation of head and neck lesions. Laryngoscope 88: 451–459, 1978

64. Warwick and Williams: Gray's Anatomy, 35th British ed. Philadelphia, WB Saunders Co., 501–509, 1973

65. Weinstein, MA, Levine, H, Duchesneau, PM, et. al.: Diagnosis of juvenile angiofibroma by computed tomography. Radiology 126: 703–705, 1978

66. Wende, S, Aulich A, Nover, A, et. al.: Computed tomography of orbital lesions. Neuroradiology 13: 123–134, 1977

67. Wortzman, G, Holgate, RC, Noyek, AM, et. al.: Otolaryngologic applications of computed tomography. Otolaryngol. Clin. North Am. 2: 501–512, 1978

68. Zimmerman, RA, Bilaniuk, LT: Computed tomography of sphenoid sinus tumors. Computed Axial Tomography 1: 23–32, 1977

Part IV

Radiography of the Pharynx and Larynx

William N. Hanafee

Chapter 1 Pharynx

Introduction

Radiologic examination can materially assist in visualizing the pharyngeal and laryngeal airways. In the pharynx most of the areas are readily accessible to the examining finger or direct vision except for the nasopharynx. Under favorable circumstances, laryngeal examinations still have blind areas regarding the subglottic space, anterior walls of the piriform sinuses, and the postcricoid regions. Poor patient cooperation will greatly expand the list of hidden areas.

Considerable information can be obtained through the use of plain films or xeroradiography of the air passages. For a more detailed study of anatomy and physiology, the techniques of tomography, barium swallow, laryngography, or nasopharyngography provide the ability to study motion as well as surface topography. Computerized tomography has provided a new dimension in the evaluation of soft tissue extensions of nasopharyngeal and laryngeal tumors. In the future, determination of operability and therapy planning may well become the perquisite of computerized tomography in malignant tumors of the head and neck.

Pharynx

Plain Views of the Pharynx

A long gray scale, wide latitude film is highly desirable for visualization of the soft tissues of the nasopharynx and larynx. Low-dose mammography film using a single intensifying screen and vacuum cassette proves most valuable in identifying the subtle differences of gray scale in the nasopharynx. The lateral projections are taken with the patient quietly breathing through the nose. This maneuver will depress the soft palate against the tongue and cause the epiglottis to become more vertical, thereby opening up the laryngeal vestibule. For the average patient 400 ma at 0.25 s (100 mAs) and 72-in distance is quite satisfactory (Fig. 1.1). In the base projection, par speed or high speed screens can be used with conventional techniques and still obtain an adequate contrast of the nasopharyngeal structures. In the nasopharynx, a base projection should be obtained with superimposition of the mandible on the anterior table of the frontal bone. In nasopharyngeal tumor suspects, the patient should be radiographed while blowing against the pinched nostrils or with the mouth open to distend the fossa of Rosenmüller. The latter two maneuvers are not uniformly successful in x-Ray filming but are more helpful during computerized tomography (CT) (Fig. 1.2). In a series of 30 consecutive patients, submentovertex views were taken with the mouth opened and the mouth closed. In 13

patients the fossa of Rosenmüller were seen better in the mouth open view, in 2 the fossa were better seen with the mouth closed, and in 15 there was no change. Nevertheless, minor asymmetries may be corrected by merely having the patient open his mouth during the base projection.

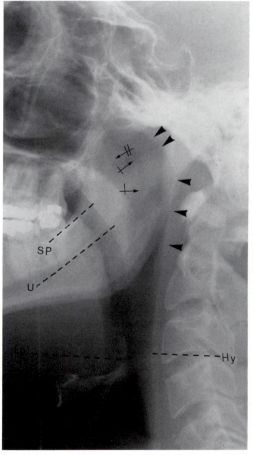

Fig. 1.1

a) Lateral projection of nasopharynx using low dose film. The posterior wall and roof of the nasopharynx and oral pharynx are clearly outlined because the x-ray beam passes tangent to the air-mucosal interface. (Adenoids area-upper two arrowheads and posterior wall of nasopharynx and oral pharynx- lower three arrowheads). The salpingopharyngeal fold projects inferiorly from the posterior margin of the opening of the eustachian tube (cross-hatched arrows). The salpingopalatine fold is less well delineated because of the enface presentation of this fold to the x-ray beam (double cross-hatched arrow). Other familiar landmarks are the soft palate (SP), the uvula (U), epiglottis (Epi) and the hyoid bone (Hy).

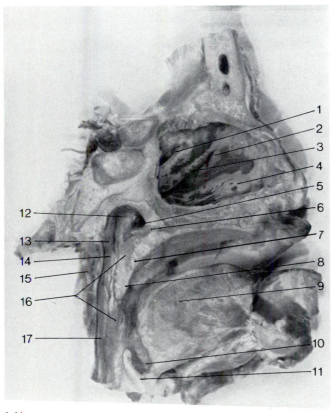

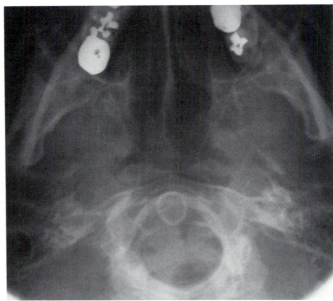

1.1 b   1.1 c

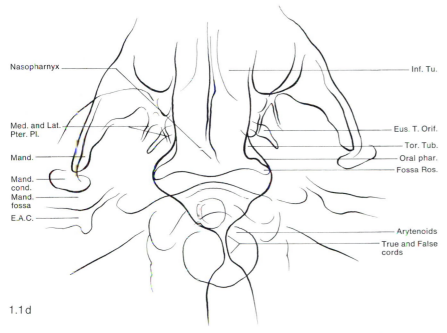

1.1 d

b) Saggital section of the nasopharynx: 1. Superior turbinate, 2. openings of the nasofrontal duct and ostium of the anterior and middle ethmoid air cells, 3. middle turbinate, 4. inferior turbinate, 5. eustachian tube orifice, 6. salpingopalatine fold region (obscured in the specimen by remaining midline structures), 7. soft palate, 8. uvula, 9. tongue, 10. vallecula, 11. superhyoid epiglottis, 12. fossa of Rosenmüller (lateral pharyngeal recess), 13. Passavant's muscle, 14. superior pharyngeal constrictor, 15. fragments of the longus colli and the longus capitis muscles, 16. salpingopharyngeal fold, 17. posterior pharyngeal wall.

c) Base projection.
d) Line drawing of the base projection. Nasopharynx – X, Medial and lateral pterygoid plates – Med. and Lat Pter. Pl., Mandible – mand., Mandibular condyle – Mand. cond. Mandibular fossa – Mand fossa, External auditory canal – EAC, Inferior turbinate – Inf. Tu, Eustachian tube orifice – Eus. T. Orif., Torus tubarius – Tor. Tub., Oral pharynx – Oral phar., Fossa of Rosenmüller – Fossa Ros., Arytenoids, True and false cords.

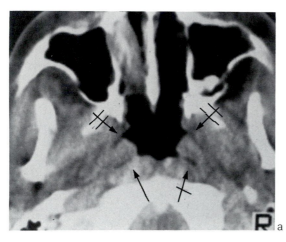

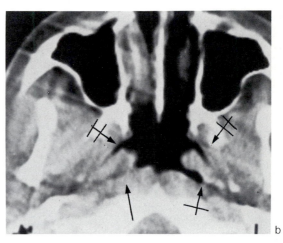

Fig. 1.2
a) Minor asymmetry of fossa of Rosenmüller due to lymphoid tissue. Axial CT scan through the level of the opening of the eustachian tube (double cross-hatched arrow). The fossa of Rosenmüller on the right (cross-hatched arrow) is slitlike and normal in configuration. On the left, there is slight irregularity of the posterior margin of the fossa of Rosenmüller (arrow). All of the deep fascial planes are entirely within normal limits in this 60-year-old female presenting with a neck node.

b) Scan through the same level with the patient instructed to blow against pursed lips and pinched nostrils. Air extends into the eustachian tube for approximately 2–3 mm (double cross-hatched arrows). The fossa of Rosenmüller on the right (cross-hatched arrow) becomes larger. On the left, the opening to the fossa of Rosenmüller distends nicely, but the deeper portion remains slitlike. The degree of pliability of the surrounding areas plus normal fascial planes would indicate this is not a malignant lesion. Biopsy of the fossa of Rosenmüller proved that the slight irregularity was due to normal lympoid tissue.

Xeroradiography

The property of xeroradiography that makes it so useful in the upper airway passages is the edge enhancement effect caused by distortions in the electric fields of the plates when exposed to x-rays. This edge enhancement effect is particularly useful because of the overall low contrast display of xeroradiography. In the lateral projection, excellent delineation of the torus tubarius and salpingopharyngeal folds are seen. On the anteroposterior projection, the density of the overlying spine interferes with fine detail. The anteroposterior view must be combined with tomography, but then patient dose and x-ray tube loading become limiting factors.

Xeroradiography exposure factors are usually in the range of 110–120 kV at 15–20 mAS and 40-in distance for the average adult. On the anteroposterior projection, tomography is used with 120 kV at 150 mAs and 40-in distance.

Tomography

When the patient is unable to cooperate for indirect or direct nasopharyngeal examination, tomography may offer useful information. Its value in demonstrating extensions of nasopharyngeal tumors or sinus cancers into the base of the skull is well recognized (33). Linear tomography of the skull base is accompanied by so many ghost shadows from the bones of the midface that it can create as many problems as it solves. The occasional lesion that is well demonstrated by linear tomography is frequently accompanied by other soft tissue densities that simulate infiltrations, thereby negating overall beneficial effects. Pluridirectional tomography with either a hypocycloidal or trispiral tube-film movement offers vastly superior results concerning the soft tissues of the nasopharynx as well as the bones of the base of the skull.

Tomography Projections

Coronal sections provide a convenient survey of the facial structures and nasopharynx. Sections are taken at 0.5-cm intervals using 180–240 mAs at 65–75 kV for the average patient. Lateral projections are most helpful for evaluating the anterior nasopharyx. The posterior wall of the nasopharynx is usually adequately evaluated without the aid of tomography. The base projection offers the opportunity for detailed visualization of the entire anatomy of the lateral and superior walls of the nasopharynx (42).

Only the very agile patients can assume a true base projection for tomography. Mechanical assistance is readily available by using a tilting tomographic device with a second table or some type of a patient support that is angulated if the tomographic unit is not tiltable (19). With these mechanical aids, highly satisfactory base tomograms of the nasopharynx can be obtained in almost every patient.

Nasopharyngogram

The usefulness of nasopharyngography is related to the availability of thorough clinical exmaination. Modern nasopharyngoscopy utilizing the Ward Berci pharyngoscope permits excellent visualization with good lighting and a minimum of discomfort to the patient. Biopsies can be obtained under direct visual control for accurately delineating the extension of tumors. If the Ward Berci scope or similar devices are not available and patient cooperation is limited, nasopharyngography offers an additional modality for evaluating blind areas (30). Premedication should consist of relatively large doses of atropine (0.8–1.2 mg) for adults and proportionally lesser amounts for children. The procedure is not painful so that analgesics are not necessary; however, local anesthesia will greatly reduce troublesome secretions. The patient is placed on the tilting fluoroscopy table on a pad with the head extended over the end of the pad so that the nasal passages lie dependent; 2–3 ml of 0.5% lidocaine are placed in each nostril and the patient told to "sniff in" and to blow his nose to distribute the anesthetic over the entire mucosa. Again with the patient in the supine position, oily propyliodone (Dionosil) is instilled into each nasal cavity and fluoroscopy performed to insure adequate filling. The fluoroscopic table should be tilted to the head down position to retain the contrast material high in the nasopharynx. The patient is instructed to flex the chin on the chest. The superior margin of the contrast material will lie against the anterior wall of the sphenoid sinus, and contrast material will flow laterally into the extremities of the fossa of Rosenmüller. Distensibility of the walls of the piriform sinus can be verified by having the patient blow against obstructed nares or by phonating (46). Films are taken in the anteroposterior and lateral projection. By keeping the chin well flexed on the chest and the head in an inverted position, contrast material can be kept in the nasopharynx and fossa of Rosenmüller for extended periods of time to allow adequate examination.

Angiography

Angiography of the pharynx can play a major role in the diagnosis and management of vascular tumors within this region. In general, the malignant tumors are poorly vascularized and the tumor vessels are not sufficiently distinctive to be diagnostic. Some benign tumors, and in particular juvenile angiofibromas, stain intensely at angiography to a sufficient extent to be almost diagnostic (43, 50). These tumors rarely remain confined to the nasopharynx, and their extensions are clearly delineated by selective external carotid angiography.

The technique of catheter carotid angiography has been well accepted because of its low morbidity and ease of performance. Various preshaped configurations of catheters have been utilized to avoid anatomic variations and pathologic conditions within the artery. The shapes are variously C-shaped, S-shaped, headhunters, and controllable tipped catheters for selectively catheterizing the common carotid and external carotid vessels from the femoral artery. At times, atherosclerotic disease may preclude catheterization of the carotid vessels from the femoral approach. Contrast studies can be performed by direct needle puncture of the neck vessels and insertion of a sheath needle such as a kornon needle or passing of a small diameter polyethylene catheter percutaneously with maneuver of the catheter into the internal and external carotid arteries as desired. Under these circumstances, only one side should be examined at a sitting.

The patients will usually tolerate the complication of a single hematoma, but bilateral hematomas require tracheostomy for management and are potentially life threatening.

In the routine study of the arteries to the face and nasopharynx, we inject 5–8 ml of a 60% meglumine iothalamate into the external carotid artery immediately distal to the bifurcation. This low position of the catheter is essential to insure filling of the ascending pharyngeal artery, which is one of the first branches of the external carotid. At times, it may originate from the common carotid artery. Films are taken in an anteroposterior, lateral, and if necessary basal projection. For vascular tumors that have extended beyond the confines of the nasopharynx, the catheter may be maneuvered into the internal carotid, vertebral artery, or thyrocervical trunks for additional contrast injections to outline the blood supply of the tumor.

Regardless of the shape of the tip of the catheter, the outside diameter of the catheter should be chosen of a material that is sufficiently small to prevent totally occluding the vessel under investigation and creating excessive spasm. Gentleness with maneuvering of the catheter is the byword. The technique of embolization will be discussed under juvenile nasopharyngeal angiofibroma.

Normal Radiographic Anatomy

Plain View of the Pharynx

The most important concept to be kept in mind when viewing plain views of the pharynx is that a soft tissue-air interface will only be visualized sharply when the x-ray beam is passing tangent to the surface. Surfaces that lie at a 45° angle to the x-ray beam will fade imperceptibly and not be seen. This explains why at times only portions of the normal roentgen anatomy can be visualized on any particular examination and tumors about the torus tubarius are not well seen on the lateral projection.

In the lateral projection, the posterior margins of the turbinates, and in particular the inferior turbinates, are seen projecting into the nasopharynx above the level of the hard and soft palate. The adenoidal pad and posterior midline of the nasopharynx and pharynx can be seen as s sharp line represented by the soft tissue-air-interface (Fig. 1.1). A fainter soft tissue-air-interface can be seen paralleling and lying 4–8 mm anterior to the posterior pharyngeal wall. This interface represents the salpingopharyngeal fold and continues down into the oral pharynx. The soft tissue thickness in the region of the adenoidal pad is quite variable (30), and elaborate statistics have been gathered. Making the diagnosis of tumor of the adenoids in an individual under 30 is frought with difficulties. Similarly, the thickness of soft tissues in the oral pharynx vary considerably with age and phase of respiration or swallowing. This is especially evident in the pediatric age group. Fortunately, the areas are readily visualized by direct mirror inspection or with a Hopkins fibro-optic rod. In general, increases in midline soft tissues of the oral pharynx of greater than 4 mm are highly suspicious of an expansive process. Increase in thickness of the salpingopharyngeal fold of greater than 8 mm, while not being diagnostic of tumor, certainly deserves direct visualization.

In the anteroposterior projection, there is considerable over lap of bony densities on the nasopharynx and upper oral pharynx so that the base projection usually gives the more optimal view. Starting at the level of the posterior margin of the turbinates, the soft palate and uvula can be seen to give increase in density to the nasopharynx with the uvula usually lying in the midline. The torus tubarius bulges into the nasal cavity on either side and contains the opening of the eustachian tube. The opening of the eustachian tube is somewhat funnel-shaped and rarely is air visible within the lumen of the eustachian tube (Fig. 1.1).

The pharyngeal recesses (fossae of Rosenmüller) are lateral extensions of the nasopharynx that are to some extent superior to the torus tubarius. At times, they are widely patent, but in children and young adults they are routinely collapsed. By having the patient blow against the obstructed nares or with the mouth open and jaw protruded during exposure in the base projection, the fossae of Rosenmüller can usually be made to distend and present greater details concerning their mucosal surfaces (33). This maneuver will also provide some information regarding pliability of the nasopharyngeal wall. Slight asymmetries between the two sides are not at all unusual. Before a diagnosis of tumor can be made, there should be further evidence of distortion of the deep fascial planes as seen on CT scanning or a mass visible on direct nasopharyngeal examination (Fig. 1.2).

The posterior nasopharyngeal wall is better visualized by angulating the x-ray tube than by having the patient hyperextend the chin. The increased angulation of the x-ray tube is more likely to provide a tangential view of the wall than if the patient is extremely cooperative and flexible. If extension of the head occurs mainly at the altanto-occipital junction, the patient may present the posterior wall as a 45 degree angle surface to the central x-ray beam and, thus, not cast a shadow. In a properly positioned base projection, the posterior wall has a "gull-winged" appearance produced by the bulging of the longus colli and longus capitus muscles lying immediately lateral to the midline. The medium raphe and the entrances into the fossae of Rosenmüller will cause a midline indentation and posterolateral outpouchings of the air columns, respectively.

The lateral walls of the oral pharynx bulge laterally in the base projection to overlap the medial pterygoid plate and should not be mistaken for the nasopharynx. They taper toward the midline to become continuous with the piriform sinuses on either side of the larynx. The air shadows of the piriform sinuses can then be seen to unite at the region of the esophageal hiatus, which is consist-

ently airless. The natural status of the cricopharyngeal muscle at the level of the lower half of the cricoid cartilage is in a contracted state. In the base projection as well as in the lateral projections, the constricted cricopharyngeal muscles serve as a termination point of the air that can be seen in the distended hypopharynx.

CT Examination of the Nasopharynx

A major advancement in examination of the nasopharynx has been possible through the use of CT scanning. Since motion is limited in the nasopharynx, the prolonged scan times of readily available CT scanners still prove adequate. CT proves to be a valuable adjunct to clinical examination since the deep structures and fascial planes are clearly demonstrated. The partial lists of indications for CT examination would include the following:

1. Persistent serous otitis media
2. Searching for occult neoplasm
3. Suspected masses of the nasopharynx
4. Directing the clinician to site of biopsy
5. Differentiation of benign from malignant tumors by patterns of deep infiltrative growth
6. Evaluation of atypical facial pain syndromes
7. Demonstration of invasion of the skull base by malignant processes
8. Treatment planning for radiation therapy or surgical procedures.

In the future, fast scanners may allow evaluation of physiologic parameters, e.g., eustachian tube function or effectiveness of pharyngeal musculature, such as the tensor palatine muscle or Passavent's ridge.

Some pitfalls in CT scanning of the nasopharynx and the methods of resolution can be outlined as follows:

Pitfalls	Suggestions for resolving
1. Adenoidal pad asymmetries	1. All deep fascial planes are symmetric
2. Asymmetric fossa of Rosenmüller	2. Re-scan with the mouth open or blowing out against pursed lips and closed nasal passages
3. Scarring post trauma	3. Search for bony distortions
4. Scarring post tonsilectomy or adenoidectomy.	4. Lack of deep infiltration or contrast enhancement may prove helpful.

At times, inflammatory responses will appear as mass lesions that are undistinguishable from malignant masses. Careful clinical evaluation and rescanning following a course of antibiotic therapy may be the only technique available; however, biopsy still remains the final determinant of benign versus malignant lesions.

Normal Anatomy

Scans are characteristically performed in the axial plane. The first section should be through the base of the skull to give a good delineation of the foramen lacerum, sphenoid sinus, and margins of the middle cranial fossa. The density of the air in the middle ear cleft should be observed as this may be a clue to eustachian tube dysfunction and serous otitis (Fig. 1.3). Subsequent sections are taken at 0.5 cm intervals with the next section usually being at the base of the medial and lateral pterygoid plates. The coronoid processes of the mandible are visible in this section. The buccinator muscle and temporalis muscle can be seen lying superficially and deep to the coronoid processes. The foramen lacerum region and clivus are usually also well demonstrated in this projection.

Subsequent levels show delineation of the medial and lateral pterygoid plates. The lateral pterygoid muscle can be traced to its insertion in the neck and condylar region of the mandible. The medial pterygoid muscle can be followed to its insertion lower on the body of the mandible and to the angle of the mandible. Both the medial and lateral pterygoid muscles have distinct fascial planes surrounding their borders, which are consistently maintained unless infiltrated by malignant tumor or aggressive inflammatory processes. The longus coli and longus capitus muscles comprise two symmetric bulging masses along the posterior pharyngeal wall. Lateral to the mus-

cle bundles lie the carotid artery and jugular vein immediately medial to the styloid processes. The carotid artery lies anterior and medial to the vein.

The torus tubarius bulges into the nasopharyngeal airway from either side immediately medial to the posterior margin of the medial pterygoid plates. A small amount of air is routinely seen in the fossa for the opening of the eustachian tube. Rarely is any air found in the eustachian tube beyond 2–3 mm from its opening.

The appearance of the adenoids is quite variable, being large and irregular in the younger age group, whereas in the older age group they tend to be more flattened and smooth in outline. Asymmetry between the two sides is not at all uncommon. This can be especially troublesome when the adenoids have a lobulated pattern. The density of the adenoids approximates that of the adjacent muscle masses, and there is not sufficient density difference between adenoids and tumors to be of diagnostic significance. With a limited experience of examining the adenoids during periods of infection, we are not certain how far lateral and posterior to the adenoids the disrupted influence of inflammatory changes will extend. In general, the separation between adenoids and the longus coli and longus capitus muscles may be obliterated, but the fascial planes between the pterygoid muscles and about the carotid vessels are always very well preserved (Fig. 1.4).

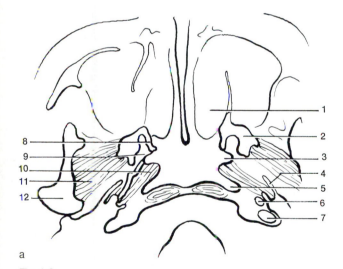

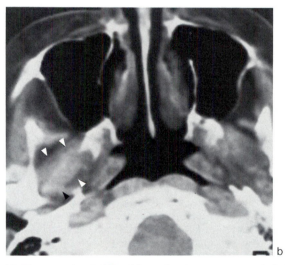

a

b

Fig. 1.3

a) Composite drawing from several scans of the midnasopharynx. 1. Inferior turbinate, 2. lateral pterygoid plate, 3. opening of the eustachian tube, 4. styloid process, 5. fossa of Rosenmüller (lateral pharyngeal recess), 6. internal carotid artery entering the skull (more inferiorly, it is adjacent to the medial border of the styloid process), 7. region of the internal jugular vein, 8. medial pterygoid plate, 9. combined shadow of the stylopharyngeus muscle and the tendon of the tensor tympani muscle, 10. levator veli palatini muscle, 11. lateral pterygoid muscle, 12. neck and condyle of the mandible.

b) The scan is slightly oblique to give a more cephalad level on the patient's left and a more caudad level on the patient's right. On the left, the lateral pterygoid muscle is seen almost in its entirety (arrowheads). The fascial planes lying medial to the muscle are always well defined. The palatine muscles may be quite slender, giving the entire parapharyngeal space a low-density appearance.

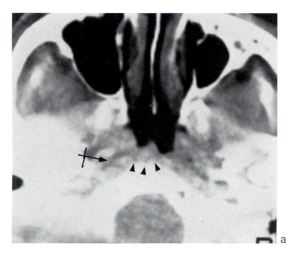

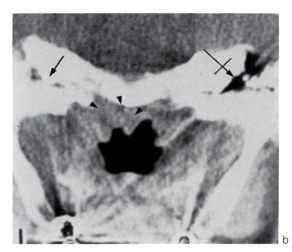

Fig. 1.4 Asymmetric adenoid enlargement.
a) Axial scan shows unilateral adenoidal enlargement on the left (arrowheads). The deep fascial planes are all intact (cross-hatched arrow). Biopsy of the adnoids show merely inflammatory reaction.
b) Coronal scan through the nasopharynx again shows the asymmetry of the adenoidal pad (arrowheads). Part of this patient's

presenting symptoms was otitis media on the left (arrow). The clouded, left middle ear cleft can be compared to the air containing right middle ear (cross-hatches arrow). The symptoms of otitis media and the major portion of the asymmetry cleared during a course fo antibiotic therapy.

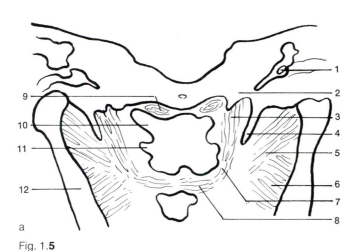

Fig. 1.5
a) Diagram of coronal scan. 1. Ossicular chain in the middle ear, 2. angular spine of the sphenoid bone, 3. superimposed shadow of the tensor veli palatini muscle and levator veli palatini muscle, 4. styloid process, 5. lateral pterygoid muscle, 6. medial pterygoid muscle, 7. tendon of tensor veli palatini muscle passing beneath the hamulus of the medial pterygoid plate, 8. soft palate, 9. combined density of the longus colli and longus capitus muscles, 10. fossa of Rosenmüller (lateral pharyngeal recess), 11. eustachian tube orifice, 12. angle of the mandible.

b) Coronal scan shows slightly more anteriorly placed structures on the left than on the right. This type of asymmetry is positional and should not be mistaken for infiltrative pathology. On the left, a portion of the pterygoid plates are in the plane of the scan as is the posterior inferior extremity of the antrum (arrowheads). The fossa of Rosenmüller on the left does not fill out due to the obliquity of the scan and also an asymmetric amount of lymphoid tissue in the fossa (cross-hatched arrow). On the right, the fossa of Rosenmüller is cut more posteriorly and is quite patulous (cross-hatched arrow). The low-density region beneath the angular spine of the sphenoid bone is the space surrounding the internal carotid artery prior to its entering the carotid canal in the temporal bone.

Coronal scanning is particularly helpful for demonstrating the extreme superior recess of the fossa of Rosenmüller and the superior surface of the soft palate (Fig. 1.5). Unfortunately, true coronal projections are difficult to obtain so that the examiner must compare different sections for the total anatomic composite.

The soft tissues of the torus tubarius should be symmetric in this projection, and air can routinely be seen in the fossa for the entrance to the eustachian tube. The soft tissues lying lateral to the pharyngo basilar fascia constitute the parapharyngeal space, which forms a continuum into the infratemporal fossa. The bony margins of the pterygoid plates are more clearly seen on axial CT scanning than on conventional anteroposterior tomography due to the angle that the pterygoid plates make with the saggital plane.

Disease Processes

Pathologic Conditions

Congenital

Choanal Atresia
The exact etiology of choanal atresia is not known; however, seveal theories have been proposed (5, 6):
1. Overgrowth of buccal pharyngeal membrane
2. Medial growth of the vertical and horizontal processes of the palatine bone
3. Failure of the buccal nasal membrane to dissolve.

None of the theories fully explain the type of tissue that blocks the posterior nares. It may be bony, membranous, or a combination of the two. The diagnosis is usually made in the delivery room or nursery when it is noted that the child has irregular breathing and intermittent cyanosis relieved by crying and aggravated by nursing. Diagnosis can be confirmed by placing methyene blue into the nose and observing the nasopharynx for passage of the material. The radiographic examination is conducted by placing a radiopaque dye in the nasal cavity with the infant supine and chin extended and obtaining a lateral view of the nasopharynx. A radiologic study will not only demonstrate the lack of continuity of the nasal lumen but will also show the thickness of any bony atritic plate to the surgeon in planning a more precise and safe approach.

The atresia is bony in 90% of the patients, while 10% have merely a membranous atresia In two thirds of the patients, the obstruction is bilateral, while in the remaining third, the obstruction is unilateral. Choanal atresia may be only part of a variety of maxillofacial dysplasias.

Cleft Palate
The diagnosis of cleft of the soft palate or hard palate is readily made by clinical examination. Radiologic examination is occasionally useful in speech problems and particularly in velopalatine closure. Barium swallow in the lateral projection will show the soft palate elevate and extend posteriorly to contact the posterior pharyngeal wall at a ridge that forms just above the anterior arch of C-1. This soft tissue ridge is spoken of as Passavant's ridge and is more prominent during swallowing than during phonation. Passavant's ridge (or muscle) is a horseshoe-shaped part of the superior pharyngeal constrictor that inserts into the soft palate. Complete closure of the velopalatine sphincter should be verified in the anteroposterior projection as well. At times, this sphincter action may be deficient in the coronal plane, and only a partial closure is accomplished. Air usually provides sufficient contrast for this study. Should the results of fluoroscopy be inconclusive, a small smount of propyliodone (Dionosil) can be instilled into the nasal cavity. The contrast installation should be avoided if possible since these children are usually distrustful of medical personnel because of their long therapeutic regimes and cooperation is rarely optimal.

Meningoceles
Midline masses within the nasal cavity of infants and young children can present a diagnostic dilemma. In the infant, the bony calvarium is largely cartilaginous so that the demonstration of defects may prove difficult. Tomography may demonstrate the communication between the mass and the central nervous system. The defect is usually in the cribiform plate but may be through the sphenoid. If the infant is older and calcification of the base of the skull has occurred, plain films as well as conventional tomography in the basal and coronal projection will usually show the defect. Metrizamide instilled into the spinal canal may be used to show the defect either on conventional filming or on CT scanning.

Cysts
The Thornwaldt cyst is a remnant of the anterior hypophyseal stalk that may occur in the midline of the nasopharynx or slightly to either side of the midline in young adults or children. It must be differentiated from meningoceles or other neoplastic processes. The lack of a bony defect of the base of the skull is extremely useful information. On CT scanning, the cysts are generally sharply outlined and do not distort distant muscle fascial planes. They cannot be differentiated from other benign tumors in the parapharyngeal and paranasopharyngeal space except that the usual parapharyngeal cyst extends much further caudad than a Thornwaldt cyst.

Functional Disorders

Functional Nasopharyngeal Obstructions

Since the classic descriptions of Dickens of the fat boy with sleep attacks, clinicians have been intrigued with the role of adenoids and nasopharyngeal soft tissues in hypersomnolence (40). The term pickwickian syndrome has been "coined" from the stories by Charles Dickens. These patients are extremely obese and exhibit excessive sleep and polycythemia. The chronic obstruction leads to chronic hypoventilation and eventually to pulmonary hypertension and cor pulmonale (34, 44). A similar type of chronic airway obstruction is said to occur in children with very large tonsils and is associated with gradual increase in daytime sleepiness.

The typical pickwickian is not necessarily cured by weight reduction. Tracheotomy is curative in the vast majority of patients but represents rather radical management.

Experimental data by Ogura (39) has shown that placing a nasal pack does alter the lower airway system on a neurological reflex basis and causes narrowing of the tracheobronchial tree. This is a reversible phenomenon that returns to normal when the nasal obstruction is relieved. The phenomenon is accompanied by a change in blood gasses with lowering of the PO_2 and a rise in the PCO_2 with the respiratory obstruction.

The role of radiology in this entity is not clear at the present time. Studies on patients with pickwickian syndromes and hypersommolence states have shown total obstruction of the nasopharyngeal airway by soft tissue masses. On CT scanning, these appear to be comprised of adenoidal type of tissue that fades imperceptively to the surrounding fascial planes (Fig. 1.6). The material is not fatty and changes very little with maneuvers that would tend to open the fossae of Rosenmüller.

Conventional roentgenograms show the soft tissue masses that appear like adenoids arising from the posterior superior nasopharynx. The masses bulge and oppose the soft palate. Surprisingly, the syndrome does not occur in some of the benign tumors that arise within the nasopharynx, such as juvenile angiofibroma or some of the neurogenic tumors. Possibly, further investigations may show that sufficient airway is present lateral to the tumors and allows nasopharyngeal breathing to take place or that the tumors themselves may interrupt the neuropulmonary reflexes that are associated with hypersomnolence states.

Neurophysiology Disturbances

The manifestations of myasthenia gravis and dermatomyocitis are quite similar in the pharynx and nasopharynx. On barium swallow, the mysthenia gravis patient will show considerable hesitancy in swallowing the bolus. The poor contractions of the pharyngeal constrictors may allow regurgitation of liquids into the nasal cavity through velopalatine incompetence. The external musculature of the larynx is generally effected, and the larynx will not elevate and rotate forcefully during the swallowing mechanism, thus permitting aspiration to take place.

Dysautonomia is also accompanied by dysphagia characterized by aspirations of large volumes of liquids into the larynx. Rather than weakness, these children also affected display a lack of coordination. The glottic chink does not close at the appropriate time so that liquids will pass into the trachea as well as into the esophagus. The total clinical picture of the patient in these disorders is so characteristic that the patients are rarely diagnosed on the basis of a roentgen examination.

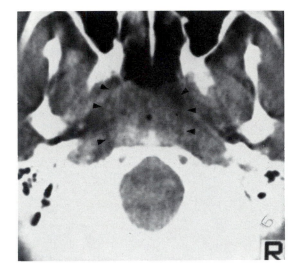

Fig. 1.6   Pickwickian syndrome. Beginning at the base of the skull and extending to the level of the lower margin of the soft palate, there is a soft tissue density totally filling the nasopharynx (arrowheads). All of the deep fascial planes are intact. The soft tissue density is not fat and not of muscle density. On clinical examination, an airway was visible. The adnoids were large but not of sufficient size to explain the density totally filling the nasopharynx. The exact explanation of the nature of this density remains obscure.

Trauma

The vast majority of midface fractures are accompanied by fractures of the pterygoid plates. Attention is characteristically directed to maintenance of an adequate bite and cosmesis so that distortions of the nasopharynx are not likely to attract the attention of the attending physician. In a single report of isolated fracture of the medial and lateral pterygoid plate, Davis (10) found the patient to experience trismis and painful chewing. Since there were no other facial fractures, the trismis was attributed to the disruption of the medial and lateral pterygoid plate on the affected side.

Computerized tomography of the facial bones provides an excellent alternative to conventional roentgen examination in demonstrating fractures in the critically injured patient (8). A survey of the intracranial injuries can be performed at the same time the facial structures are being visualized. The airway can be confirmed, both in the nasopharynx and in the larynx. In general, encroachment upon the pharyngeal airway is readily apparent on clinical examination. Bilateral fractures of the angle of the mandible are particularly worrisome because they allow the tongue to sublux posteriorly. Pterygoid plate fractures may produce trismis but usually do not reach sufficient displacement to encroach upon the airway. The laryngeal CT scanning of trauma is discussed in the subsequent chapter on the larynx.

Puncture wounds about the nasopharynx and pharynx may produce air in the soft tissues, abscesses, and distorted airways. Passage of an endoscope or catheter for tracheal suction has been shown to perforate the pharynx, especially in the newborn (36). Diagnosis of these pharyngeal perforations is again made by the presence of air in the soft tissues or the associated inflammatory changes. On occasion, gastrograffin swallow has shown a defect in the mucosa with contrast material entering the parapharyngeal soft tissues.

Thorium injuries (27) to the pharynx represent a special type of trauma. Thorium is radioactive, emitting α-, β-, γ-rays. The major tissue damage is believed due to the α particles. The patient will usually succumb to either the induced malignancy or the combination of vasculitis and cellulitis. Thorium dioxide (Thorotrast) was used as a contrast agent for cerebral angiography. Once administered, thorium is not easily eliminated from the body and has a half-life of 1.39×10^{10} years. Since 1945 clinical use has been prohibited. If carotid angiography was attempted by needle puncture of the common carotid and the thorium injected paravascularly, granulomas formed in the neck. The radiopaque thorium will be visualized for life in the facial planes and may cause sarcomas of the soft tissues (Fig. 1.7). The chronic radiation of the carotid artery wall leads to the envelopment of the artery by dense sclerotic tissue that causes narrowing and eventual occlusion of its lumen. In the avascular regions, chronic infections develop that may lead to fatal hemorrhages from adjacent vascular beds. The patients usually present with either localized pain, dysphagia, or cranial nerve deficiencies. Major vascular occulsions may lead to strokes despite wide resection of the granulomas and devitalized tissues. If they do not die from radiation-induced malignancy, they succumb to infection and hemorrhage after a 20 to 30-year latency period.

Infections

The usual patient with upper respiratory infection does not present for roentgen examination or CT scanning of the nasopharynx. Occasionally, inflammatory responses in hypertrophied adenoids may simulate tumor and lead to further investigation by CT scanning. The swelling of the adenoids is usually symmetric but may be asymmetric and closely simulate a malignant process. The inflammatory response stays relatively superficial and does not extend into the more distal fascial planes as one would expect from an infiltrating neoplasm. Malignancies characteristically infiltrate deeply. As in any head and neck lesion, biopsy is mandatory before embarking on a therapeutic regimen (Fig. 1.8).

Mucor infections begin in the nasopharynx and invade the sphenoid sinus and paranasopharyngeal space. The fungus *Mucorales* is normally saprophytic with branching. Most cases are reported in patients with uncontrolled diabetes but may occur in any debilitated state, such as carcinoma, extensive burns, or in the immunosuppressed patient. The disease spreads throughout the nose and paranasal sinuses and eventually invades the orbit. Intracranial extensions occur through the superior orbital fissure, foramen rotundum and foramen lacerum, and through the cribiform plate. Not uncommonly, the carotid artery is directly invaded, and the fungus can be found within the lumen of the carotid artery. This arteritis can lead to carotid artery occlusion.

Therapy is directed to the local disease as well as the systemic debilitating illness. Routine views and tomography may show the soft tissue swelling of the nasopharynx and sinus involvement. CT scanning is extremely helpful in demonstrating the local nasopharyngeal disease as well as orbital extension. At times, the infection spreads to the inferior surface of the temporal bone in the region of the carotid canal. Osteomyelitis and sequestrum formation may occur due to the virulent nature of the infection and its ability to occlude blood vessels. CT scanning should be performed in the axial as well as the coronal plane to demonstrate more completely the lateral extensions into the base of the pterygoid plates and inferior surfaces of the temporal bones (Fig. 1.9). CT scanning also allows an evaluation of treatment response. Adequacy of debridement can be verified by coronal and axial CT scanning.

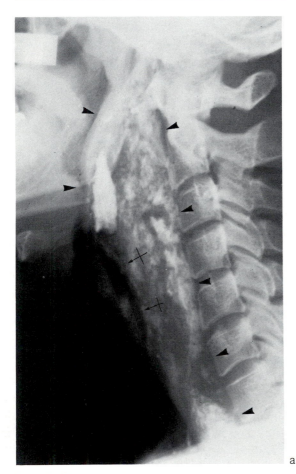

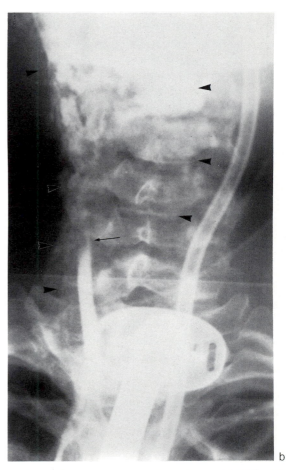

Fig. 1.7 Thorium-induced necrosis of the pharynx in a 32-year-old man who had received a carotid angiogram at age two. The thorium dioxide contrast agent had been injected perivascularly.
a) On the lateral projection of the pharynx, the thorium retained in a granuloma is visible throughout the entire pharynx and lower cervical region (arrowheads). This granuloma had become infected with fistula formation, abscess, and anterior displacement of the larynx (cross-hatch arrows).

b) Although the internal carotid artery was totally occluded on angiography (arrow), the patient still bled profusely from the ulcerating granulomatous mass due to collaterals from the opposite carotid, the vertebral, and the thyrocervical trunk. The retained thorium is deposited diffusely over a wide area (arrowheads).

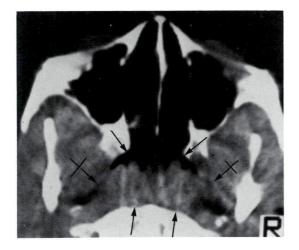

Fig. 1.8 Thirty-year-old male with infected adenoids. The lobulated pattern to the surface of the adenoids in a young person is not at all unusual. There has been obliteration of the fascial planes between the adenoids and the longus colli and longus capitus muscles (arrows). Despite the large size of the "mass", the fascial planes about the pterygoid muscles are very well preserved (cross-hatched arrows). Air is also seen entering the openings of the eustachian tubes bilaterally.

Malignant External Otitis

A special form of otitis of the external auditory canal occurs in diabetics or debilitated patients that has been termed malignant external otitis (7). The causative organism is *Pseudomonas aeruginosa,* which spreads in the soft tissue beneath the temporal bone leading to cranial nerve palsies, mastoiditis, septicemia, and osteomyelitis of the base of the skull. Prior to the availability of carbenicillin and gentamicin, the inflammation was almost invariably fatal. At the present time, the patients are hospitalized and given intravenous carbenicillin and gentamicin for prolonged periods of time while carefully following the progress of disease. The visible disease in the external auditory canal usually clears promptly, but the infection may smolder in the mastoid, along the inferior surface of the petrous bone, and in the paranasopharyngeal space. CT scanning of the nasopharynx can provide vital information for patient management. The degree of soft tissue swelling in the paranasopharyngeal space can be followed carefully, and the osteomyelitis of the temporal bone can be monitored for sequestrum formation. Should osteomyelitis occur, it is usually accompanied by cranial nerve palsy involving the 7th, 9th, 10th, or 11th nerves. Surgical débridement and aggressive antibiotic therapy produces a high salvage rate despite cranial nerve involvement. Conventional films and pluridirectional tomography may show the soft tissue swelling of the nasopharynx but do not allow early diagnosis of sequestra formation to the degree that can be achieved with CT scanning.

Granulomatous Infections

A group of granulomatous inflammatory diseases may involve the nasopharynx, producing exuberant masses or ulcerations about the fossae of Rosenmüller. These include TB, blastomycosis, rhinoscleroma, and sarcoid. Rhinoscleroma and sarcoid are easily diagnosed by additional lesions that invariably occur in more accessible areas of the nasal cavity. The lesions of sarcoid are exophytic and frequently affect the paranasal sinuses (11). Bone destruction is quite common, which may involve the sinus walls or nasal septum.

Rhinoscleroma is caused by *Klebsiella rhinoscleromatis,* a gram-negative rod, and is endemic in Latin and South America. The early lesions are commonly in the nasal cavity and appear as beefy-red granulation tissue. As healing takes place, scarring, strictures, and webs form. Deformity of the nasopharynx will vary with the maturity of the lesions. Biopsy and culture must be relied upon for final etiologic diagnosis since the roentgen changes are nonspecific.

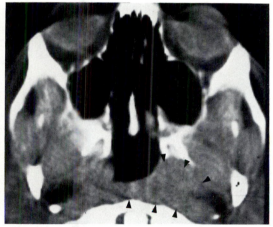

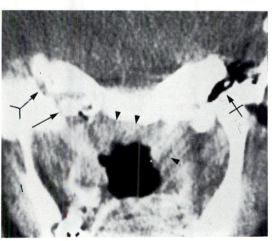

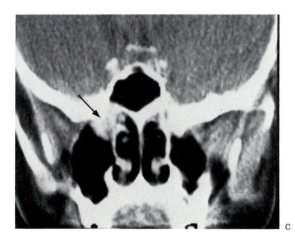

Fig. 1.9 *Mucor* mycosis in a previously undiagnosed diabetic.
a) Axial scan shows the aggressive inflammatory process on the posterior wall of the nasopharynx extending laterally on the right and through the parapharyngeal space (arrowheads).
b) Coronal scan through the posterior portions of the antrum show a fungus ball on the right (arrow). With a different window setting, a small amount of bone destruction could be seen at this level.
c) Coronal scan more posteriorly shows a sequestrum that has formed in the inferior surface of the temporal bone surrounded by a relatively low-density area (arrow). The middle ear cavity on the right is clouded (Y-shaped arrow) by comparison to the normal air-containing middle ear cavity on the left (cross-hatched arrow). Inflammatory process in the vault and right parapharyngeal space is shown to cross the midline (arrowheads).

Tumors

Benign

Benign tumors of the nasopharynx are unusual but not rare. They may be divided into pedunculated types presenting as rounded masses in the nasopharynx or submucosal and parapharyngeal tumors that bulge into the airway.

Choanal polyps, inflammatory polyps inverting papillomas, and juvenile angiofibromas are the most common pedunculated lesions, while neuromas, fibromas, lipomas, and cysts are more likely to be found in the parapharyngeal space (16). The latter group must be differentiated from lymphadenopathy in the retropharyngeal space or extensions of tumor masses originating in the base of the skull or intracranial lesions that have extended inferiorly. Parotid tumors arising from the deep lobe may bulge into the paralaryngeal space causing medial displacement of the tonsilar pillars.

Venous malformations may produce swellings in the paralaryngeal space, however, these are usually obvious by clinical examination although radiology may play a significant role in delineating the extent of the malformation.

Choanal Polyps

Choanal polyps are benign polyps that originate from the maxillary sinus at its ostium and protrude into the nasal cavity. As the polyp enlarges, it presents posteriorly through the choana and into the nasopharynx. The mass may reach considerable size with a surprisingly few symptoms. Frequently, the mass is discovered by the patient when he looks in the mirror with his mouth open. Radiographic examination will usually show evidence of sinus disease and the offending antrum may be totally opaque. The posterior nasal airway will be filled with tumor, but diagnosis is usually suggested on the lateral projection (Fig. 1.10). The choanal polyp will present as a smoothly outlined mass projecting posteriorly above the level of the soft palate and uvula. The inferior pole of the mass will present at about the level of the soft palate in the average patient. Characteristically, there is no evidence of bone expansion or bone destructive changes with choanal polyp. The meatus of the antrum may be enlarged but is usually not demonstrable on roentgenograms. Occasionally, the nasal septum may deviate to the opposite side due to the mass of the polyp; however, this change is more common with inverting papillomas. Additional polyps may be present in the nasal cavity, and there may be additional evidence of sinus disease. The mass must be differentiated from angiofibromas since the latter are exceedingly vascular and require more careful management (Fig. 1.10b).

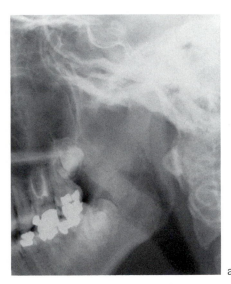

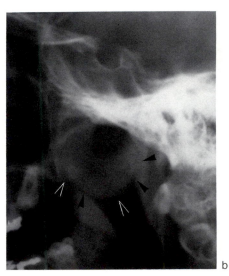

a

b

Fig. 1.10 Benign pedunculated tumors.
a) Choanal polyp arising from the antrum and presenting in the mesopharynx. The inferior pole of the tumor (arrowheads) is characteristically elongated and produces some depression of the soft palate as it presents through the nasal choana into the nasopharynx. There was no visible roentgen evidence of bone erosion on the remainder of the roentgen findings.

b) Juvenile angiofibroma presenting into the nasopharynx. The more rounded appearance of the angiofibroma as it presents into the mesopharynx (arrowheads) is strikingly different from the choanal polyp as shown in Fig. 1.10a). There is also widening of the pterygopalatine fossa on the side of the tumor. Tumor has extended into the sphenoid sinus.

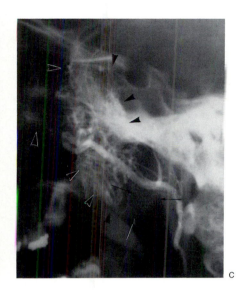

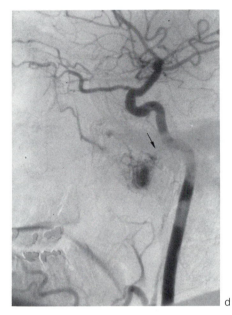

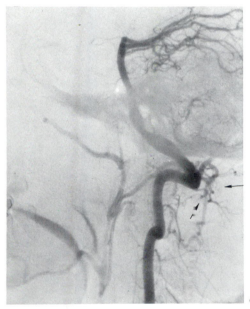

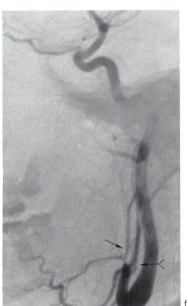

c) The same patient as in Fig. 1.10 b) during contrast angiography. This patient exhibits all of the mistakes in the radiologic management of juvenile angiofibromas. A rather large catheter is in position high in the internal maxillary artery. Contrast view shows the characteristic hypervascularity (arrowheads), but note that the inferior pole of the tumor is not opacified (arrow). This is the portion that is supplied by the ascending pharyngeal. The tumor was embolized from this catheter position, and there was excellent obliteration of the internal maxillary. The catheter was too large to fit into the ascending pharyngeal, and no attempt was made to embolize that vessel.

d) Same patient postoperative. The patient bled approximately 12 000 ml at surgery, and bleeding was finally controlled with nasal packing and tying off both external carotid arteries. This repeat angiogram with common carotid injection was performed ten days later, which shows that vascularity has already reoccurred through branches of the internal carotid system (arrow) and collaterals from the opthalmic artery.

e) Same patient postoperative. Vertebral angiography shows collaterals filling the external carotid system from the first and second segmental branches of the vertebral artery (→).

f) Same patient postoperative. Common carotid injection of the opposite side shows that the ligated external carotid artery (↣) has recanalized and fills the internal maxillary artery (→).

Inflammatory Polyps

Inflammatory polyps of the nasopharynx are exceedingly rare but may arise from the roof of the nasopharynx (16). They present as rounded masses within the nasopharynx and require clinical examination to be differentiated from the choanal polyp. They closely simulate fibromas of the nasopharynx. Unless there is a confirming clinical history of long-standing chronic inflammation, surgical removal may be the only method of providing a final diagnosis.

Juvenile Angiofibroma

Juvenile angiofibroma is the most common benign tumor of the nasopharynx. It characteristically affects teenage males although the reported age range has been 7–32 years. The most common complaint is nasal obstruction associated with spontaneous epistaxis. The tumor has been reported in females but the incidence is extremely low. Juvenile angiofibromas are said to regress after the age of 20–25; however, persistance is all too frequently the case. Juvenile angiofibromas have the unique property of extending along natural foramina and fissures. The tumor grows very slowly and produces pressure distortions of natural bony septa. Contrary to common opinion (38), the tumor may originate in the pterygopalatine fossa and gain access to the nasopharynx through the sphenopalatine foramen. Once in the pterygopalatine fossa, the tumor may extend into the subtemporal space through the sphenomaxillary fissure. As the tumor expands, it produces characteristic anterior bowing of the posterior margin of the maxillary sinus. The latter finding is so constant as to be almost diagnostic of a juvenile angiofibroma (24). The tumor may extend from the pterygopalatine fossa through the inferior orbital fissure into the floor of the orbit. Posteriorly, the tumor may gain access into the middle cranial fossa from the inferior orbital fissure via the superior orbital fissure. The tumor may extend anteriorly into the nasal passages and present as a mass from the nares or may extend posteriorly into the sphenoid sinus. Once the angiofibroma is in the sphenoid sinus, it may erode into the cavernous sinus.

Radiology plays a major role in diagnosis as well as therapy of juvenile angiofibroma. Biopsy is not recommended because of the tendency to severe hemorrhage following any manipulation. Selective angiography will show such intense staining of the tumor mass as to be practically diagnostic of juvenile angiofibroma in the proper clinical setting (50). Angiography has also been used to identify the blood supply of the vessels for surgical management or embolization prior to surgical extirpation (47).

More recently, CT scanning has shown considerable specificity in identifying the tumor spreads and characteristic bony deformities associated with juvenile angiofibromas (49). The pertinent findings of CT scanning as well as conventional tomography can be predicted from a knowledge of the previously described spread of this tumor. In the axial projection, the following findings can be elicited:

1. Rounded mass within the nasopharynx
2. Tumor extension into the nasal cavity
3. Widening of the pterygopalatine fossa on the side of the tumor
4. Distortion of fascial planes in the subtemporal space
5. Indentation of the posterior wall of the antrum by pressure erosion from the tumor mass
6. Possible invasion of orbit, sphenoid sinus, or middle cranial fossa.

Contrast enhancement should be administered to differentiate the extensions of juvenile angiofibromas from normal adjacent tissues or secondarily occluded sinuses. This is particularly helpful in determining invasions into the sphenoid sinus and ethmoid sinuses. The juvenile angiofibromas will frequently obstruct the sinuses, producing fluid and debris-filled sinus cavities that closely simulate the density of an angiofibroma. By administering contrast material, the enhancement of the contents of paranasal sinuses permits a definite diagnosis of invasion. Particular attention should be paid to the sphenoid sinus since tumor invasions of the sphenoid sinus gain access to the cavernous sinuses. If the cavernous sinus has been invaded and surgery is attempted, fatal hemorrhage has been reported when the tumor is extracted from the sphenoid sinus (48). Invasions into the pterygopalatine fossa and subtemporal space can be better delineated with contrast enhancement. In general, the distortions of the fascial planes are quite obvious, but the relationships of the tumor to the medial and lateral pterygoid might not be as precise without contrast enhancement.

Invasions into the orbit are usually quite obvious since the orbital fat is grossly different in density from the angiofibroma. On the other hand, once the orbit has been invaded, the next logical area of spread is through the superior and inferior orbital fissures into the middle cranial fossa. Juvenile angiofibromas are quite similar in density to the brain so that contrast enhancement to demonstrate these infiltrations along the medial wall of the cranial fossa can be quite valuable. The intracranial extensions are extremely difficult to see on the conventional axial projection and can be much better appreciated by coronal scanning.

The angiographic evaluation of nasopharyngeal angiofibroma is somewhat related to the size of the tumor, any previous surgical procedure, whether surgery is contemplated, and evidence of ocular signs.

For a small lesion that is being considered for surgical extirpation, the minimun studies should include a bilateral selective internal and external carotid angiogram. Transfemoral catheterization of the carotid vessels can be performed by transfemoral technique using 0.045 radiopaque polyethylene caster material (50). In the young patient, this material is easily maneuvered into both common carotid arteries sequentially so that selective studies can be made of both internal and external carotid arteries. Bilateral studies should always be performed since approximately half of the tumors receive blood supply from the contralateral arterial systems. Use of 6–8 ml of a 60% meglumine iothalamate solution proves ideal, and the filming sequence should extend over a 6–8 s period to include the late venous phase during which the juvenile angiofibroma stains intensely.

When indicated, the catheters should be maneuvered into the vertebral arteries selectively and 6 ml of 60% meglumine iothalamate injected for each side. The filming sequence should include at least 8 s since contrast material that reaches the tumor will usually be passing through a collateral circulation that adds 1–3 s to the circulation time. These collateral pathways will be through segmental branches of the 1st, 2nd, and possibly the 3rd cervical vertebrae. Collateral pathways intracranially are usually about the circle of Willis.

The thyrocervical trunk may contribute to very large juvenile angiofibromas, especially if there has been previous surgery and ligation of some of the carotid vessels. The thyrocervical trunk arises from the subclavian vessels distal to the vertebral artery along its posterior superior wall. The cervical profunda branch (deep cervical) of the thyrocervical trunk is the contributing supply to the juvenile angiofibroma, usually by collaterals with the internal maxillary and ascending pharyngeal artery. The angiographic findings are characterized by marked hypertrophy of the internal maxillary artery. The angiofibroma will derive blood supply from any vessel in the area of spread. The palatine and alveolar branches are notable supply vessels.

Great care should be exercised in performing the external carotid angiogram to keep the tip of the catheter low in the external carotid artery during contrast injection. A careful search should be made to make sure that the ascending pharyngeal artery has been opacified since this branch supplies the posterior and inferior portion of juvenile angiofibromas. The ascending palatine and the terminal branches of the internal maxillary are the vessels most likely to be involved with contralateral supply of the tumor.

A rich arterial anastomosis occurs in the floor of the middle cranial fossa from the arterial supply of the dura. These vessels include the middle meningeal artery from the external carotid, the cavernous branches of the carotid syphon, and the recurrent meningeal branch of the opthalmic artery. All may hypertrophy and form collateral pathways to an angiofibroma, especially if there has been previous surgery with ligation of the external carotid artery (32).

After the filming sequences have been completed and while the catheter is still in place in the femoral artery, a careful search should be made of the margins of the tumor as outlined. Juvenile angiofibromas grow very slowly and do not invade wildly like a malignant tumor. The margins of the tumors should be smooth and sharply delineated. If any of the margins of the tumor are shown to be ragged in outline, or the contrast material seems to fade off imperceptibly, additional vessels should be studied. The lack of sharp margins is caused by nonopacified blood supplying a portion of the tumor that has not been visualized. This is especially worrisome with an anomalous origin of the ascending pharyngeal artery. The ascending pharyngeal may arise from the common carotid below the level of the bifurcation. Under these circumstances, the ascending pharyngeal will frequently supply the posterior and deep portions of the tumor, making any surgical extirpation hazardous and extremely bloody (Fig. 1.10)

Embolization

In general, the juvenile angiofibroma that has not as yet invaded intracranially or into the orbit is best managed by surgical means. Preoperative embolization has a definite role to play in reducing the bleeding and complications of surgical procedures (47). Whether an absorbable gelatin sponge (Gelfoam), latex, or detachable balloons are used for embolization is a matter of the individual angiographer. In general, embolization should be performed within 24 h of surgery as a separate procedure from the diagnostic study and preferably the morning of surgery. In an experience with nine patients, blood loss was reduced to under 1000 ml in eight and generally was in the range of 200–350 ml. These embolizations were performed with Gelfoam and in all instances bilateral embolization was performed except in the single case where bleeding was 800–900 ml (2). The catheter tip should be placed well into the internal maxillary artery to avoid embolization of the skin. This does not prove troublesome with Gelfoam but may lead to permanent skin damage if latex or one of the other polymers is used. Care should also be exerted as progressive emboli are being injected and the tumor begins to show slowing of circulation. Eventually, when the blood supply to the tumor has been totally occluded, the emboli will tend to flow retrograde in the external carotid system and may gain access to the internal carotid artery. The use of a Seldinger guide wire to "gently tap the Gelfoam pledgets and pack them in place" adds to the safety of the procedure.

Embolization of the middle meningeal artery may prove hazardous if it happens to be the blood supply for the anterior genu of the facial nerve within the temporal bone. Facial paralysis of a temporary nature has occurred during embolization of this vessel for meningiomas (3).

The role of embolization should not be aimed at occluding every minute vessel but merely reducing the risk of hemorrhage during surgical extirpation. Embolization will not cure the tumor. As a matter of fact, the decreased vascularity due to embolization is quite temporary, and collateral circulation will develop rapidly if surgery is not performed promptly (Fig. 1.10)

Neurogenic Tumors

Lesions arising from the vagus nerve constitute the most common benign parapharyngeal tumors. Neuromas of the vagus, trigeminal and occasionally the hypoglossal nerve present as rounded tumor masses bulging into the nasopharynx. They are relatively slow growing and produce pressure on the 9th, 10th, and 11th nerves. Generally, the neurological manifestations are quite minimal, and the patient merely notices a swelling or fullness in the posterior pharynx. Plain views of the pharynx are indicated to rule out more aggressive lesions or tumors beginning within the skeletal structures or central nervous system. CT scanning may show the homogeneous nature of the mass and in particular the sharp delineation of the mass from surrounding normal tissues. The vertical extent of the lesion is usually evident from the clinical examination but can be ascertained from CT scanning as well. The principal use of CT is differentiating these benign tumors from the more commonly occurring regional metastases or direct extensions of malignant lesions of the nasopharynx or deep lobe of the parotid. CT will show that the surrounding fascial planes are well preserved except around the carotid artery. The great vessels can be identified if contrast is infused. The jugular vein is usually displaced posteriorly by the mass. The absence of adenopathy in the posterior jugular chain will give added confidence to the surgeon that he is dealing with a benign process (Fig. 1.11).

Glomus Tumors

Glomus jugulare and intravagale and carotid body tumors may present as soft tissue bulgings of the pharyngeal wall (9). All arise from paraganglionic cells that are derived from the primitive neurocrest. They produce catecholamines-ephineprine and norepinephrine.

The glomus jugulare and the carotid body tumors are the more common lesions, while approximately 45 cases of glomus intravagale have been reported (9). The tumors are very slow growing and show a familial tendency, especially for carotid body tumors. Approximately one fourth are said to be bilateral, and many glomus tumors affect multiple sites, such as the jugular fossa and carotid bifurcation. Less than 10% are malignant.

The carotid body tumors and glomus intravagale may have a bruit that would differentiate them from other benign cystic or neurogenic tumors of the parapharyngeal area. CT scanning will show contrast enhancement because of their exceedingly vascular nature. Bone erosion only accompanies the glomus jugulare tumor, whereas the glomus intravagale and carotid body lesions are free to expand in the carotid sheath and parapharyngeal space (Fig. 1.12).

Angiography may play a significant role in the management of carotid body tumors and the glomus intravagale tumors by delineating the site of origin as well as the extent of the tumor. Glomus intravagale tumors cause anterior displacement of the internal carotid artery immediately distal to the carotid sinus (4). The carotid body tumors, on the other hand, cause the internal and external carotid vessels to spread apart, and the tumor mass will produce posterior displacement of the internal carotid artery and carotid sinus. The tumor masses tend to spread in the carotid sheath surrounding the internal carotid artery; however, their blood supply is derived primarily from the external carotid system. Very large lesions may derive a blood supply from the vertebral artery and the thyrocervical trunk. Preoperative information of the blood supply of the tumor will greatly reduce the blood loss encountered in these very vascular lesions (21).

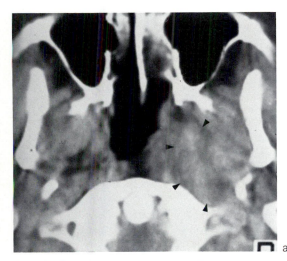

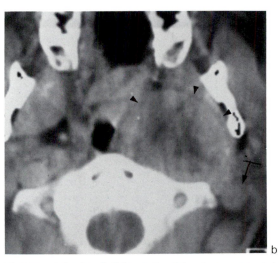

Fig. 1.11   Neuroma parapharyngeal area.
a) Midnasopharynx shows a well-circumscribed mass in the right paranasopharyngeal area (arrowheads). The lesion distorts but still does not obliterate the pterygoid muscle fascial planes and does not cross the midline.

b) Scan at the level of the soft palate shows a much larger mass (arrowhead) but no evidence of deep infiltration. Following contrast administration, this mass does not enhance. The jugular vein is displaced posteriorly (cross-hatched arrow). Some relatively low-density areas within the tumor probably represent areas of necrosis and hypovascularity.

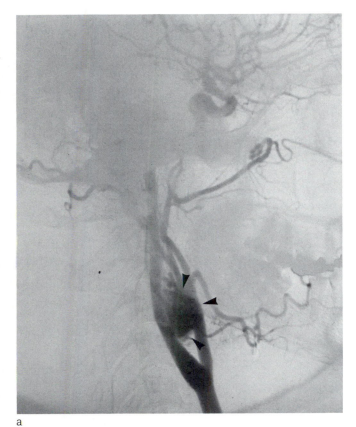

a

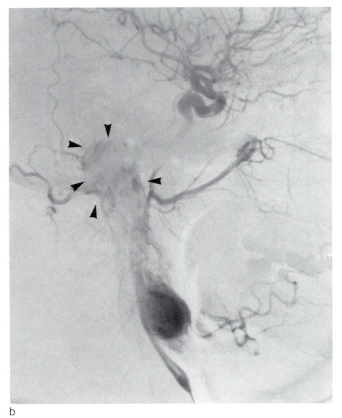

b

Fig. 1.12   Carotid body tumor and glomus jugulare tumor. Eight years previously, this patient had been operated on the opposite side for a carotid body tumor. She now presented with tinnitus and was being investigated for glomus jugulare tumor on the left.
a) Early arterial phase of the left carotid angiogram shows a densely staining tumor at the carotid bifurcation that was not suspected clinically. This staining and location is characteristic of a

carotid body tumor. Subsequent selective studies showed the tumor to be fed by branches of the external carotid artery.
b) During the late arterial phase of the same study, early staining of the suspected glomus jugulare tumor (arrowheads) was present. This tumor was fed almost exclusively by the greater occipital artery. At a later date, embolization was performed in the early morning prior to surgical extirpation.

Nasopharyngeal Tumor-Malignant

Nasopharyngeal malignancies account for 2%–5% of all head and neck cancers. In whites, the rate of occurrence of cancer is between 0.25%–3%, whereas in southern Chinese, nasopharyngeal epidermoid carcinoma was listed as the leading cause of death from malignant disease. The high incidence of nasopharyngeal carcinomas is also found in Eskomos, Kenyans, and the Maltese (2). It is found in all ages, and the youngest known patient reported to have an epidermoid carcinoma was four years of age (Fig. 1.13) (12, 14, 18, 31, 45). The radiologic appearance of the tumors has little relationship to the cell type (25, 28). Most of the tumors are epidermoid carcinomas, folowed by lymphoepitheliomas and lymphosarcomas arising from the lymphoid tissue of the roof of the nasopharynx. The rare adenocarcinoma arises from mucous glands, while occasionally tumors arising from minor salivary glands may be encountered in the nasopharynx. Tumors of the adjacent clivus and the base of the skull will bulge into the airway and invade the nasopharynx. Plasmocytomas and melanomas may arise from the nasopharynx or extend to the nasopharynx from the adjancent nasal cavity or paranasal sinuses.

The clinical diagnosis of tumors of the nasopharynx is based on local pain, metastatic neck nodes, or nasal obstruction interfering with eustachian tube function.

The tumor spreads may be lymphatic, direct extension, or hematogenous.

The lymphatic spreads are to the retropharyngeal nodes or to the more laterally placed upper posterior cervical nodes. The tumors may spread to deep upper jugular chains producing pressure on cranial nerves IX, X, XI, and XII in or near the jugular fossa. By the time paralysis of the above-listed cranial nerves occurs, the tumor spread is usually advanced.

Lymphadenopathy to the posterior cervical chain brings up the clinical entity of the "unknown primary" (Fig. 1.13). This particular group of patients represents an entity that requires precision radiographic techniques as well as thorough clinical examination and extensive biopsies. The usual rules of immediately biopsying any mass for diagnosis can be extremely harmful in the case of the unknown primary. The sine qua non of adequate cancer surgery in the head and neck is to remove the primary along with any metastases in block. This means that if biopsy of the lymph node has been performed and proves to be a head and neck cancer, future definitive surgical procedures will require that surgeons remove all of the skin and subcutaneous tissues violated during the biopsy. Removal of this much skin plus the lymphatic chain and primary tumor may produce such a defect that it will be impossible to close without extensive grafting and flap formation due to the unwarranted lymph node biopsy.

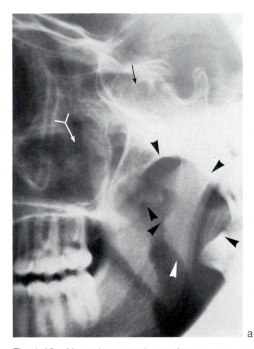

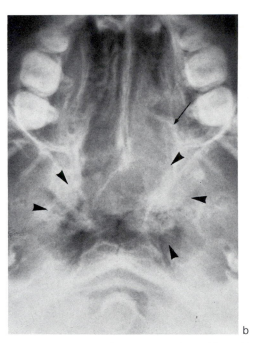

Fig. 1.13 Nasopharyngeal carcinoma on a 16-year-old boy whose presenting symptom was cervical adenopathy.
a) Lateral view of the sinus series shows opacification of the sphenoid sinus (arrow) and a polypoid lesion in the right antrum (Y-shaped arrow). The nasopharyngeal airway is irregularly constricted by a circumferential type of carcinoma (arrowheads).

b) Base projection of the same patient with total loss of the normal air shadows and surface anatomy of the nasopharynx due to the presence of the circumferentially growing carcinoma (arrowheads). The tumor has extended anteriorly into the nasal cavity, producing obstruction of the sphenoid sinus and posterior ethmoid sinuses, especially on the left (arrow).

In approximately 70% of the patients with a single palpable malignant lymph node in the mid or upper cervical chain, the site of primary tumor will be as follows:

1. Nasopharynx   25%
2. Tonsil   11%
3. Base of tongue   10%
4. Thyroid   33%
5. Extrinsic larynx 21%

By performing triple endoscopy, nasopharyngoscopic washings, blind biopsies of all mucosal surfaces together with careful radiographic investigation, the site of any head and neck primary should be diagnosed in 100% of the patients. The rate of cure of the true unknown primary should be 0% since this would mean that the site of the primary is either in the chest, abdomen, or skeletal structures and the disease is already far advanced. Conceivably, there may be a rare tumor arising in a branchial cleft remnant. Biopsy of the palpable lymph nodes should only be performed after the radiographic examinations of the head and neck and the extensive clinical and pathological survey outlined above.

Direct Extensions

The bony margins of the sphenoid sinus, the first and second cervical vertebrae, and the lateral walls of the nasopharynx are covered by thin but tough fascial plane that tends to prevent early deep infiltration of nasopharyngeal tumors. Initially, sinus spread is usually through the natural ostium. They tend to penetrate perivascular and perineural spaces so that extensions may occur through the foramen lacerum surrounding the carotid artery or through the foramen rotundum or foramen ovale. Tumors that have spread around the carotid artery will involve the cranial nerves within the cavernous sinus, mainly III, IV, and VI.

Direct extension along the mucosa may occur to involve the opening of the eustachian tube. The dysfunction of the eustachian tube either by direct blockage or interference with muscular function of the tensor veli platini muscles; all contribute to formation of serous otitis media. The superficial spreads may occlude the natural ostium of the sphenoid sinus or extend anteriorly into the nasal cavity. Hematogenous spread of nasopharyngeal tumors does occur although it is rather unusual. They may spread to the lungs, and bony metastases have been reported.

Roentgen Findings

The roentgen findings of nasopharyngeal carcinomas are related to the site of origin and general growth characteristics. At times, it is impossible to tell the site of origin; however, approximately 37% are said to arise from the fossa of Rosenmüller, 32% from the roof, 15% from the posterior wall, and 8% are central in origin. They may be exophytic or ulcerative. A particularly difficult variety to diagnose is the occult infiltrative type. In a series of 31 necropsies, 2 patients were reported in whom the surface epithelium of the nasopharynx appeared to be intact and only slight irregular thickening of the submucosa was visible in the posterior wall. In another report (28), 30% of 90 cases studies were of the occult infiltrative type of nasopharyngeal carcinoma.

Plain Film Findings

In searching for nasopharyngeal tumor, examination should consist of a lateral projection and a non rotated base projection with the mandible superimposed on the frontal bone. The base projection, can be made with the mouth opened and the mouth closed to give maximum visualization of the change in configuration of the fossae of Rosenmüller. The fossae of Rosenmüller will be slit-like in the closed mouth projection but will open up as the mouth is opened to allow better appreciation of symmetries. If questions still exist as to the symmetry of the fossae of Rosenmüller, the patient can be instructed to blow against the pinched nostrils, and a repeat base projection is performed. By these two maneuvers of nasopharyngeal physiology, between 20%–50% of the patients will exhibit better filling of the fossae of Rosenmüller and will correct any minor asymmetries. In approximately 5% of the patients, there will be less visualization in the fossae of Rosenmüller, and in somewhere between 50%–70% there will be no real change in the appearance of the fossae of Rosenmüller.

The bony architecture of the sphenoid should be carefully evaluated on both the base and lateral projections. Sclerosis has been reported by Potter (41) and others as one of the early manifestations of nasopharyngeal tumors. The sclerosis or destruction may be in the dorsum sellae, body of the sphenoid, and clivus region. The sclerosis may extend out into the floor of the middle cranial fossa involving the greater wing of the sphenoid. Destructive lesions may also be found in the sphenoid secondary to the direct spread of nasopharyngeal tumors. If the tumor has invaded the midline, it may extend into the arch of C-1 or into the body of C-2 vertebral bodies. Since sclerotic reaction of these bones can be caused by radiation therapy, it is important to have a good pretherapy baseline for any future patient management.

The plain lateral view of the nasopharynx taken with a wide latitude film should clearly demonstrate several gradations of gray corresponding to the various walls and folds of the nasopharynx. Most posteriorly should be the sharp delineation of the posterior nasopharyngeal wall and the air-containing nasopharynx. This shadow can be followed superiorly where it will be deflected away from the bone by the adenoidal pad. There is tremendous variation in the volume of adenoidal tissue in the teenager and young adult, but this adenoidal pad shadow should greatly diminish after the age of 35. No good measurement appears to be available at the present time to differentiate adenoidal hypertrophy from a malignant new growth with respect to the configuration of the adenoidal pad.

The next gradation of gray scale with an interface should appear between 4–10 mm anterior to the posterior pharyngeal wall. This fold represents the salpingopharyngeal fold and continues inferiorly into the oral pharynx. Tumors that arise in the fossae of Rosenmüller and extend along this fold may obliterate the shadow or may cause the shadow of the fold to be displaced anteriorly. Since the salpingopharyngeal folds are paired structures, obliteration of the fold on one side will not be appreciated in the lateral projection. One must constantly be reminded that nasopharyngeal tumors that begin along the lateral wall, about the fossa of Rosenmüller, or on the anteriorly placed salpingopalatine fold will be totally missed on the lateral projection unless the tumor growth pattern is pedunculated and the tumor projects into the air space of the nasopharynx (Fig. 1.14). Soft tissue structures can only be visualized radiographically when the x-ray beam passes tangent to a soft tissue-air interface about the periphery of an exophytic tumor. It is extremely difficult to pick up a gentle curve of a mound of tissue that does not allow the x-ray beam to

pass tangent to the surface. For this reason, even in the normal patient the salpingopalatine fold is rarely seen in its entirety.

Contrast Nasopharyngography

Contrast nasopharyngography is relatively easy to perform, is noninvasive, and yields helpful information concerning the blind areas of the nasopharynx. It has not received wide reception probably because of the rarity of nasopharyngeal tumors and lack of familiarity with the procedure. With the more widespread availability of fiberoptic nasopharyngoscopic examination and the use of CT scanning of the nasopharynx, positive contrast nasopharyngoscopy will probably remain a seldomly utilized diagnostic technique. The type of tumor growth can be identified whether it is exophytic or ulcerative. The infiltrative type of lesion will show a relative immobility of the nasopharyngeal wall involved. Unfortunately, the usefulness of contrast nasopharyngoscopy is in direct competition with clinical examination. The bulky exophytic tumors that are readily demonstrable by

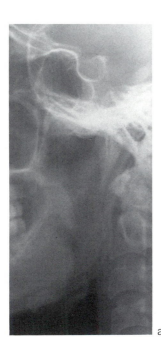

a

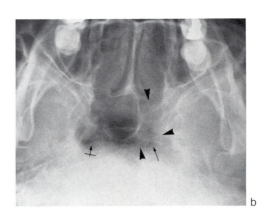

b

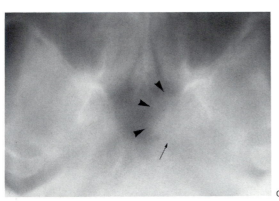

c

Fig. 1.**14** Pedunculated anaplastic carcinoma of the lateral wall of the nasopharynx.
a) In the lateral projection, the posterior pharyngeal wall soft palate and salpingopharyngeal folds are all fairly well seen and appear grossly normal. One could question a slight increase in density of the nasopharyngeal air shadow, but this is extremely minimal.
b) Base projection shows a normal fossa of Rosenmüller on the right (cross-hatches arrow), while on the left the fossa is partially obliterated and obscured (arrow). The soft tissue mass arising from the left lateral wall of the nasopharynx is poorly seen but causes an increase in density (arrowhead).
c) Base tomogram shows the pedunculated mass projected into the nasopharynx (arrowheads) and encroachment upon the fossa of Rosenmüller (arrow).

contrast nasopharyngoscopy are also readily visible on mirror or fibro-optic examination. The infiltrating tumors that have an intact mucosa escape detection unless CT scanning or multiple blind biopsy are used.

CT Scanning

CT scanning of the nasopharynx is the radiologic procedure of choice to delineate the origin of a tumor mass, especially if axial and coronal views are obtained. In general, contrast enhancement has not proved helpful for local disease because the muscles seem to enhance to the same degree as the tumor masses. If the tumor has extended, intracranial contrast enhancement is extremely valuable to show changes in the adjacent brain. Small amounts of air in the fossae of Rosenmüller or in the opening of the eustachian tubes are easily seen, and fascial planes obliterated by tumor masses become quite evident.

The most important feature of CT scanning in nasopharyngeal malignancy is the demonstration of deep infiltration. Disruptions of the lucent fascial planes surrounding the pterygoid muscles, the low density areas lateral to the tensor and levator palatine muscles and the sheaths of the carotid vessels all give clues to the malignant nature of nasopharyngeal tumors. The deep infiltra-

tions as demonstrated on the coronal plane may be partially obscured by the overlying pterygoid plates. Regardless, changes in density of tissues below the temporal bones can prove quite helpful. In a review of 20 consecutive nasopharyngeal malignancies, the overall pattern of growth would be described as follows:

Flattened 9
Bulging mass 4
Exophytic or pedunculated 4
Circumferential 3

All of the tumor masses showed deep infiltration with loss of fascial planes surrounding muscle bundles near the site of tumor. The margins of the nasopharynx tend to become fixed as one might expect in the region of the tumor. Having the patient blow against closed nostrils or assuming the open mouth position do not appreciably change the contours of the fossae of Rosenmüller or walls of the nasopharynx near the regions of deep infiltrations. Neither did the histology of the tumor seem to dictate the pattern of growth to any reliable extent. Some of the more anaplastic tumors and lymphomas tend to grow with a much more circumferential mucosal type of spread (Fig. 1.15). The adenocystic carcinomas that are noted for their perineural lymphatic invasions did not show any characteristic changes on the CT. The major

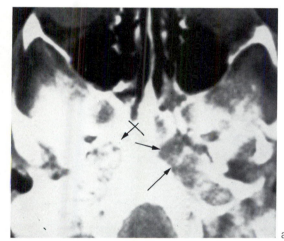
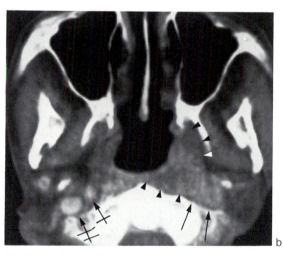
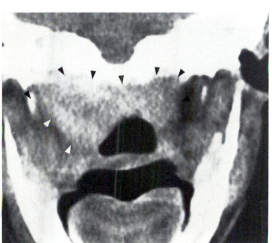

Fig. **1.15** Circumferential growing squamous cell carcinoma of the nasopharynx with early invasion about the foramen lacerum region.
a) Scan through the base of the skull shows asymmetry of the region of the foramen lacerum with destructive changes on the right (arrows) as compared to the more normal bony architecture on the left (cross-hatched arrow).
b) Section through the midnasopharynx with extensive infiltration extending anteriorly to the medial pterygoid plate and posteriorly to the base of the skull and crossing the midline (arrowhead). Contrast material was administered, and a normal carotid artery (cross-hatched arrow) and jugular vein (double cross- hatched arrow) are demonstrated on the left. The carotid sheath region on the right is totally enveloped in tumor (arrows).
c) Coronal scan at the level of the soft palate shows the circumferential growth of the tumor extending across the vault of the nasopharynx and up to the base of the skull (arrowheads). The undersurface of the right petrous bone is partially eroded.

nerves that surround the nasopharynx could not be visualized nor could any localized changes in densities near the orifices of the foramen rotundum or foramen ovale be suggested that would indicate perineural invasion. The overall densities of the tumor masses all appeared approximately the same.

The site of origin of the tumors could be suggested from the CT scan, but at times the advanced nature of the lesions was such that the nasopharynx could only be described as diffusely involved by tumor. As best can be determined, the site of origin of the 20 tumors are listed as follows:

Fossa of Rosenmüller	9
Lateral wall	3
Posterior wall	2
Superior wall	2
Diffuse	4

The tumors that arose in the fossa of Rosenmüller were not necessarily still confined to the fossa of Rosenmüller at the time of the CT examination. The center of the expansivity of infiltration merely seemed to be arising from that location. There did not seem to be any relationship of cell type to the site of origin although lymphosarcomas are said to occur more commonly from the superior wall of the nasopharynx.

No chordomas were encountered in this small group. Chordomas characteristically originate in the midline. In one third of the patients, the tumors start from within the clivus and present as nasopharyngeal masses. On CT scans, chordomas may show calcification within the tumor mass that usually bulges in the midline. Because of their slow-growing nature, they tend to reach larger size by the time the patients seek medical attention.

The common spreads of nasopharyngeal tumors are apparent on coronal and axial tomography. Invasion about the carotid artery within the cavernous sinus cannot be seen directly but is diagnosed by the indirect evidence of demineralization about the foramen lacerum (Fig. 1.16). Bone destruction is seen on the coronal sections about the lateral body of the sphenoid, and cerebral changes after contrast infusion also give clues to cavernous sinus involvement.

The syndrome of tumor spread to the highest jugular node is readily apparent on CT scanning because of loss of the normal low-density areas around the carotid sheath. If contrast enhancement is used, the carotid artery and jugular veins are well opacified and can be shown to be displaced by tumor masses within the lymph nodes. In advanced lesions, bony invasion of the temporal bone and occipital bone can frequently be demonstrated on axial scanning.

Otitis media is a well-known presenting symptom of patients with nasopharyngeal tumors. The tumor may interfere with eustachian tube physiology by producing a mechanical blockage of its ostium or by interfering with the function of the tensor veli palatini muscles and to a lesser extent the levator veli palatini muscles. The tensor muscle takes origin from the cartilaginous portion of the eustachian tube and causes the eustachian tube to open, while the levator veli palatini muscle in its action causes the eustachian tube to close. In a review of 24 tumors involving the nasopharynx, 14 patients were found to have otitis media as part of the clinical picture (20). All of the patients with serous otitis had tumor involving the ostium of the eustachian tube. Many of the patients with serous otitis had tumor involving the tensor veli palatini but not all of the otitis media patients had muscle involvement. In addition, many of the patients without

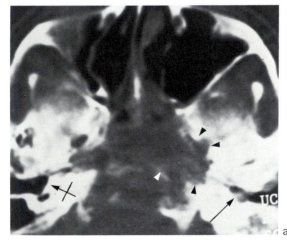

a

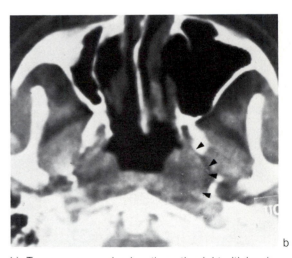

b

Fig. 1.16 Invasion of the base of the skull with 3rd, 4th, and 6th nerve paresis.
a) Axial scan through the base of the skull shows extensive destruction centering about the foramen lacerum and extending laterally to the region of the foramen ovale (arrowheads). The middle ear cavity on the side of the bone destruction shows some increase in density (arrow) by comparison to the air-containing middle ear cavity on the left (cross-hatched arrow).

b) Tumor mass predominantly on the right with involvement of the right eustachian tube orifice and tumor extending posteriorly into the longus collis muscle plane (arrowheads). The tumor also involves the wall to a considerable extent on coronal sections (not illustrated).

serous otitis also demonstrated involvement of the muscle about the eustachian tube. It would seem that mechanical obstruction of the ostium of the eustachian tube is the dominant factor in the formation of serous otitis in patients with nasopharyngeal tumors (Fig. 1.17). The differentiation of tumor spreads to the sphenoid sinus and blockage of the sphenoid sinus with secondary infection may be difficult. The density of material within the sinuses is identical, and unless there is extensive bone destruction, one cannot be certain whether the superficial mucosal spreads of tumor have caused sinus block-age or actual invasion has taken place. Biopsy may be the only reliable means for differentiation.

Tumor spreads to the nasal cavity are readily apparent and frequently cause blockages of the paranasal sinuses. If the tumor has invaded laterally about the pterygoid venous plexus, it may spread intracranially through the floor of the middle cranial fossa. The pterygoid plexus has venous channels that go directly through the inferior portion of the greater wing of the sphenoid, through the foramen ovale, and occasionally may accompany the middle meningeal artery through the foramen spinosum. The tumors may then produce central nervous system disturbances in the subtemporal gyri and changes about the temporal horn.

A very important feature of nasopharyngeal tumors that bears direct relationship to radiation therapy is the demonstration of spread to deep cervical and jugular lymph nodes. The distortion of fascial planes and displacement of vascular structures may serve as clues to the radiotherapists for planning of treatment ports. At the present time, it is not possible to differentiate between reactive nodes and tumor-bearing nodes; however, the loss of discrete outlines of lymphadenopathy and changes in density of the fascial planes about the great vessels are highly suspicious of the presence of malignant lymphadenopathy or direct tumor extension (Fig. 1.18). In summary, it would seem that CT offers the ability to study the deep structures of the pharynx, including the nasopharynx. The patterns of tumor growth, while not being exacting, allow a fairly accurate appraisal of benign versus malignant processes, especially when coupled with adequate clinical history.

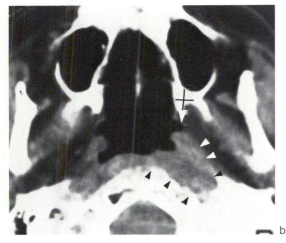

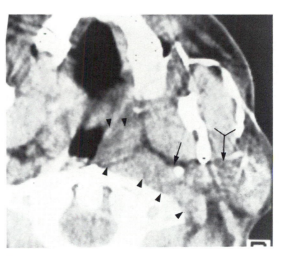

Fig. 1.17 Tumor disturbance of eustachian tube physiology.
a) Adenocarcinoma of the nasopharynx, which has infiltrated the ostium of the eustachian tube on the left and spread deeply into the paranasopharyngeal space (arrowheads). The eustachian tube on the left does not open (arrow) despite the patient performing the maneuver of blowing against the occluded nostril that has opened the eustachian tube on the right (double cross-hatched arrow). Serous otitis was a presenting symptom.
b) Deeply infiltrating squamous cell carcinoma obliterating the posterior wall of the fossa of Rosenmüller on the right and extending toward the base of the skull (arrowheads). The shadow of the tensor veli palatini and levator veli palatini muscles are enveloped in the tumor extension. The eustachian tube orifice is widely patent (cross-hatched arrow) on the right as well as on the left in this patient who had no evidence of middle ear inflammatory disease.

Fig. 1.18 Carcinoma lateral pharyngeal wall at the level of the soft palate with extensive lymph node metastases. CT sialography was performed, which showed nonfilling of the deep lobe of the parotid ←, presumably due to metastases from the pharyngeal carcinoma. The tumor mass extends by both direct extension and lymphatic spread to the region of the carotid sheath (arrowheads). The carotid artery can be identified (arrow) by the calcification in its wall as it lies immediately medial to the densely calcified stylohyoid ligament. The jugular vein is deformed and displaced posteriorly (most posterior arrowhead) by tumor extension.

As fast scanning and highly detailed scanning become available, we can look forward to meaningful studies of physiology of the nasopharynx, eustachian tube function, and possibly disturbances of muscle balance that may affect temporal mandibular joints and the entire upper respiratory and gastrointestinal systems.

References

1. Barnes EL, Zafar Tasneem: Laryngeal amyloidosis-clinicopathologic study of seven cases. Ann Otol 86: 856–863, 1977
2. Bentson John MD-personal communication.
3. Bentson J, Rand R, Calcaterra T, Lasjaunas P: Unexpected complications following therapeutic embolization. Neuroradiology 16: 420–423, 1978
4. Black FO, Myers EN, et al: Surgical management of vagal chemodectomas. Laryngoscope 87: 1259–2368, 1977
5. Calderelli D, Friedberg S: Transnasal microsurgical correction of choanal atresia. Laryngeoscope 87: 2023–2030, 1977
6. Carpenter RJ, Neal HB: Correction of choanal atresia in children and adults. Laryngoscope 87: 1304–1311, 1977
7. Chandler JR: Malignant external otitis: further considerations. Ann Otol 86: 417–428, 1977
8. Claussen CD, Lohkamp FW, Krastel A: Computed tomography of trauma involving brain and facial skull (craniofacial injuries). J Comput Assist Tomogr 1: 472–473, 1973
9. Conley J, Clairmont A: Glomus intravagle. Laryngoscope 87: 2096–2100, 1977
10. Davis David MD – personal communication.
11. Delaney P, Henkin RI, Manz H, Satterly A, Bauer H: Olfactory sarcoidosis. Arch Otolaryngol 103: 717–724, 1977
12. Deutsch M, Mercado R, Parsons JA: Cancer of the nasopharynx in children. Cancer 41: 1128–1133, 1978
13. Eisenberg L, Wood T, Boles R: Mucormycosis. Laryngoscope 87: 347–356, March 1977
14. Fernandez C, Cangir A, Samaan N, Rivera R: Nasopharyngeal carcinoma in children. Cancer 37: 2787–2791, 1976
15. Firoonia H, Pinto RS, Lin JP et al: Chordoma: radiologic evaluation of 20 cases. Am J Roentgenol 127: 797–805, 1976
16. Fletcher GH, Jing BS: The Head and Neck. Year Book, Chicago 1968
17. Gould LV, Cummings CW, Rabuzzi DD, Reed GF et al: Use of computerized axial tomography of the head and neck region. Laryngoscope 87: 1270–1276, 1977
18. Greene MH, Graumeni JF, Hoover R: Nasopharyngeal cancer among young people in the United States: racial variations by cell type. J Natl Cancer Inst 58: 1267–1270, 1977
19. Hanafee WN, Gussen R: Correlation of basal projection tomography in clinical problems. Radiol Cl in North Am 12: 419–430, 1974
20. Hanafee WN, Mancuso AA, Jenkins H et al: CT scanning of the temporal bone. Ann Otol, Rhinol, Laryngol 1979
21. Hanafee WN, Von Ledon H: Angiography in management of carotid body tumors JAMA 191: 499–502, 1965
22. Hawkins DB: Glottic and subglottic stenoisis from endotracheal intubation. Laryngoscope 87: 339–346, 1977
23. Ho JHC: An epidemiologic and clinical study of nasopharyngeal carcinoma. Radioat Oncol Biol Phys 4: 183, 1978
24. Holman CB et al: Juvenile nasopharyngeal fibroma- roentgenologic characteristics. Am J Roentgenol 94: 292, 1965
25. Hoppe RT, Williams J, Warnke R et al: Carcinoma of the nasopharynx-the significance of histology. Radiat Oncol Biol Phys 4: 199–205, 1978

26. Jereb B, Anggard A, Baryd I: Juvenile nasopharyngeal angiofibroma; a clinical study of 69 cases. Acta Radiol (Ther) 9: 302–310, 1910
27. Kamijo A, Okabe, Kazuhiko, Hirose, Takeshi: Thorium Dioxide Granuloma of the neck with resultant fatal hemorrhage. Arch Otolaryngol 105: 45–47, 1979
28. Kaseff LG: Early x-ray diagnosis of occult infiltrating nasopharyngeal carcinoma. Ann Otol 86: 864–870, 1977
29. Khoo FY, Chia KB, Teo AT, Osman MBH, Kanagasuntheram R: Radiology of the eustachian fossa. Clin Radiol 28: 151–160, 1977
30. Khoo FY, Kanagasuntheram R, Chia KB: Variations of the lateral recesses of the nasopharynx. Arch Otolaryngol 86: 122–128, 1967
31. Lanasa JJ, Putney JF: Nasopharyngeal malignancy in childhood. South Med J 67: 1363–1364, 1974
32. Lasjaunias P, Moret J, Vignaud J: External carotid supply to orbit. In: Orbit Roentgenology, ed by Arger P, Wiley and Sons, New York 1977
33. Mancuso AA, Bohman L, Hanafee WN, et al: CT of the nasopharynx: normal, variations of normal and pathologic correlations. Exhibit presented at the American Roentgen Ray meeting. Canada, March 1979
34. Mangat D, Orr WC, Smith RO: Sleep apnea, hypersomnolence, and upper airway obstruction secondary to adenotonsilar enlargement. Arch Otolaryngol 102: 383–386, 1977
35. Methney JA: Dermatomyositis- a vocal and swallowing disease entity. Laryngoscope 88: 147–161, 1978
36. Meyers AD, Lillydahl P, Brown G: Hypopharyngeal perforations in neonates. Arch Otolaryngol 104: 51–54, 1978
37. Moss WT, Brand WN, Therapeutic radiology: rationale, technique, results. Mosby, St. Louis 1969
38. Neal HB, Whicker JH, Devine KD, Weiland LH: Juvenile angiofibroma- a review of 120 cases. Am J Surg 547–556, 1973
39. Ogura JH: Fundamental understanding of nasal obstruction. Laryngoscope 87: 1225–1232, 1977
40. Pahor AL: Charles Dickens and the ear, nose, and throat. Arch Otolaryngol 105: 1–5, 1979
41. Potter GD: Sclerosis of the base of the skull as a manifestation of nasopharyngeal carcinoma. Radiology 94: 35–38, 1979
42. Rizzuti RJ, Whalen JP: The nasopharynx – roentgen anatomy and its alteration in the base view. Radiology 104: 537–540, 1972
43. Rosen L, Hanafee W, Hahum A: Nasopharyngeal angiofibroma, an angiographic evaluation. Radiology 86: 103–107, 1966
44. Simmons FB, Guilleminault C, Dement WC, et al: Surgical management of airway obstruction during sleep. Laryngoscope 87: 326–338, 1977
45. Snow JB: Neoplasms of the nasopharynx in children. Otolaryngol Clin North Am 10: 11–24, 1977
46. Tada S, Kino M, Yamamotot W, Harada J: Contrast nasopharyngography. Clin Radiol 28: 569–662, 1977
47. Thibaut A, Callignon J: Nasopharyngeal angiofibroma. Neuroradiology 16: 419, 1978
48. Ward PH, Thompson R, Calcaterra TC, Kadin M: Juvenile angiofibroma: a more rational therapeutic approach based upon clinical and experimental evidence. Laryngoscope 84: 2181–2194, 1974
49. Weinstein MA, Levine H, Duchesneau PM, Tucker HM: Diagnosis of juvenile angiofibroma by computed tomography. Radiology 126: 703–705, 1978
50. Wilson GH, Hanafee WN: Angiographic findings in 16 patients with Juvenile nasopharyngeal angiofibroma. Radiology 92: 279–284, 1969

Chapter 2 Larynx

Introduction

The larynx is truly a remarkable organ that coordinates the functions of breathing, speech, deglutition, heavy lifting, and "abdominal straining." In lower animals, the respiratory system is anatomically separated from the gastrointestinal tract to facilitate the above-listed functions. In man, precision neuromuscular control and structural adaptations permit these functions to proceed with only split-second intervals between successive physiologic events.

The anatomic foundation of the larynx is the cricoid cartilage, which is shaped like a signet ring with the large signet being posterior and thin ringlet lying anterior. The remaining supporting structures of the larynx are mostly paired structures consisting of two pyramidal cartilages called the arytenoid cartilages lying on the superolateral margins of the signet of the cricoid cartilage (Fig. 2.1). A projection arises from the anterior inferior margin of the arytenoid cartilages, which serves as the support for the vocal ligament. The anterior and lateral boundaries of the larynx are formed by the paired thyroid cartilages that form a shield and supporting structure for both intrinsic and extrinsic musculature. The vocal ligament is attached to the inner surface near the inferior margins of the thyroid cartilage. The single remaining unpaired cartilage is the epiglottis, which consists of an upper free margin, a body, and a wedge-shaped inferior point called the petiole that attaches by the thyroepiglottic ligament to the same point of attachment as the anterior extremity of the vocal cords. The petiole is continuous with the midportion of the epiglottis or body of the epiglottis that separates the lumina of the larynx from a fat-filled space anterior to the epiglottis called the preepiglottic space. The upper margin of the epiglottis is a free margin with mucosal surface on both sides of the epiglottis. Folds from the free margin of the epiglottis pass out laterally to a lateral pharyngeal wall and are called the pharyngeal folds. Additional folds pass from the posterior margins of the epiglottis to the arytenoid cartilages forming the aryepiglottic folds. They delineate the space anterior to the free margins of the epiglottis, which is called the vallecula, from spaces that lie lateral and posterior to the laryngeal vestibule and medial to the thyroid cartilage, which are the piriform sinuses. The piriform sinuses conduct fluid and solid boluses from the oral pharynx to the esophagus. The second fold that passes from the posterolateral free margin of the epiglottis to the arytenoid cartilages serves to prevent aspiration of liquid or solid food particles from the piriform sinuses into the laryngeal vestibule. Four small cartilages lie in the aryepiglottic folds. Paired corniculate cartilages sit on top of the arytenoid cartilages and immediately lateral are the cuneiform cartilages in the free margin of the aryepiglottic folds.

The true and false vocal cords function to close off the airway during deglutition and straining, and the true cords partially oppose each other during phonation. Both true and false cords are attached anteriorly at the midline and posteriorly to the arytenoids and lateral wall of the larynx. Radiologic investigation of the larynx becomes more sophisticated as the more esoteric functions and anatomic details are being studied. The examinations consist of plain views, tomography, positive contrast laryngography, and computerized tomography. All have advantages and limitations that must be weighed in the light of patient discomfort and radiation exposure for the simpler procedures to a possibility of morbidity due to anesthesia and contrast reactions with positive contrast laryngography (Table 1).

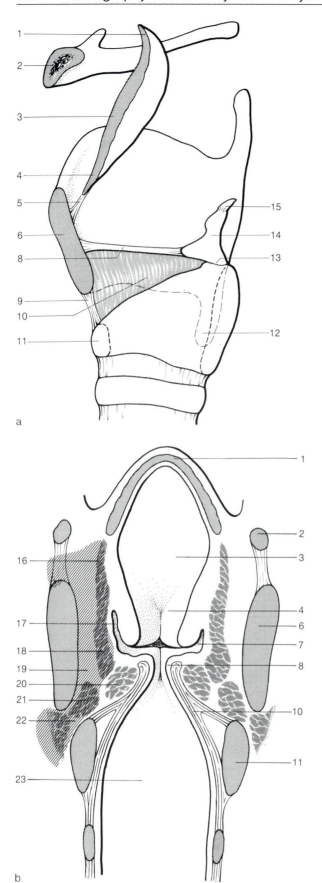

Table 1   Choices of Roentgen Examinations

	Advantages	Limitations
Plain views	1. Gross extent of airway 2. Demonstration of advanced cartilage destruction 3. Occasional demonstration of cartilage distortion	1. Information limited 2. Serves for screening only
Tomography	1. Noninvasive 2. Economical 3. Some idea of tumor bulk possible 4. Subglottic airway well demonstrated	1. Subtle deformities easily missed 2. Irregular surfaces poorly demonstrated 3. Good patient cooperation imperative
Positive contrast laryngography	1. Physiology clearly demonstrated 2. Mucosal surfaces can be studied in minute detail 3. Subglottic area well delineated 4. Excellent for piriform sinuses and laryngeal ventricles	1. Invasive procedure 2. Deep infiltrations not directly shown 3. Duplicates information of direct laryngoscopy
Computerized tomography	1. Excellent for cartilages 2. Excellent for airway 3. Ideal for deep infiltrations 4. Noninvasive	1. Mucosal surfaces poorly delineated 2. Vertical spatial arrangements not completely accurate 3. Equipment expensive 4. Shows morphology not histology 5. Study of physiology limited

Fig. 2.1 Diagrammatic representation of laryngeal cartilages and paralaryngeal space.
a) View of the right half of the larynx on midsaggital cut.
b) Midcoronal view of the larynx looking from behind. 1. Suprahyoid epiglottis, 2. hyhoid bone, 3. body of epiglottis, 4. petiolus of epiglottis, 5. thyroepiglottic ligament, 6. thyroid cartilage, 7. laryngeal ventricle, 8. vocal ligament, 9. cricothyroid membrane, 10. conus elasticus, 11. cricoid cartilage, 12. inferior cornu of thyroid cartilage, 13. cricoarytenoid joint, 14. arytenoid cartilage, 15. corniculate cartilage, 16. aryepiglottic muscle, 17. appendix of the laryngeal ventricle, 18. the lateral thyroarytenoid muscle, 19. paralaryngeal space (shaded area), 20. vocal muscle, 21. lateral cricoarytenoid muscle, 22. inferior extension of the paralaryngeal space, 23. trachea.

Larynx-Radiologic Techniques

Plain Views

The lateral view of the larynx should be performed during quiet respiration to give maximum contrast of the air-filled passages and soft tissues (14). A wide latitude gray scale film, such as single emulsion film using a single vacuum-packed screen, is most helpful to delineate cartilage as well as air and soft tissue. Technical factors vary but average about 40 MAS, 65 kV (range 60–70 kV) at a 40-in distance. The relationship between the thyroid cartilage and cricoid cartilage will be of considerable interest in evaluating the distortions by malignancy, trauma, and any evidence of localized destructive lesions (Fig. 2.2). Plain anteroposterior views are best performed during quiet respiration to show the maximum airway possible. A second anteroposterior view with the patient phonating may be of help to accurately locate the position of the true cords and demonstrate the subglottic space. Unfortunately, small mass lesions can easily be missed during phonation. Their bulk is best demonstrated when the true and false cords are maximally abducted during quiet inspiration. The limitation of any mass in the transglottic airway will be clearly visible.

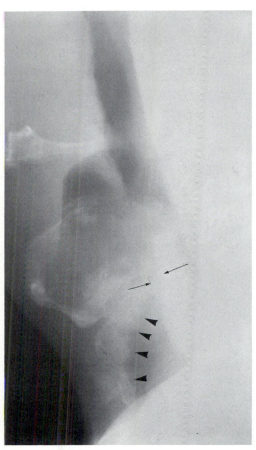

a

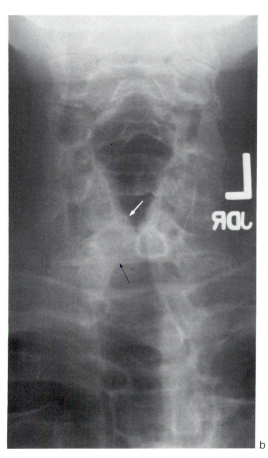

b

Fig. 2.2   Carcinoma of the larynx with subglottic extension.
a) Lateral projection. The striking feature of this study is the lobulated mass that extends inferior beyond the level of the cricoid cartilage to the region of the first tracheal ring (arrowheads). The airway is narrowed to a slitlike passage near the posterior commissure (arrows). There has been partial destruction of the cricoid cartilage, and the thyroid cartilage has rotated anteriorly to narrow the space between the remaining superior rim of the cricoid and thyroid cartilages.

b) In the anterior posterior projection, the major portion of the mass is on the right in the region of the true and false cords (arrows) with lesser swelling present on the left. The major portion of the subglottic mass is anterior and does not cast a shadow because the x-ray beam does not pass tangent to the surface of the tumor mass.

Tomography

Tomography of the larynx can be performed rather successfully with linear tomography when pluridirectional tomography is not available. Examination may prove useful in patients who are too ill to withstand positive contrast laryngography and information is needed regarding webs of scarring in the sublgottic region or upper trachea (Fig. 2.3). The procedure has largely been supplanted by CT scanning for examination of endolaryngeal lesions. Tomography is performed during quiet respiration with films being taken at 2–3 mm intervals through the larynx in both anteroposterior and lateral projection. Factors average 55–60 kV, 25–35 MA for a 6 s exposure using cronex 6+ (or comparable film) and high-speed screens. In addition, tomography is performed at 2-mm intervals in the anteroposterior projection when the patient is phonating E.

Positive Contrast Laryngography

Advances in conservation surgery for carcinoma of the larynx and precision radiation therapy have required a reappraisal of our diagnostic methods in carcinoma of the larynx (26, 29, 45, 55). Some obvious blind areas to clinical examinations are the inferior borders of bulky tumors, inferior poles of the piriform sinuses, lateral walls of the laryngeal ventricles, and to a considerable extent the subglottic space. Laryngography has proved to be reliable in evaluating the above areas as well as accurately depicting alterations in normal physiology.

Total laryngectomy introduced in 1874 by Bilroth had been the mainstay of surgical management of laryngeal cancer. Similarly, early radiation therapy was directed to the entire larynx and lymph nodes drainage in the neck using large fields. Since the entire area was either going to be removed or irradiated, there was little need for

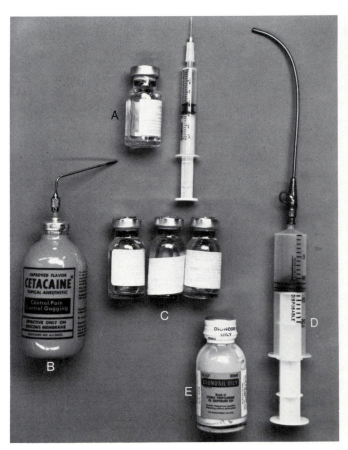

Fig. 2.3 Laryngeal scarring and subglottic web secondary to prolonged intubation. Tomography in the lateral projection shows a thick web in the subglottic space (arrows). Considerable scarring is present within the larynx as evidenced by the anterior position of the arytenoid cartilage (Y-shaped arrow) even though the patient is slowly inspiring during the tomographic exposure.

Fig. 2.4 Laryngography equipment. Twenty minutes prior to the study, between 0.8 and 1.2 mg of atropine (A) are given intramuscularly. Cetacaine (B) or similar local anesthesia is sprayed into the pharynx to reduce the gag reflex. Either 0.5% or 1% of lidocaine (C) is used for anesthetizing the larynx, trachea, and carina region. The syringe and cannula demonstrate the Abraham cannula (D), which is used for dripping the lidocaine over the posterior surface of the tongue. Oily propyliodone (Dionosil) (E) is first heated and shaken for 3–4 min to insure adequate suspension of the contrast material. The propyliodone is allowed to cool to room temperature to provide the proper viscosity to the contrast agent.

precision delineation of the extent of the disease other than for prognostic pruposes. Principles of modern radiation therapy of the larynx emphasize small fields with sparing of the normal surrounding structures. It was natural that the radiation therapist first became interested in laryngography. Very little change in the basic technique has occurred since it was first introduced by Powers in 1957 (48).

Technique

Three inseparable prerequisites for successful laryngograms are: 1. thorough instruction of the patient, 2. adequate anesthesia, and 3. filming during physiologic maneuvers that will test laryngeal functions. All are equally important, and absence of either will negate the study. Prior to any anesthesia, the patient should be instructed on the maneuvers that will take place during actual filming. This conversation can take place very conveniently while awaiting the effects of 0.3–1.2 mg of atropine given intramuscularly. This rather high dose is necessary to diminish laryngeal secretions. The patient is also told that there will be a slight sensation of desiring to "clear the throat" or swallow due to the instilled contrast material. To prevent this, the patient is told to constantly keep his mouth open since swallowing cannot be initiated with an open mouth and protruded tongue. Preoperative sedatives are not indicated and will only diminish the patient's power of concentration.

Anesthesia is accomplished with 1% lidocaine, an Abraham cannula, and a 10-ml syringe (Fig. 2.4). Fluoroscopic capabilities with an image intersifier is an indispensable adjunct to the careful topical anesthesia. The patient is examined in a seated position.

With 10 ml of 1% lidocaine in the syringe connected to an Abraham cannula, the patient is instructed to take a rapid deep breath on the count of "3" while at the same time the anesthetic material is injected just over the base of the tongue. In the preinstruction, the patient has been warned that he is attempting to aspirate the anesthetic material into his windpipe, which will naturally cause some coughing. This initial injection of lidocaine is to anesthetize the trachea, corina, and to some extent the laryngeal and pharyngeal structures.

A second 10 ml of lidocaine is injected while the patient is phonating E. The purpose of phonating E is to adduct the true vocal cords and cause any injected anesthetic material to be retained in the laryngeal vestibule. Anesthesia is accomplished by the direct contact of lidocaine

with the laryngeal vestibule. Making sure the lidocaine flows to the proper place is accomplished by fluoroscopy in the lateral projection. The examiner will see the non-radiopaque anesthetic materials flow into the vallecula and later into the piriform sinuses. A distinct air fluid level will be visible in the piriform sinuses that will gradually rise until the level reaches the upper border of the arytenoids (Fig. 2.5). The anesthetic will then flow into the larynx, and the gradual expiration of air through the adducted cords while the patient is saying E will cause air bubbles to flow through the anesthetic material. A second or third injection of anesthetic material during phonation may be necessary if the patient has encountered any difficulty in performing the maneuver. At least two installations of lidocaine into the laryngeal vestibule are helpful in assurring adequate anesthesia of the extreme lateral portions of the laryngeal ventricle. A second function of the anesthetic material is to wash out any retained secretions that may be adherent to the tumor around the glottic region. The patient is now ready for the contrast instillation, and all assistants should be alerted to make the procedure go rapidly since the anesthesia is only effective for 10–12 min.

At the present time, oily propyliodone (Dionosil) is the contrast material of choice. It should first be warmed to slightly above body temperature and vigorously shaken for 3–5 min. After thorough mixing, the contrast material should be allowed to cool to room temperature. A very warm contrast material will flow rapidly into the trachea and not coat the laryngeal structures. During installation of the contrast material, the patient is fluoroscoped in the lateral projection. Initially, he is instructed to breathe in and out through the mouth while the contrast material flows into the vallecula and into the piriform sinuses. After 3–4 ml of contrast material has been injected, the examiners will see the contrast material spilling from the piriform sinuses into the laryngeal vestibule. The patient is instructed to say E in order to hold the contrast material in the larynx by the opposed cords. He is then told to blow out the cheeks or strain to insure adequate coating of all laryngeal and pharyngeal structures. This maneuver is followed by immediately panting to prevent the urge of swallowing. Within a few seconds, the patient will become more relaxed and the procedure can begin. Should any surface of the larynx not be coated, the patient's head and shoulders can be tilted to make the material flow to the dependent portions of the larynx or pharynx.

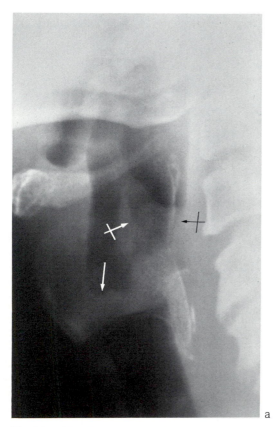

a

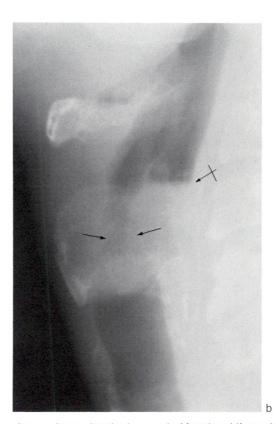

b

Fig. 2.**5**   Anesthesia levels in the larynx.

a) Lateral view of a patient with a true vocal cord lesion involving the anterior commissure (arrow) prior to the installation of anesthesia. Note the air-containing piriform sinuses (cross-hatched arrows) superimposing on the aryepiglottic folds.

b) The patient is instructed to say E, which forces the true vocal cords to become opposed. The anesthetic material is seen to first fill the vallecula and then an air-fluid level forms in the piriform sinuses (cross-hatched arrows). After the piriform sinuses fill, the contrast material flows over the aryepiglottic folds into the larynx. The opposed true cords hold anesthetic material in the larynx, and at fluoroscopy air bubbles can be seen rising through the liquid (arrows). The anesthetic can be held in the larynx for as long as the patient can continue to say E, thus assuring good anesthesia of the mucosa including the laryngeal ventricles.

Radiologic Anatomy

Five basic maneuvers are utilized to test the integrity of the larynx. They are performed in the following sequence:

1. Quiet inspiration
2. Phonating E
3. Modified Valsalva's maneuver
4. True Valsalva's maneuver
5. Phonation during inspiration or 'reverse E."

All of the above maneuvers are accompanied by extensive changes in configuration of the larynx. An attempt is being made to list some specific sites that are tested by the maneuver; however, one should bear in mind the demonstration of normal structures and their function is equally important to the demonstration of the tumor.

Quiet inspiration – the patient is instructed to slowly breathe in through the mouth. PA projection demonstrates the maximum amount of abduction of the true and false cords and therefore the maximum airway. The arytenoids are rotated laterally, and hence the widest angle possible of the intra-arytenoid notch is demonstrated (Fig. 2.6). Quiet respiration lateral projection – the absence of tension on the true cords will allow maximum visualization of the anterior commissure without

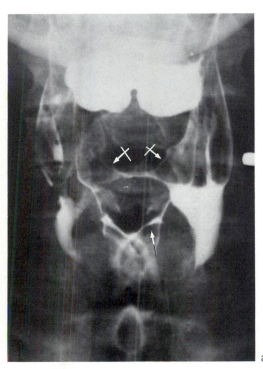

a

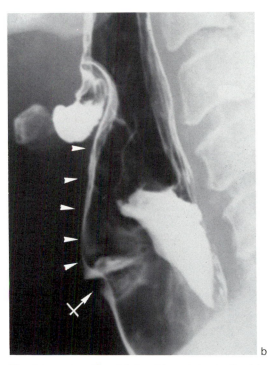

b

Fig. 2.6 Figures 2.6 through 2.10 are from the laryngogram on a patient with a very early carcinoma of the junction of anterior and middle third of the left true cord without evidence of spread beyond the immediate vicinity of the mucosa. There was no clinical or radiologic evidence of impaired physiology.

a) Anteroposterior view in quiet respiration. The (arrow) indicates the bulging superior surface of the left true cord at the site of the tumor. In the midline, medial to the arrow, is the anterior commissure where the true cords are attached to the thyroid cartilage. Lateral to the arrow is a line of contrast material marking the posterior margin of the true cord when the cord is in full abduction.

The interarytenoid notch is widened due to the lateral position of the arytenoid cartilages (cross-hatched arrows').

b) Lateral projection in quiet respiration. The anterior commissure (cross-hatched arrow) is smooth and there is no evidence of tumor mass. The tumor of the middle third of the true cord cannot be visualized in the lateral projection because of the superimposition of the normal right side. The infrahyoid portion of the epiglottis, which attaches to the anterior commissure area by the thyroepiglottic ligament (lower arrowhead), can be traced superiorly to the junction of the body with the free margin of the epiglottis at the level of the hyoid bone (upper arrowhead).

mucosal distortion. The epiglottis will assume a more vertical angle, and the thyroid cartilage will descend showing the minimum amount of space in a preepiglottic region.

Phonation E – the patient is told to attempt to softly say E for a prolonged period of time, realizing his disease and the contrast material will distort the sound. During phonating E in anteroposterior projection – the true cords are adducted to the midline indicating their mobility and configuration. The false cords become paramedian in position. The laryngeal ventricles are filled with contrast material. Since air is flowing upward between the opposed true cords, their superior surfaces will be maximally coated with contrast material. The interarytenoid notch will assume a V configuration. The piriform sinuses will be in a slightly distended position (Fig. 2.7).

Phonation E-lateral projection – the laryngeal vestibule will open slightly; however, there may be a slight posterior bowing of the body of the epiglottis. There is also a slight elevation of the thyroid cartilage, giving some indication of the amount of mobility of the epiglottis and preepiglottic space. The junction of the inferior margin of the epiglottis with the true cords marks the superior surface of the anterior commissure. It should appear as a sharp point.

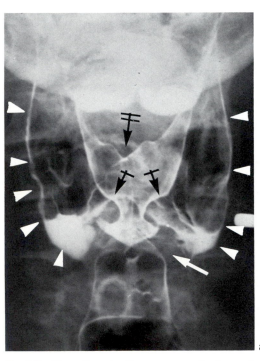

a

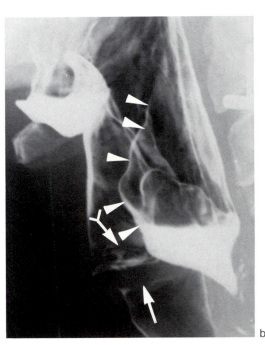

b

Fig. 2.7 Phonation in the same patient as demonstrated in Fig. 2.6.

a) Anteroposterior projection shows the interarytenoid notch is now almost totally obliterated (double cross-hatched arrow) because the arytenoid cartilages have rotated to their more medial positions. The false cords (cross-hatched arrow) are separated, and the true cords are in apposition during phonation (arrow). The very small tumor of the left vocal cord is hidden by the contrast-filled laryngeal ventricle.

b) A small amount of contrast material outlines the undersurface of the true cord (arrow), and the opposed true cords present as a radiolucent transverse band. Air can be seen in the laryngeal ventricle (Y-shaped arrow). Although there is some irregularity of the superior surface of the true cords, a tumor cannot be diagnosed because of all of the overlapping structures. Air can be seen in the piriform sinuses (arrowheads), and their anterior margins cross the aryepiglottic folds.

True Valsalva's maneuver-PA projection – in this maneuver, the patient strains as if lifting a weight. The false cords and true cords come forcefully together in the midline squeezing the contrast material out of the laryngeal ventricles (Fig. 2.8). The subglottic space changes in configuration from an arched cathedral-type of roof to a flattened roof beneath the anterior half of the true cords. Any disparity between the two sides becomes highly significant.

True Valsava's maneuver – lateral projection – the thyroid cartilage elevates to approximate the hyoid bone, and the epiglottis bows markedly posteriorly. Some assessment of the overall infiltration of the preepiglottic space and mobility of the epiglottis is now possible. At the level of the true cords, the inferior surfaces of the true cords bow inferiorly and are smooth. Any alteration of the configuration is significant for subglottic extension of tumor.

The modified Valsava's maneuver is performed in a manner similar to blowing a trumpet. By expiring against pursed lips with a little bit of air being exhaled, the true

and false cords are paramedian and the neck structures become distended. The piriform sinuses are greatly distended by the modified Valsava's maneuver, and any irregularities of the mucosa or stiffening of the walls is readily apparent on the PA and oblique projections. At times, the laryngeal ventricles will become distended by the increased pressure within the laryngeal vestibule and afford some degree of delineation of the lateral extension of true cord lesions. The oblique views also give an unobscured view of the aryepiglottic folds (Fig. 2.9).

Modified Valsava's maneuver – lateral projection – the suprahyoid epiglottis tilts posteriorly, and there is anterior ballooning of the piriform sinuses as well as the valleculae. In all previous maneuvers, it has been difficult to separate the anterior wall of the piriform sinuses from the aryepiglottic folds. As the piriform sinuses become distended, their anterior margin will become rounded and project anterior to the aryepiglottic folds. The posterior surface of the cricoid and arytenoid regions can usually be well delineated in this lateral view.

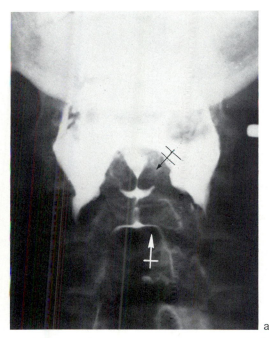
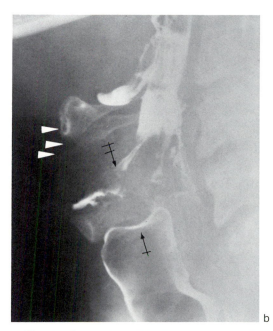

Fig. 2.8   True Valsalva maneuver in same patient described in Fig. 2.6.
a) The true cords and false cords are forcefully adducted, squeezing out the contrast material in the transglottic area. The undersurface of the true cords assume a right angle with lumen of the trachea (cross-hatched arrow) The false cords (double cross-hatched arrow) are visible above the level of the laryngeal ventricle.

b) The inferior surface of the true cords bow inferiorly; note that the anterior margin of the true cords is at a much more caudad level than the posterior margin. The region of the false cords (double cross-hatched arrow) is visible as a radiolucent zone. The thyroid cartilage elevates to approximate the hyoid bone (arrowheads), giving some appreciation of the pliability of the preepiglottic space.

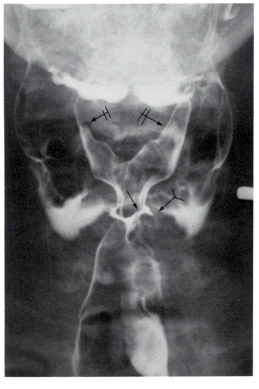

a

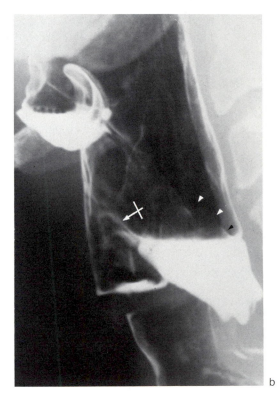

b

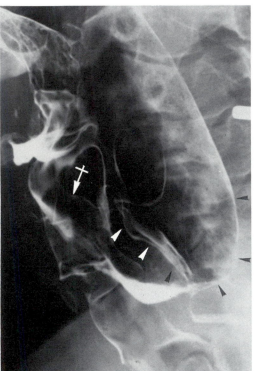

c

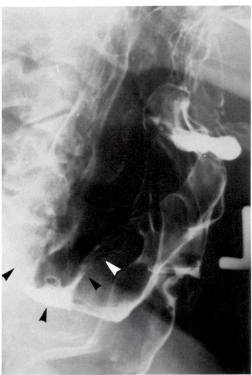

d

Fig. 2.9 Modified Valsalva maneuver in same patient as Fig. 2.6.
a) Anteroposterior projection showing the tumor bulging from the superior surface of the left true vocal cord (arrow). The extreme lateral portion of the laryngeal ventricle is sharp, and one connot be certain whether there is tumor extending to the lateral wall of the ventricle or not (Y-shaped arrow). With the piriform sinuses distended laterally, the aryepiglottic folds become clearly visible on the AP projection (double cross-hatched arrow). The post-cricoid line is obliterated because the postcricoid region does not touch the posterior pharyngeal wall during this maneuver.

b) Lateral projection. The distended piriform sinuses permit visualization of the upper postcricoid and postarytenoid region (arrowheads). The posterior pharyngeal wall should be smooth without indentations.
c and d) Oblique projections with the modified Valsalva maneuver specifically taken to visualize the inferior poles of the piriform sinuses (arrowheads). The posterolateral margins of the postcricoid region can be clearly identified from this projection through the distended piriform sinuses. The oblique view also permits visualization of the aryepiglottic folds (cross-hatched arrow in Fig. 9c).

Phonation during inspiration or reverse E maneuver – since most patients have difficulty with this maneuver, it is saved for last (28). He is instructed to try to make a noise (any noise) while breathing in slowly. By lowering the air pressure beneath the level of the opposed true cords, they are made to descend and there is lateral distension of the laryngeal ventricles. This lateral distensibility is exceedingly important in deep infiltration of true cord tumors. Excess contrast material is "sucked" from the superior surface of the true cords into the trachea. Mucosa irregularities are better defined. To a lesser extent, the piriform sinuses descend, which may be helpful in evaluation of limited pliability (Fig. 2.10). The information obtained in a lateral reverse E phenomena is insufficient to warrant the maneuver.

Fluoroscopy during laryngography will already give the examiner some impression of laryngeal mobility and pliability. Cine-techniques or video tape recordings are excellent methods of recording these physiologic functions; however, each have their drawbacks. Cines cannot be developed and viewed while the patient is still anesthetized to be assured of the adequacy of the study. Video recording requires viewing equipment that might not be available in clinical areas other than the radiology department.

Spot films taken during the laryngogram are carefully scrutinized to be sure the patient has correctly performed the maneuvers and adequate coating and detail is available. If additional films are required, the larynx will have to be reanesthetized as well as recoated since surface anesthesia only lasts 10–12 min. Mucous is constantly being formed despite the high dosages of atropine, which will cause a clumping of the contrast material if the procedure becomes prolonged. For an average laryngogram, 8–10 ml of contrast material may be used with approximately 4 ml of this being swallowed sometimes during the procedures. If more than one coating is required, a brief fluoroscopy of the chest will give the examiner some appraisal of the amount of contrast material that flows into the tracheobronchial tree. If the bronchi are well filled bilaterally, it may prove prudent to "toilet" the tracheobronchial tree by placing the patient prone with the head down-feet up at a 15°–20° angle for 3–4 min. The patient is allowed to expectorate some of the contrast material before proceeding with the study.

Contraindications to Laryngography

The contraindications to laryngography are similar to those of bronchography as well as local anasthesia. Patients with respiratory distress due to airway

encroachment may be further compromised by the coating of contrast material and injected anesthetic substances. Although more scientific methods are undoubtedly available, a useful criteria can be called the "two flight of stairs test," that is, if the patient can climb two flights of stairs without undue shortness of breath, in all probability there will be no difficulty with contrast laryngography.

Small amounts of lidocaine are absorbed from the mucosal surfaces, but anesthetic that is swallowed is readily detoxified and does not appear to produce harmful reactions. Elderly patients should be watched carefully for signs of excitability or confusion as a manifestation of drug toxicity.

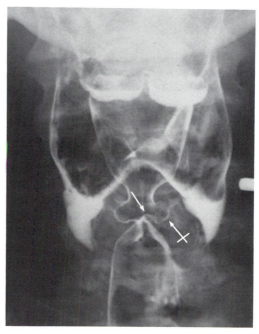

Fig. 2.10 Same patient as in Fig. 2.6. Reverse E maneuver is only performed for the AP projection. The tumor mass of the left true cord is visible as a small exophytic growth (arrow). The lateral walls of the laryngeal ventricles are well distended and are shown to be free of tumor (cross-hatched arrow). Both the true cords and the inferior poles of the piriform sinuses have descended slightly from the resting position.

Computerized Tomography

Computerized tomography has proved to be a valuable adjunct to the clinical examination of the larynx. The examination is noninvasive and can be performed with relative ease even in the most severely debilitated patient. The maximum use of CT scanning is to provide information concerning the status of the laryngeal cartilages and the soft tissues deep to the mucosal surface. Other examinations, such as positive contrast laryngography, tend to compete with the information obtained at direct laryngoscopy. Both positive contrast laryngography and direct laryngoscopy are excellent for delineation of mucosal detail and motion physiology. Unfortunately, the evidence for deep infiltrations of tumors or inflammatory processes must be derived by indirect means, i.e., relative fixation or increased bulk of intrinsic structures. CT examination shows the disturbance of normal fascial planes and direct invasion of a pathological process.

The cartilages of the larynx calcify in an irregular fashion. Destruction of thyroid or cricoid cartilage is extremely difficult to diagnose by routine views unless far advanced. Computerized tomography is five to ten times as sensitive in picking up minute amounts of calcium so that the diagnosis of early destruction is distinctly possible.

The configuration of the cartilages, and in particular the thyroid cartilage, is very susceptible to distortions by adjacent bulky lesions, muscular pull, or negative pressures generated by the velocity of passage of adjacent gases. This type of information is not obtainable by other presently known techniques.

In the acutely ill patient, the airway as visualized by CT scanning correlates more closely with the appraisal obtained at clinical examination. This airway appraisal is particularly helpful in the acutely traumatized patient where neck injuries or other fractures may prevent a detailed clinical examination.

Lastly, CT examination of the neck has shown considerable promise in the demonstration of lymph node metastases or more distant spreads of tumors adjacent to the carotid sheath. The latter infiltrations have serious prognostic significance and directly affect patient management.

Some of the disadvantages of CT scanning are related to the state of the art, which will undoubtedly be corrected with future generation scanners. Unfortunately, the major problem of equipment cost shows no real signs of abating. Scan times of less than 3 or 4 s are highly desirable but not generally available. With presently available scan times of 20 s, motion artifacts cause image distortions. The 8–13 mm thickness of scan slices also causes problem with partial volume effects. Part of this difficulty can be eliminated by overlapping scans. The long scan times prevent the use of any physiologic maneuvers that would allow an appraisal of laryngeal function. Lastly, CT scanning does not give histology but merely shows altered density and morphology. Edematous changes and cellular responses adjacent to tumors are impossible to differentiate from actual tumor spreads.

Radiologic Techniques

The scans demonstrated in this material were performed on an EMI 5005, utilizing 20-s scan times and a 360 × 360 matrix. For scanning, the patient is placed supine and instructed to quietly breathe, preferably without any delay at the peak of inspiration or expiration. Some individuals tend to close their true and false vocal cords at the peak of inspiration and expiration with a very slight delay in air movement. This produces motion artifacts that can be eliminated with a little prescanning practice. The notch at the inferior margin of the thyroid cartilage is carefully palpated in the midline, and the first scan is obtained 1 cm below this level. The scan is viewed for technique and to be sure that the anterior ring of the cricoid cartilage has been visualized. If the level is not sufficiently inferior, successive scans are obtained at 5-mm intervals until the anterior ring of the cricoid cartilage is clearly demonstrated. As mentioned earlier, the cricoid cartilage is the basis of the larynx, and its integrity must be verified for any future patient management. In some individuals, the shoulder may interfere with the lower scans, and the cricoid cartilage can be made to move cephalad by elevating the patient's chin. After the lower limits of the larynx have been visualized, the scanning table is returned to the region of the inferior notch of the thyroid cartilage, and scans are obtained cephalad at 5-mm intervals until the hyoid bone has been clearly demonstrated. Extensions of tumors into the base of the tongue have proved difficult to depict and are probably better demonstrated by physical examination.

CT scanning of the larynx introduces a concept of anatomy that may be foreign to all except those individuals involved with whole organ sectioning. The major advantage of CT scanning is outlining the areas deep to the mucosa that comprise the paralaryngeal space, the preepiglottic space, and the region of the conus elasticus (Fig. 2.11).

The conus elasticus is the tough membrane that originates at the free margin of the true vocal cord and extends inferiorly to insert along the free margin of the cricoid cartilage (8, 42). The conus elasticus is thickest anteriorly and fuses to the thyrocricoid ligament (Fig. 2.1). The conus elasticus defines a mucosal region caudad to the true cords and is spoken of as the subglottic space. Lateral to the conus elasticus is a freely communicating space that extends between the thyroid and cricoid cartilages posteriorly and contains an articulation between the inferior cornu of the thyroid cartilage and the signet of the cricoid cartilage. This space is the inferior extension of the paralaryngeal space (Fig. 2.1). The paralaryngeal space is the region lateral to the conus elasticus and mucosa of the laryngeal vestibule and contains the vocal muscle, the thyroarytenoids, and cricoarytenoid muscles (54). The lateral extent of this space is limited by the thyroid cartilage. Posteriorly, the space is rather loosely arranged and allows for bulging of the piriform sinuses into this space during the swallowing act. The laryngeal ventricle and appendices of the laryngeal ventricles bulge into this space from its medial margin. The paralaryngeal space is rich in blood vessels and contains branches of these superior and recurrent laryngeal nerves with accompanying vessels. The nerves and vessels provide a ready pathway from the paralaryngeal space to the space surrounding the carotid artery and internal jugular vein. Anteriorly, the paralaryngeal space is a continuum into the preepiglottic space, providing free communication between the two sides. On CT scanning, the paralaryngeal space is of relatively low density and can be readily identified by the high density of surrounding structures, such as the thyroid cartilage and vocal ligament in the free margin of the true vocal cord. Anteriorly, this space diminishes as the mucosa of the larynx lies in opposition to the thyroid cartilage and in the subglottic space the mucosa is immediately beneath the cricothyroid ligament.

The preepiglottic space is low in density due to the high fat content. Some transverse fibers of high-density connective tissue can be seen stranding through the midportion of the preepiglottic space, but there is always a layer of lowdensity fat immediately anterior to the epiglottis and deep to the ala of the thyroid cartilages. Superiorly, the hyoid bone and the vallecula form a roof to the preepiglottic space.

The characteristic configurations of the thyroid cartilage, cricoid cartilage, and hyoid bone greatly facilitate the orientation on CT scanning. In the midportion of the larynx, the shield-like pattern of the thyroid cartilages are readily apparent, and the extrinsic musculature along their external surfaces should not be mistaken for infiltrations or inflammatory processes (Fig. 2.11). The inferior thyroid notch as well as the superior thyroid notch will create a characteristic "dehiscence" of the thyroid cartilage, again identifying levels of the cuts. Inferiorly, the inferior cornua of the thyroid cartilage are invariably identified as rounded, dense shadows lying posterolaterally to the subglottic space with their density lying outside the confines of the ring of the cricoid cartilage. The signet of the cricoid cartilage calcifies first along its anterior and posterior surface at the posterola-

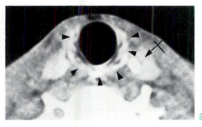
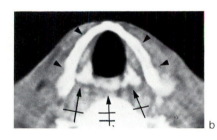
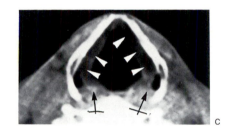
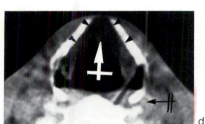
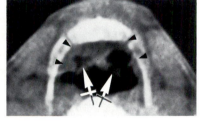
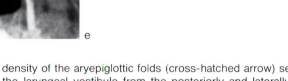

Fig. 2.11 Level of the cricoid ring.

a) The inferior cornu of the thyroid cartilage (cross-hatched arrow) is visible lateral to the cricoid ring (arrowheads), which establishes the low level of the cut. The cricoid ring surrounds the air column, and characteristically no soft tissue can be identified between the inner lamina of the cricoid and the air column. The cricoid contains a medulary cavity that is low density, while calcification tends to begin along the surfaces of the posteriorly placed signet of the cricoid and then extends anteriorly (arrowheads).

b) True cord level. Approximately 1 cm cephalad to Fig. 2.11 a) shows the thyroid cartilages form a wishbone appearance protecting the anterior and lateral surfaces of the larynx (arrowheads). The paired arytenoid cartilages (cross-hatched arrow) are seen resting on top of and slightly lateral to the signet of the cricoid cartilage (double cross-hatched arrow). The true vocal cords extend anteriorly from the arytenoid cartilages to attach to the thyroid cartilage. No soft tissue should be visible immediately in the midline beneath the thyroid cartilage.

c) False cord level. Approximately 5 mm cephalad to Fig. 2.11 b). The false cords are visible and can be identified by their wavy free margin and the soft tissue crossing the midline immediately inferior to the thyroid cartilages (arrowheads). The soft tissue

density of the aryepiglottic folds (cross-hatched arrow) separates the laryngeal vestibule from the posteriorly and laterally placed piriform sinuses lying to either side of the aryepiglottic folds.

d) Body of the epiglottic level. Approximately 5 mm cephalad to Fig. 2.11 c one sees the thyroid cartilages becoming deficient in the midline anteriorly, indicating the superior thyroid notch. In the midline, the body of the epiglottis is partially volumed with the petiolus, which bulges into the laryngeal vestibule (cross-hatched arrow). Rarely does the epiglottis contain sufficient calcification for identification. The preepiglottic space is low density and extends laterally beneath the thyroid cartilages as the paraepiglottic space (arrowheads). Posteriorly, the superior cornua of the thyroid cartilages are visualized as dense, rounded structures (double cross-hatched arrows).

e) Hyoid bone level. The hyoid bone, which can be identified because of its three segments. Posteriorly, the free margin of the epiglottis (cross-hatched arrows) separates the entrance to the laryngeal vestibule from the valleculae (arrowheads). The two valleculae are separated in the midline by a frenulum, and the base of the tongue is partially volumed in this section lying adjacent to the hyoid bone.

teral margins of the signet. Surface calcification proceeds medially to the midline and anteriorly into the anterior arch of the cricoid cartilage. A good way to get orientated to the cricoid cartilage is to think of the cricoid as having a medullary cavity that is filled with low-density material. Since the signet is highest posteriorly, the cartilage will appear as a flattened oval with calcification on its surface and a radiolucent center. The more inferior the CT levels are obtained, the more complete the ring of the cricoid cartilage will appear. The arytenoid cartilages are usually quite densely and irregularly calcified. They lie along the superior borders of the signet of the cricoid cartilage. When the patient is quietly breathing, they are laterally positioned. The hyoid bone at the upper limits of the preepiglottic space of the larynx can be readily recognized because of its three segments consisting of two lateral horns and a midline synthesis.

Within the larynx, the true cords can be seen arising from the vocal process of the arytenoids and extending to the anterior inferior border of the thyroid cartilage just above the inferior thyroid notch. The true cords have a dense vocal ligament along the free margin and relatively low-density material composing the body of the true vocal cords. This density is supplied by the vocal muscle. The junction of true and false vocal cords is marked by the air in the laryngeal lumen forming a diamond-shaped contour. The lateral points of the diamond are caused by air in the partially filled laryngeal ventricles. The next most cephalad cut is through the false vocal cords (Fig.2.11). Differentiation from true vocal cords is readily apparent by the configuration at the anterior commissure. Tissue of 3–4 mm can be seen crossing the midline that is not present at the level of the true vocal cords. This tissue is a combination of petiolus of the epiglottis and the thyroepiglottic ligament. Posteriorly, the arytenoid cartilages are usually partially volumed with the false cords, and an excellent view of the upper portion of the posterior commissure is available. The posterolateral limit of the laryngeal vestibule is made up by the aryepiglottic folds. They are usually seen as rather thick structures at the level of the false cords and become much more delicate with the next most cephalad cut.

As one continues taking scans more cephalad, the body of the epiglottis is encountered anteriorly, and the aryepiglottic folds and piriform sinuses can be seen posteriorly and laterally. The preepiglottic space, as mentioned earlier, is of low density, and infiltrations by tumor or inflammatory process are readily visualized by a change in density. The epiglottis is extremely flexible and readily distorted by extrinsic pressure. The piriform sinuses should be relatively symmetric. They become widened during phonation or whenever the arytenoid becomes adducted (Fig. 2.11).

The most cephalad slice usually goes through the hyoid bone, which is visualized anteriorly as a three-segmented bone. The free margin of the epiglottis separates the space of the laryngeal vestibule from the anteriorly placed valleculae.

Pathologic Conditions

Congenital

Abnormalities of the larynx in the infant and newborn may produce varying degrees of dyspnea and cyanosis. Inspiratory stridor is characteristic of lesions of the larynx and immediate subglottic space. Expiratory wheezing is characteristic of tracheal obstruction within the mediastinum. Radiology of congenital lesions of the larynx is quite limited since all of the cartilages are uncalcified. Sophisticated special studies cannot be performed due to the lack of patient cooperation or patient movement with respect to CT scanning. On the other hand, by careful timing of roentgen exposure during inspiration, a great deal of information can be obtained regarding the patency of airways and to some extent physiologic function of the upper airways. The newborn and infant larynx and trachea undergoes distortions that are totally unheard of in the adult patient. During expiration, there is normally a buckling of the subglottic trachea with a deviation of the trachea to the left due to the mediastinal vessels (Fig. 2.12). The retropharyngeal soft tissues will enlarge greatly during expiration, giving a spurious impression of a retropharyngeal abscess. Because of these variations in air shadows and because of the possibility of pulmonary or cardiac disease mimicking upper airway obstruction, roentgen examination of the larynx should be merely one part of the radiologic work-up of a dyspneic child.

Part of the examination of a neonate should include fluoroscopy of the larynx and trachea. Hypopharyngeal ballooning (32, 57) occurs due to the obstructions at the laryngeal level with the attempt of "sucking" air into the trachea against a partial obstruction. Fluoroscopy may reveal the "cleft larynx" or unilateral or bilateral paralysis of the true vocal cords. Partial collapse of the trachea occurs during inspiration. In tracheomalacia, collapse of the trachea during expiration may be localized to the lower neck, upper mediastinum, or may involve the entire trachea (15, 23, 53, 58, 60).

Vocal cord paralysis of the newborn may be due to central nervous system (CNS) deformity or related to peripheral nerve injury. The central nervous system lesions associated with bilateral vocal cord paralysis are located in the pons and brain stem. Arnold-Chiari malformation with cervical meningomyelocele is a common finding, but any brain stem insult may precipitate vocal cord paralysis or paresis (16, 21). The spontaneous cases have been associated with birth trauma, and occasionally cytomegalovirus has been a suspected etiology (59). Fluoroscopy provides a convenient method of following the progress of these children. The vast majority will return to normal or near normal without specific treatment, providing there is no CNS anomaly.

The cleft larynx is characterized by inspiratory stridor and redundant aryepiglottic folds that impinge upon the airway. The interarytenoid muscles are absent and allow the arytenoids to deviate laterally and forward. In a rapidly breathing infant with respiratory distress, some of these changes may be extremely difficult to visualize. Careful direct laryngoscopy becomes indispensable for a definitive diagnosis.

Congenital tumor masses within the larynx include polyps, angiomatous polyps, hemangiomas, and congenital cysts (21). Radiology plays a significant role in identifying a mass lesion as a cause of respiratory obstruction as compared to a physiologic disturbance, such as vocal cord paralysis. If a tumor mass can be identified, this is an indication for further clinical work-up. Hemangioma

of the larynx may be associated with other hemangiomas of the face or central nervous system giving a clue to the etiologic diagnosis (Fig. 2.13). On the other hand, polyps or cysts will only show mass lesions. The subsequent clinical management will be vastly different since surgical correction will probably be undertaken at an early date if nutrition and respiratory function show significant impairment. On the other hand, elaborate roentgen procedures for histologic diagnosis are not warranted since the dictates of therapy are primarily directed to maintenance of physiologic functions.

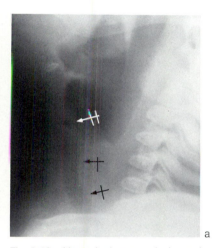

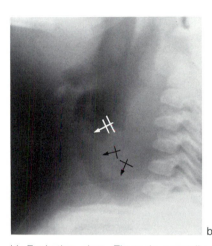

Fig. 2.**12**   Normal pharyngeal airway in an infant-inspiration and expiration.

a) Inspiration view. The hypopharyngeal air space is rather generous. The trachea shows a bulge along its posterior wall (cross-hatched arrows) due to the bulk of the cricopharyngeus muscle and opening of the cervical esophagus. A small amount of air can be seen in the laryngeal ventricle (double cross-hatched arrow), indicating the upper level of the true vocal cord.

b) Expiration view. There is normally anterior buckling of the trachea due to the bulk of the cricopharyngeus muscle and cervical esophagus (cross-hatched arrows). This view was taken at the end of expiration, and the infant had momentarily closed the true vocal cords (double cross-hatched arrow).

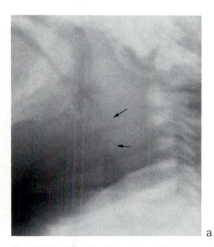

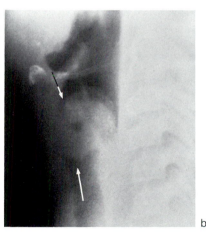

Fig. 2.**13**   "Benign" tumors of childhood.

a) Hemangioma of the larynx. This two-month-old child had multiple hemangiomas of the face and scalp and showed signs of respiratory embarrassment. Lateral view of the larynx shows encroachment on the airway (arrows). Due to the more chronic nature of the obstruction, the marked hypopharyngeal distension is not present. This child died of laryngeal hemorrhage.

b) In an older child, more discreet rounded defects in the larynx are seen that proved to be papillomas (arrows). The chest x-ray was of considerable importance since it showed the overexpansion of the lung fields consistent with papillomas extending throughout the tracheobronchial tree. This child had not yet developed cor pulmonale.

Functional Disorders

Spastic Dysphonia

Spastic dysphonia is a speech disorder characterized by a voice that is jerky, hesitant, and somewhat strangulated in quality (13, 47). The disorder was originally thought to be psychological in origin, but more recent sutdies prove that the disease is related to a nervous system disorder that may be central or peripheral in origin. Cineradiographic studies of the larynx will show clonic movements of the pharynx and laryngeal structures. The vocal cords may undergo tonic-type movements with the cords adducted or abducted. If fluoroscopy is performed during speaking and the cords become tonic in adduction, the speech will become arrested and be followed by an explosive quality when the cords finally separate. If the cords are tonic in abducted position, the speech quality becomes breathless and is accompanied by a sudden drop in pitch (33). Since the true etiology of this disorder was not realized until recently, many of these patients still carry a diagnosis of psychogenic voice disturbances, and radiologic examination can be an extremely useful tool in convincing clinicians of the "Parkinson disease-like nature" of spastic dysphonia.

Paralytic States

The neuromuscular weaknesses, such as myasthenia gravis, dermatomyositis and multiple sclerosis, are but a few of the conditions that may interfere with laryngeal and pharyngeal function based on generalized muscular or nervous system involvement (34). Aspiration is a common feature that seems to be more closely related to involvement of the superior laryngeal nerve supply to the extrinsic muscles of the larynx. The intrinsic musculature seems to remain functional for a longer period of time. The radiologic changes are characterized by the larynx remaining in a vertical position with very little elevation of the larynx during the swallowing act. The arytenoids will usually move forward, but the epiglottis will not forcefully invert and appose the arytenoids to prevent secretions from entering the laryngeal vestibule.

The recurrent laryngeal nerves supply the intrinsic laryngeal musculature and tend to be preserved for a longer period of time in these generalized muscular and central nervous system disorders. When the swallowing act is initiated, fluoroscopy will show contrast material or secretions entering the laryngeal vestibule, and only a small amount will pass through the glottic chink into the trachea. When the swallowing act is completed and the true vocal cords relax, the contents of the laryngeal vestibule are then free to flow into the trachea. Recurrent nerve paralysis may occur following surgery of the thyroid or mediastinum. Paralysis of the vocal cords can be simulated by the Riley-Day syndrome (dysautonomia) in which the disordered autonomic nervous system prevents coordination of the swallowing act and contrast material or injected food will immediately pass into the trachea causing aspiration pneumonias.

Voice Abuse Granulomas

Singers' nodules and voice abuse granulomas are varying degrees of the same problem, i. e., abnormal vocal function together with excessive use of the voice. The pathologic changes on the cord consist of the epithelial "warty" overgrowths or even granulomas that cannot be distinguished radiologically from other mass lesions. They may closely simulate a very early mucosal carcinoma on both laryngography and CT scanning. Since the radiologic appearance is identical to malignancies, the diagnosis of mass lesions will be discussed under tumors.

Trauma

The patterns of deformity of the larynx following trauma are surprisingly predictable depending on the mechanism of injury (31). A classification may be listed as follows:
I. Iatrogenic
    A. Voice abuse
    B. Intubation injuries
        1. Immediate
            a. Arytenoid dislocation
            b. Hematomas
        2. Late effects
            a. Glottic scarring
            b. Webs
            c. Subglottic scarring and webs
    C. Radiation therapy effects
        1. Acute
            a. Edema
            b. Cartilage softening
        2. Late
            a. Chondronecrosis
II. Blunt trauma
    A. Acute
        1. Hematoma and airway encroachment
        2. Cartilaginous fractures
        3. Ligamentous disruptions
    B. Late
        1. Scarring
        2. Web formation
        3. Vocal cord distortions.

The ability of CT to accurately depict the status of the cartilages and laryngeal airway make this examination ideal in the acutely injured patient. There is no discomfort involved, and patients who have spinal or intracranial injuries may be examined without endangering vital structures through movement. The laryngeal examination can even be performed at the same time that CT is used for studying facial fractures or intracranial injuries. The examination technique for laryngeal injuries does not vary from the standard technique used in patients harboring laryngeal tumors. Sections are taken at 5-mm intervals from the anterior arch of the cricoid cartilage to the level of the hyoid bone. Again, the patient is instructed to quietly breath throughout the examination, thus insuring CT recording of the maximum transglottic airway.

Intubation Injuries

Edema, mucosal lacerations and small hematomas following endotracheal intubation are quite common and usually resolved without the need of elaborate roentgen examination. Rarely is there sufficient injury to produce airway encroachment.

Arytenoid dislocation represents an unusual cartilaginous injury that may closely mimic vocal cord paralysis (50). This is particularly worrisome if the injury follows thyroid or mediastinal surgery. In the typical arytenoid dislocation, the patient awakens following anesthesia with a hoarse voice and a minimum of laryngeal pain. Indirect laryngoscopy may be quite difficult due to the previous surgery. The examiner will note a flaccid appearance to the involved cord. CT studies will show the involved vocal cord to be paramedian in location, with the arytenoid cartilage displaced anteriorly and somewhat laterally compared to the normal side (Fig. 2.14). This diagnosis cannot be made by other radiographic examinations as the cartilages are incompletely visualized even on high quality tomographic studies. The clinical management of this disorder is relatively simple. At direct laryngoscopy, the tip of the laryngoscope is used to reduce the arytenoid dislocation, and the patient will make an uneventful recovery.

Late Intubation Injuries

The late effects of prolonged endotracheal intubation represents a challenging clinical problem that will test the patience and persistence of any laryngeal surgeon (19. 61). The radiologic studies must not be thought of as a separate clinical examination but only in the context of adjunct information to the direct laryngoscopic examination. Information concerning the function of the false cords, true cords, and any endolaryngeal webs is obtained via the clinical examination. Radiology, while being perfectly capable of demonstrating vocal cord mobility, does not materially add to the information obtained by clinical examination. On the other hand, the subglottic space usually requires a minimum of plain films to accurately appraise the length of any subglottic narrowing and the configuration of residual airway. Some of this information can be obtained from clinical examination if the patient has a tracheostomy stoma in place that allows for a mirror examination of the undersurface of the true cord. If webs are present, they more frequently occur along the anterior surface of the larynx between the vocal cords. They form in response to denudation of the surface epithelium. The very presence of the web prevents good visualization of the subglottic space. Information concerning the thickness of the web is vital since they are managed by placement of a "stent", which consists of prosthetic material that is inserted to cover the raw surfaces of the webs after they are cut (40). The synthetic material is usually held in place by wire sutures placed through the larynx until healing has taken place. The more extensive granulations in the subglottic space that narrow the airway are treated by excision of the scar tissue and at times resection of the involved tracheal rings. Should subglottic stenosis be present, caution should be used in performing positive contrast laryngography if the patient has any stridor or breathlessness. The addition of contrast material and anesthetic to the already compromised airway may be sufficient to throw the patient into acute respiratory decompensation.

If a tracheostomy is in place, positive contrast examination is relatively simple. The patient is placed supine on the roentgen examining table and tilted into a Trendelenburg position; 2–3 ml of 1% lidocaine can be instilled into the tracheostomy's stoma, which will provide entirely adequate anesthesia for the study. Oily propyliodone (Dionosil) can then be instilled with the patient still in a Trendelenburg position and the larynx filled in a retrograde fashion. Filming will outline the full extent of any stenotic lesions and provide a record of the amount of functioning larynx in the preoperative state (Fig. 2.15).

Radiation Injuries

The reaction of the laryngeal mucosa to radiation therapy is well known and documented (2.17). The edema and radiation mucositis usually appears from 21–35 days after the instigation of radiation therapy. It may persist for six weeks to three or four months following the termination of a course of radiation therapy. Clinical problems associated with the edema in radiation mucositis are usually managed without the need of roentgen examinations. Rarely, there may be acute respiratory embarrassment, possibly associated with cartilage softening (30). Plain views of the larynx will not identify the cartilage softening, and positive contrast studies are contraindicated in view of the radiation mucositis. CT scanning is exceedingly helpful in showing the configuration of the thyroid cartilages as well as any airway encroachment (Fig. 2.16). This type of an "inbuckling" of the thyroid cartilages is probably a combination of the Venturi effect of air passing through a narrowed glottic chink, intrinsic and extrinsic laryngeal muscular pull, and cartilage softening. The increased velocity of air through the narrowed airway will cause a "sucking in" of the walls of the larynx. In addition, there may well be an associated acute chondritis that contributes to the weakening of the thyroid cartilages. These speculations are an attempt to explain the appearances of the CT scan.

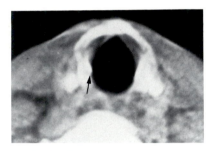

Fig. 2.**14** Post-traumatic dislocation of the arytenoid. Section at the level of the undersurface of the true cords shows that the arytenoid on the left is displaced anteriorly (arrow). The arytenoid on the right is not visible in this section. Because of the dislocation, the two arytenoids are not on the same level.

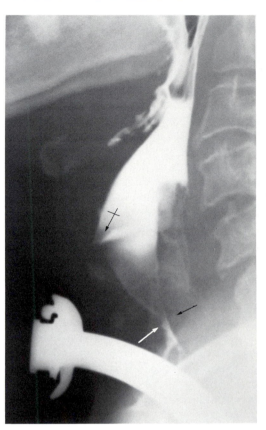

Fig. 2.**15** Subglottic stenosis secondary to prolonged intubation. After anesthetizing the larynx by instilling lidocaine through the tracheostomy tube, contrast material was instilled in the routine manner over the base of the tongue. Contrast material fills the laryngeal vestibule and the subglottic space. The level of the true cords can be identified (cross-hatched arrow). The lumen is approximately 3–4 mm in diameter (arrows), and the narrowing extends to the region of the tracheostomy stoma.

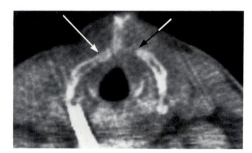

Fig. 2.**16** Acute "inbuckling" of the thyroid cartilages approximately six weeks post radiation. Scan at the level of the true cords shows a marked amount of edema of the soft tissues. The patient presented with progressive respiratory obstruction that required tracheotomy. The thyroid cartilages bow inward at their weakest point, which is immediately lateral to the symphysis.

Late Radiation Injuries

Persistent edema of the larynx following radiation therapy is an ominous fact and is more likely due to residual tumor in the deeper structures of the larynx. In the absence of tumor, some factors contributing to residual edema include continued smoking or some type of irritating environment, residual laryngeal distortions following cure of advanced lesions, and repeated deep biopsies of already "marginally viable" cartilaginous structures. The edema of the glottic chink with airway encroachment can be demonstrated by routine films, tomography, or on CT scanning. Since CT scanning can also show the status of the cartilage, it becomes the procedure of choice. Demonstration of cartilage injuries may be quite troublesome on routine films since the minerali-

zation of the thyroid cartilage and cricoid cartilage is always irregular. If the structural support of the cricoid cartilage has been compromised or the thyroid cartilages are disintegrating, there may be disruption of the normal alignment of the larynx with overlapping of the thyroid cartilage on the cricoid ring. This advanced type of cartilage change can be diagnosed by routine views (Fig. 2.17). CT scanning of the larynx will give a much more accurate appraisal because fragments of the cartilage may inbuckle or overlap, producing masses in the paraglottic region. Despite an intact mucosa, these masses may closely simulate recurrent deep tumor masses, leading the clinician to repeated deep biopsies that will further aggravate the already degenerating cartilages.

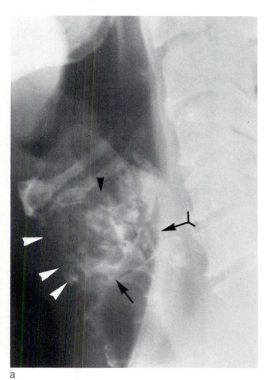

a

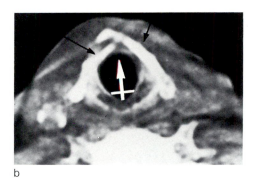

b

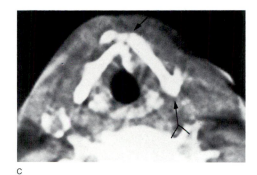

c

Fig. 2.**17** Chondronecrosis 11 months post radiation therapy.
a) Lateral view of the larynx shows extensive destruction and distortion of the thyroid cartilages (arrowheads). The destruction of the thyroid cartilage has allowed the entire larynx to shift forward on the cricoid (Y-shaped arrow). This forward shift causes a narrowing of the space between the inferior margin of the thyroid cartilage and the superior border of the cricoid (arrow). The entire airway is narrowed by soft tissue thickening anteriorly.

b) Scan at the level of the inferior margin of the true cords shows the thyroid cartilages overlapped anterior (arrows). The lack of support allows the soft tissues to bulge into the lumen in what would normally be the subglottic space (Y-shaped arrow). The signet of the cricoid is intact lying posteriorly.
c) Scan at the level of the true cord shows the thyroid cartilages overlapped anteriorly (arrow). The anterior displacement of the right ala of the thyroid is strikingly shown by its change in relationship to the cricoid and arytenoid on the right (Y-shaped arrow).

Blunt Trauma

The direction of the force striking the larynx is more important than whether the injury was due to strangulation, flying object, striking the larynx with a steering wheel or fist, etc. Xeroradiography or routine films of the larynx will show a small percentage of the cartilaginous injuries and give some appraisal of the airway. In general, the information obtained from these examinations is so fragmentary that the studies may even be misleading in patient management.

CT examination of the traumatized larynx not only demonstrates the status of the airway and cartilages but also allows for an excellent correlation of the mechanism of injury to the radiologic findings.

Trauma to the larynx can come from a blow directed anteriorly, which will compress the larynx between the offending instrument and the cervical spine. The second type of injury is from the anterolateral surface of the larynx, which will partially compress the larynx against the spine (Fig. 2.18). Remembering that the cricoid cartilage is a ring and a major support of the larynx, it follows the same rules of fracture of any ringed structure and must be disrupted in more than one place. The thyroid cartilages form a shield to the larynx, and their site of junction in the midline appears to be quite strong. The posterior margins of the thyroid cartilage are capable of "spreading" to accomodate the trauma, and the weakest portion of the cartilage seems to be anterolaterally in the "parasymphyseal region".

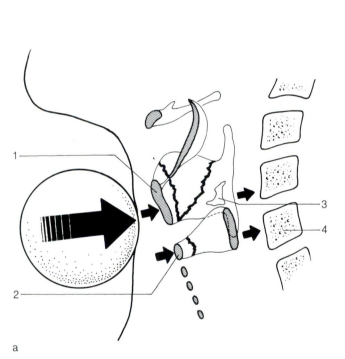

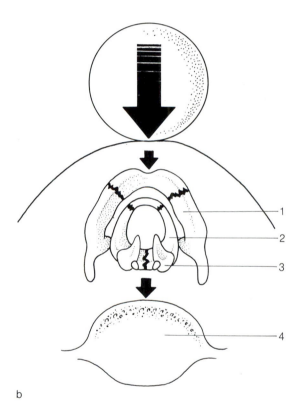

a

b

Fig. 2.**18**   Distribution of force to the larynx.

a) Diagrammatic lateral projection of a ball striking the anterior surface of the larynx and b) the view from above. The larynx is trapped between the force of the ball and the vertebral bodies posteriorly. The thyroid cartilages may shatter with an oblique fracture, vertical fracture, or combination of both to allow posterior displacement of the symphysis. The cricoid fracture must occur in two places since the cricoid is a ring. A bilateral anterior fracture may displace a segment of the ring posteriorly. The major impact may be with the signet of the cricoid against the spine. One or two fractures through the signet are accompanied by an anterior ring fracture allowing both halves to be displaced laterally.

1. Thyroid cartilage, 2. cricoid cartilage, 3. arytenoid cartilage, 4. cervical vertebral body.

Trauma to the larynx from directly anterior may cause the anterior ring of the cricoid to break in one or even two places with posterior displacement of the ring should bilateral fractures occur. The signet posterior portion of the cricoid will be impinged against the cervical vertebral bodies and any osteophytes arising from the intervertebral disk spaces. The signet of the cricoid will split in a vertical line, with the two lateral fragments being displaced laterally and even rotating to further disrupt the support of the larynx (Fig. 2.19). The thyroid cartilages may fracture vertically on either side of the symphyseal region, and the midportions of the larynx may be displaced posteriorly.

If the injury comes from the anterolateral surface of the larynx, the cricoid ring fractures are usually not midline fractures. They occur on either side, either anterolaterally or posterolaterally. The cricoid signet may become comminuted into multiple fragments. The thyroid cartilages may have oblique linear fractures or become shattered into multiple fragments lying within the soft tissues of the neck (Fig. 2.20).

Regardless of the direction of force, the cartilage disruptions may be accompanied by massive hematomas, avulsion of the attachment of the epiglottis to the thyroid cartilage, dislocations of the arytenoids, and even complete transections of the cricoid cartilage from the upper trachea (1, 36, 39). As yet, the full impact of CT scanning of the acutely traumatized larynx has not been appreciated in the planning of surgical management of these injuries.

Late Effects

If the fractures of the cricoid, thyroid, and laryngeal disruptions are not corrected, extensive scarring and web formation may ensue (11, 18, 40). Reconstructions and replacements of cartilage dislocations are exceedingly difficult after scarring has taken place (35). CT scanning shows many times that a distorted larynx is in reality, due to lack of the supporting cartilaginous architecture rather than vocal paralysis, or secondary to nerve injury. The clinician once armed with CT scanning surveys may be encouraged to pursue restorative operative procedures.

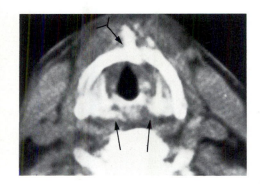

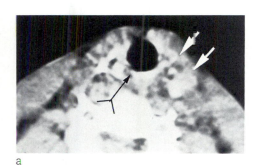

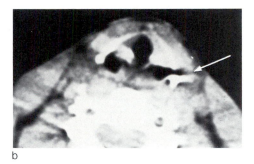

Fig. 2.**19** Fractured cricoid ring. Scan through the level of the inferior margin of the true vocal cords shows that the signet of the cricoid ring has been fractured in two places (arrows) and the lateral portions of the cricoid rings on either side are rotated laterally. The anterior ring of the cricoid and the inferior margins of the thyroid cartilages are displaced posteriorly (Y-shaped arrow). Both inferior surfaces of the true cords show soft tissue thickening secondary to the distortion and foreshortening of the true vocal cords.

a

b

Fig. 2.**20** Shattered thyroid cartilage.
a) Scan at the level of the true vocal cord shows the right thyroid cartilages totally shattered, and multiple fragments are displaced posteriorly (arrows). In addition, the signet of the cricoid cartilage is fractured posterolaterally on the left (Y-shaped arrow) causing distortion of the ring. The anterior portions of the left thyroid cartilages are also fractured inferiorly and are no longer recognizable.

b) Scan at the level of the false cord and aryepiglottic folds shows the fragment of the right thyroid cartilage being rotated and lying posterior in the soft tissues of the neck (arrow). The paralaryngeal space is high density secondary to scarring and distortions following healing of the fractures.

Inflammatory Lesions

Inflammatory lesions of the larynx may be thought of as acute or chronic. The acute inflammations that present as acute respiratory distress require radiologic investigation to insure an adequate airway. The chronic inflammatory lesions are mainly granulomatous diseases that closely mimic tumor masses. The radiologist must be constantly reminded that roentgenograms only delineate morphology and not histology. Neither the clinician nor the radiologist should attempt a final diagnosis of malignancy based on appearance of the lesion (56). Bacteriologic or histologic confirmation is essential in every instance.

Acute Infections

Laryngotracheal bronchitis, commonly known as croup, is of viral origin and affects children 6 months to 6 years of age (58). Since the transglottic and subglottic regions are the narrowest portion of the respiratory system in this age group, radiologic examination of the larynx becomes a vital diagnostic tool in determining the causes of upper respiratory obstruction.
The children have a characteristic brassy cough that usu-

ally follows a few days of low-grade fever. The respiratory difficulty is characterized by an inspiratory as well as expiratory stridor. On anteroposterior views of the larynx, the normal cathedral curve of the airway beneath the level of the true cords is exaggerated and prolonged due to the edema of the mucosa overlying the conus elasticus and extending into the upper trachea (15). The pathologic changes are easier to demonstrate on the lateral projection (Fig. 2.21). The subglottic edema causes exaggerated inspiratory effort. The entire larynx descends, causing a ballooning of the hypopharynx. Because of the distension of the lateral wall of the hypopharynx, the tonsils become more prominent in the air column and should not be confused with acute tonsilitis. Since the inflammatory condition is part of a generalized tracheobronchitis, complete evaluation of the thorax must accompany the laryngeal study (60). Other considerations in the differential diagnosis of croup include congenital tumors and aspirated foreign bodies. The clinician should be especially alerted to the possibility of alternative diagnoses if the symptoms of croup occur prior to the age of six months.

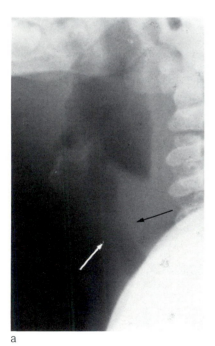

a

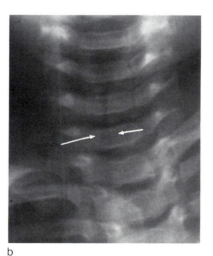

b

Fig. 2.**21**   Croup (laryngotracheobronchitis).
a) Lateral projection shows the narrowing of the trachea in the immediate subglottic area (arrows). The hypopharynx is greatly distended secondary to the "air hunger" that these children exhibit.

b) Anteroposterior projection. Arrows indicate the narrowing of the air column immediately below the level of the true and false cords. If this narrowing were due to physiologic apposition of the true cords, the configuration would be more of a right angle between the tracheal lumen and the undersurface of the true cords.

Acute epiglottitis is characterized by an infection of the epiglottis and aryepiglottic folds (Fig. 2.22). The degree of respiratory obstruction may be severe, and the offending organism is almost invariably *Hemophilus influenzae* (51). The peak of acute epiglottitis is in the three to seven year age group but has been found as early as three months and may even be the cause of respiratory distress in adults.

On roentgen examination, the pharynx and hypopharynx are distended on the inspiratory film in a manner similar to that in croup. The characteristic swelling and enlargement of the epiglottis should be readily apparent on the lateral projection. CT scans are impossible to obtain due to movement and rapid respiration. Positive contrast is contraindicated and may interfere with bronchoscopy.

The differential diagnosis should include trauma with hemorrhage, edematous states, and foreign body aspiration. Inflammatory lesions of the lingual tonsils, lingual thyroid tissue, or cysts about the base of the tongue may simulate enlargement of the epiglottis on the roentgen examination.

Chronic Infections

Radiologic investigation of the larynx in patients with tuberculosis, coccidioidomycosis, blastomycosis, histoplasmosis, and other granulomas of the larynx are usually performed because of a mistaken belief on the part of the clinician that a malignancy exists. They all produce mass lesions that interfere with laryngeal physiology. Their radiologic manifestations are those of granuloma formation with the morphology determined by type III immune response. If the lesions are investigated early in the illness and the host reaction is less effective, edema and inflammatory cell response will predominate the roentgen picture. The larynx shows diffuse swelling of the mucosa. This type of pattern is most predominant in the active phase of rhinoscleroma that affects the larynx. The diagnosis of rhinoscleroma is usually based on concomitant lesions being present in the nasal cavity since the disease characteristically begins in the nose and spreads inferiorly.

Blastomycosis within the larynx is more likely to be exuberant and exophytic in its appearance. The body response is somewhat variable, but in general the blastomycosis forms tumor masses quite indistinguishable from malignant lesions.

Tuberculosis and coccidiodomycosis lesions are more of an intermediate type of response with some elements of edema and some granulomas causing mass-like expansions within the paralaryngeal space. If the diagnosis is suspected clinically, there is little need for roentgen examination. Ward (56) reported on four patients with coccidiodomycosis, one of whom developed subglottic stenosis with airway narrowing.

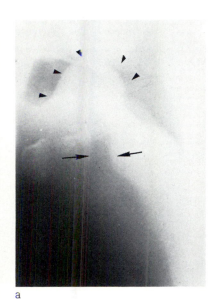

a

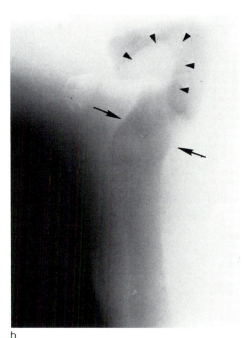

b

Fig. 2.**22**   Acute epiglottitis. Four-year-old with acute respiratory distress.
a) Shows marked edema of the free margin of the epiglottis (arrowheads) and swelling in the preepiglottic space. The posterior commissure region has caused narrowing of the AP diameter of the airway (arrows).

b) One week following the preceding examination, the respiratory symptoms have largely abetted. There is only minimal swelling of the free margin of the epiglottis (arrowheads). The laryngeal vestibule is now widely patent (arrows).

Miscellaneous Disorders

A group of chronic granulomas or deposits within the larynx, such as amyloid, may produce roentgen changes that resemble malignancies. They produce hoarseness by interfering with vocal cord function. Amyloid may be deposited as a tumorlike nodule resembling a papilloma or may be present as a diffuse infiltrating variety. The localized nodule may also occur deep within the larynx (4).

The deposits of amyloid, whether primary or secondary, within the larynx will closely mimic deep infiltrating tumors and in particular carcinomas arising within the appendices of the laryngeal ventricle. Amyloid, some chronic granulomas, and the deeper infiltrating cancers may spread for great distances with an intact mucosa. Plain views of the larynx, positive contrast laryngography, and CT scanning will show the distorted anatomy, but usually the cartilages are intact in all three conditions. It is rare to identify cartilaginous destruction in malignancies without advanced mucosa lesions as well. On positive contrast laryngography and CT, the infiltrations characteristically involve the true cords, laryngeal ventricles, and generally involve the paralaryngeal space deep to the false cords. Motion is preserved until the disease is advanced.

Laryngeal Tumors

Benign Tumors

Benign tumors of the larynx are quite rare and as a rule, the role of radiology in their management is limited. They may arise from the mucosa and appendages or supporting cartilages and vessels. In a series of 5000 primary laryngeal neoplasms seen in a 30-year period at the Massachusetts Eye and Ear Infirmary, Huizenga found only ten cartilaginous tumors. The more commonly encountered lesions lie in the borderline area between true tumors or distorted normal tissues. Polyps and laryngoceles fall into the latter category. True laryngeal adenomas are exceedingly rare, and some feel that they do not exist (41). The benign glandular lesions that appear as adenomas show cell types consistent with adherrent salivary gland tissue (52). The oncocytoma has been called oncocytic papillary cystadenoma and Warthin's tumor of the larynx. Some investigators draw a fine line of differentiation between the two lesions based on whether lymphatics are found within the tumor mass. Radiologically, the pattern is the same, and a mass lesion is found within the larynx that interferes with phonation. Oliveira (41) collected 68 such patients from the literature and showed that many of the cysts of the larynx were indeed lined with oncocytes. The lesions are benign and respond favorably to surgical extirpation.

Clinical examination will demonstrate the mass lesions in the vast majority of benign tumors. Some pedunculated papillomas may "flop back and forth" between the superior surface of the true vocal cords and the subglottic space during phonation or respiration. If the mass happens to be located subglottically beneath the anterior commissure region during indirect examination, visualization may be difficult. The rounded mass is usually of low density and difficult to see on conventional lateral and anteroposterior projections. The lesion must be suspected because of hoarseness, and tomography or positive contrast laryngography will reveal the lesion and its mobile nature (Fig. 2.23).

Laryngoceles, although not tumors, present as benign expansive processes. They represent extensions of the normal appendices of the laryngeal ventricle (saccule) that are visible in about 40% of the positive contrast laryngograms (5). The appendices (saccules) are outpouchings arising from the anterior third of the laryngeal ventricle (Fig. 2.24). They are directed superiorly into the false cord region and extend posterolaterally and superiorly into the lateral wall of the larynx (20). The appendices secrete a very fine mucus to lubricate the true vocal cord. They may extend as far cephalad as the aryepiglottic fold. If the natural ostium becomes occluded, secretions may "back up" in the appendix, and the condition called mucocele of the appendix is formed. This entity is frequently referred to as a cyst of the aryepiglottic fold but in reality originates from the laryngeal ventricle. The diagnosis of benign cyst should be made with extreme caution since carcinomas may occlude an appendix and secondarily produce a mucocele. If the appendix becomes distended secondary to voice abuse, the lumen may extend into the aryepiglottic fold and then bulge into the laryngeal vestibule producing an "internal laryngocele." If the major portion of the expansion of the cyst is lateral and anterior to the piriform sinus, it is spoken of as an "external laryngocele." Plain films or tomography with the patient performing a modified Valsalva will frequently outline the air-filled cavity and permit accurate evaluation of the lesion (Fig. 2.25).

True cysts of the larynx do occur and are related to occluded mucous and serous glands. They appear as rounded masses on routine views of the larynx and, again, are generally diagnosed by clinical examination rather than radiologic techniques.

The hemangiomas of childhood or lymphangiomas of the neck and mediastinum as found in infants are entirely a different problem. Radiologically, the mass lesions can be demonstrated, but a histologic diagnosis cannot be made. If the lesion bleeds and is accompanied by cutaneous manifestations of hemangioma elsewhere, little doubt will occur in the minds of the clinician or radiologist concerning the nature of the lesion (Fig. 2.13).

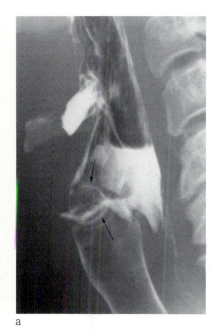

a

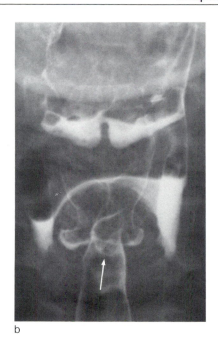

b

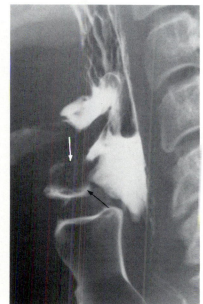

c

Fig. 2.**23**   Laryngeal polyp.
a) Lateral projection during quiet respiration shows the polyp (arrows) to lie with its inferior border resting on the free margin of the true vocal cord.
b) Reverse E maneuver causes the polyp to be "sucked" inferiorly to lie between the vocal cords (arrows). The laryngeal ventricles are distended, and the true cords descend during this maneuver preventing complete inferior prolapse of the polyp.
c) True Valsalva maneuver with the true cords forcefully adducted. The polyp (arrow) has been pushed superiorly to rest between the false vocal cords.

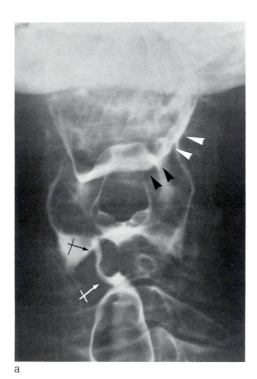

a

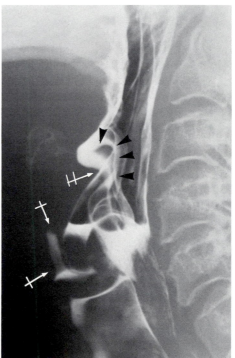

b

Fig. 2.**24** Appendix of the laryngeal ventricle in a patient with carcinoma of the left pharyngoepiglottic fold.

a) PA projection. The appendix of the laryngeal ventricle is seen filling from the superolateral margin of the right laryngeal ventricle (cross-hatched arrow). The appendix extends in the paralaryngeal space anteriorly and laterally. The appendix on the left does not fill, which is of no clinical significance. The patient's tumor involving the vallecula, pharyngoepiglottic fold, and lateral pharyngeal wall (arrowheads) stops at the entrance to the piriform sinus.

b) Lateral projection shows the appendix extending anteriorly with the tip being at about the level of the superior margin of the false vocal cord. When the appendix is longer than the one demonstrated, it will turn posteriorly at approximately this level to extend to the region of the aryepiglottic fold. The patient's tumor of the pharyngoepiglottic fold causes asymmetry of the two sides with the side of the tumor (arrowheads) being slightly higher than the patient's normal right side (double cross-hatched arrow).

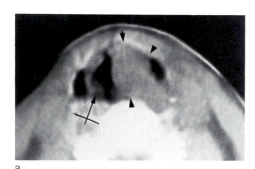

a

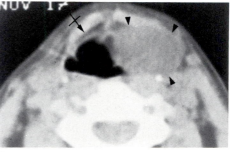

b

Fig. 2.**25** Laryngocele.

a) Soft tissue density extending in the aryepiglottic fold on the right (arrowheads). The normal aryepiglottic fold is visible for comparison on the left (cross-hatched arrow). Air is visible lateral to the laryngocele lying in the piriform sinus.

b) Section through the upper body of the epiglottis shows a normal preepiglottic space on the left (cross-hatched arrow). The laryngocele bulges outside of the larynx laterally (arrowhead), giving this lesion an internal and an external component. The CT numbers of the laryngocele were of water density indicating its fluid-filled nature at the time of this examination.

Malignant Tumors

A classification of tumors of the larynx based on laryngography and CT scanning is not warranted. A comparison of the findings of CT and laryngography may prove helpful since both give clues to tumor extensions that greatly affect patient management. As high resolution, rapid CT scanners become more widely available, the trend will definitely swing to CT as the more superior method of evaluating extent of disease.

The host responses to malignancies within the larynx vary greatly and are reflected in the roentgen appearance. This is especially evident when the host responds with exuberant fibrous tissue reaction or edema that on CT and laryngography appears as an extension of tumor far beyond the limits of malignant cells. At the present time, CT examination does not differentiate the density of the physiologic tissue responses. Even histologic examina-

tion can at times be confusing since the fibrous tissue will assume a bizarre quality that has been termed "pseudosarcoma" (Fig. 2.26).

Some grouping of the tumors as to site of origin is helpful for discussion to allow the examiner to concentrate on those maneuvers that are most likely to yield clinical findings. Nevertheless, all five basic maneuvers of laryngography are performed in every instance, and the CT examination is always conducted from the anterior arch of the cricoid cartilage to the hyoid bone. Tumors may be grouped as follows:

1. True cord tumors
2. False cord and aryepiglottic fold
3. Infrahyoid epiglottis
4. Suprahyoid epiglottis
5. Piriform sinus (not truly laryngeal carcinoma)
6. Postcricoid and esophageal hiatus.

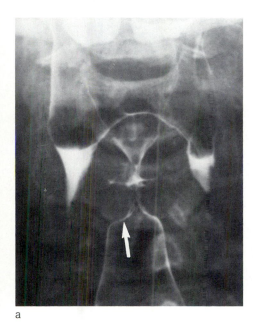

a

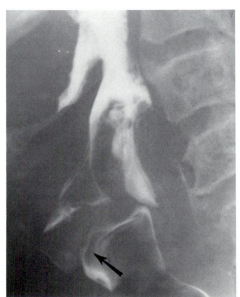

b

Fig. 2.**26** Pseudosarcoma of the larynx.
a) Sparce nests of tumor cells were found on the right vocal cord extending across the anterior commissure to involve the left vocal cord and paralaryngeal space bilaterally. The excessive fibroblastic cell response to the carcinoma is manifest on the laryngogram by markedly thickened true cords with swelling of the false cords and slit-like laryngeal ventricles. The inferior surface of the right true cord is slightly lower than the left (arrow).

b) Valsalva maneuver shows that the larynx is able to elevate, but the anteroinferior margins of both true cords are distorted due to the involvement of the anterior commissure and undersurface of the true cords (arrow). This pattern of growth is not radiologically characteristic and could be interpreted as diffuse edema, extensive tumor, or an inflammatory response.

True Cord Tumors

True cord tumors that begin in the anterior third of the true cord have a propensity for spreading to the anterior commissure region and across to the opposite true cord (49). They tend to involve and grow in a circumferential pattern and involve the inferior surface of the anterior commissure (25). Inferiorly, the thick conus elasticus forms a barrier to their deep spread, and they stay in the mucosa for a prolonged period of time (43, 44, 46). Anteriorly, they may directly invade the thyroid cartilage. They also spread in the paralaryngeal space and accompany the entering vessels and nerves (Fig. 2.27). Tumors that begin in the middle or posterior third of the

true cord spread in all directions. As they spread laterally into the lateral extent of the laryngeal ventricle, they gain access to the paralaryngeal space. Direct extension occurs posteriorly and inferiorly into the space between the thyroid and cricoid cartilages. The more posteriorly placed tumors grow posteriorly into the arytenoid cartilage and involve the cricoarytenoid joint. The tumors may also spread posteriorly into the intra-arytenoid area where they tend to grow aggressively in the mucosa and even rapidly become circumferential about the subglottic space (Fig. 2.28). Tumors that have gotten into the cricoarytenoid joint may destroy portions of the signet of the cricoid and invade widely from the posterolateral

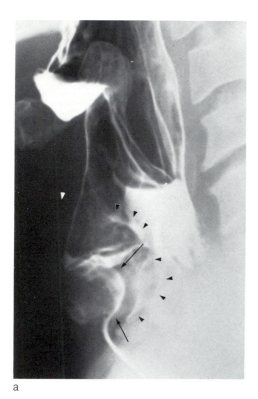

a

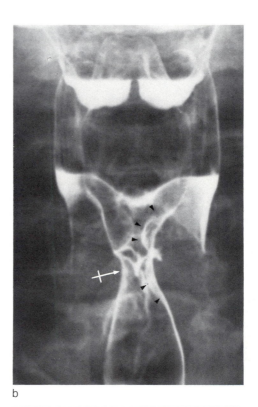

b

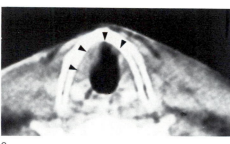

c

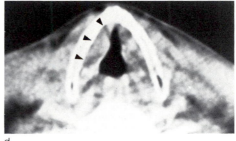

d

Fig. 2.27 Left true cord carcinoma extending subglottically and crossing the anterior commissure.

a) Lateral projection during quiet respiration shows the bulky tumor mass on the left involving the left false cord (upper arrowheads) and extending subglottically with involvement of over two thirds of the left true cord (lower arrowheads). The tumor also extends across the anterior commissure to involve the right true cord (arrows).

b) PA view in quiet respiration shows the bulky tumor mass on the left involving false cord, true cord, and subglottic space (arrowheads). The knotty appearance to the right true cord due to is the

spread across the midline, which is confined to the anterior portion of the cord leaving the posterior margin relatively normal (crosshatched arrow).

c) CT scan at the inferior margin of the true cords shows involvement of the undersurface of the left true cord, which crosses the midline and is also present on the right (arrowheads). The cartilages are all intact.

d) Scan at the level of the false cord shows an increase of density in the lateral portion of the left false cord (arrowheads). The right false cord appears entirely normal.

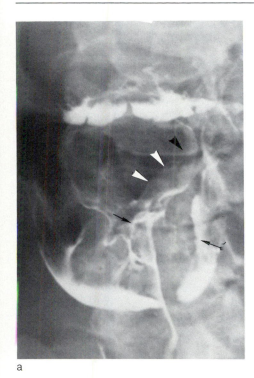

a

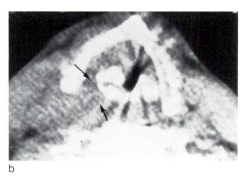

b

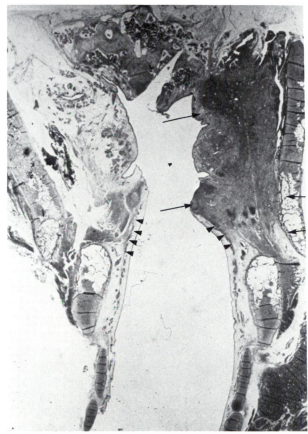

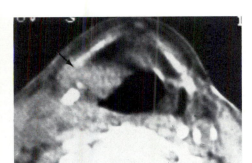

c

d

Fig. 2.28 Left true cord carcinoma extending posteroinferiorly and through the thyroid cartilage.

a) Posteroanterior modified Valsalva maneuver in the laryngogram. The bulky tumor of the left true cord has produced fixation (arrow). There is infiltration of the aryepiglottic fold (arrowheads) and distortion of the lateral wall of the larynx. The medial wall of the piriform sinus is displaced laterally due to the posterior inferior extension of the tumor (Y-shaped arrow).

b) CT scan at the level of the upper true cord shows the bulky tumor mass with extension of the tumor posteriorly between the cricoid cartilage and thyroid cartilage (arrows). The tumor mass has extended posterior to the ala of the thyroid cartilage causing the larynx to rotate. The posterior portions of the larynx have been

spread apart, changing the contour of the thyroid cartilages at the symphysis.

c) The upper extensions of the tumor in the paralaryngeal space produces a loss of the normal low-density material. The tumor has extended through the thyroid cartilage laterally into the soft tissues of the neck (arrow).

d) Whole organ section from another patient but with similar subglottic spread of tumor (arrows) (courtesy of Dr. Bohna). The tumor mass extends inferiorly between the thyroid and cricoid cartilage. The conus elasticus (arrowheads) is clearly shown and tends to serve as a barrier to tumor growth. In this instance, tumor is present in the mucosa of the true cord but peripheral to the conus elasticus in the subglottic space.

border of the larynx. The increase bulk of tumor tissue lying posterolaterally causes the thyroid cartilages to "spread" posteriorly and to rotate on the verticle axis from their support on the cricoid cartilage. Plain film examination of the larynx may demonstrate a bulging mass arising from the true cords. This may be visible on either the anteroposterior or lateral projection. Most important is the lateral projection in quiet respiration to see if there is a mass in the subglottic region bulging into the airway. Destruction of thyroid cartilage may be present in advanced lesions. Unfortunately, less than 20% of the patients having cartilaginous invasion can be demonstrated on routine roentgen examinations. The accuracy of CT scanning has been so impressive that this author no longer performs routine views or xeroradiography for cartilage invasion. The indication for CT scan versus positive contrast laryngography is not an easy question to answer. The very early mucosal lesion can be studied equally well by either technique provided direct laryngoscopy has been performed. If clinical examination has been limited, positive contrast laryngography provides a better survey.

During positive contrast laryngography for true cord lesions, the most important maneuver is quiet respiration. Obtaining good respiration views is the most neglected view despite the fact it gives the most accurate delineation of crucial clinical areas. The condition of the anterior commissure and the immediate undersurface of the true cords at the anterior commissure level must be determined preoperatively. When doing a vertical hemilaryngectomy, meticulous care is taken not to cut through tumor-bearing areas (7,37). Good quiet respiration lateral views of the larynx will show the degree of mucosal thickening lying immediately deep to the thyroid cartilage. Contrast material outlining the tracheal mucosa anteriorly should form a straight line to the undersurface of the thyroid cartilage. If the mucosa bulges posteriorly, anterior commissure invasion should be suspected. Since the true cords are attached in the midline, any edema or limited mobility may cause them to be tightly opposed. Contrast material will be displaced from their surfaces at the anterior commissure much like one would squeeze toothpaste from a tube. Cinefluorography can be helpful to show fleeting moments of true cord separation during quiet respiration. On the anteroposterior projections, the amount of bulk to the tumor mass lying along the lateral wall of the larynx will give appreciation of the amount of deep infiltration in an indirect way.

CT examination in the anterior third of the true cords will show if the tumor mass is grossly confined to one true cord, but the thickness of cut with present scanners makes evaluation of the inferior extent not quite as precise. On the other hand, CT scans will show the position of the conus elasticus, and most importantly CT will show the cricoid cartilage ring anteriorly and the relationships of inferior spreads of tumor to the cricoid ring. Since the integrity of the anterior cricoid ring must be maintained in any conservative laryngeal surgery, this information can be vital in patient management (Fig. 2.29) (3). CT examination of bulky lesions has

another distinct advantage since it can determine accurately whether the bulk of the tumor is due to exophytic growth or whether the bulk is due to a deeply infiltrating tumor that is forming a large mass. This type of differentiation can be implied from direct laryngoscopy and contrast laryngography by the degree of mobility or lack of same once the vocal muscle has been infiltrated. Cartilaginous invasion can easily be identified on CT scanning, and this type of information is not readily obtainable or is frought with gross inaccuracies when attempted by any other means. It is surprising how frequently the surgical pathologist will miss cartilaginous invasion unless he is performing serial whole organ section (Fig. 2.30) (45).

Tumors of the middle and posterior third of the true cord can be shown very nicely on quiet respiration views during laryngography. On the anteroposterior projection, the lumen of the trachea should be traced from inferiorly toward the true vocal cords as a straight line. Any deviation would indicate invasion extending inferiorly for varying distances. Posteriorly, a similar straight line should continue up from the trachea to the intra-arytenoid area during quiet respiration. Distortions due to tumor in the posterior commissure region are difficult to evaluate during phonation and require maximum abduction of the arytenoids in quiet respiration. CT scanning shows the mucosal thickening between the two cricoarytenoid joints (Fig. 2.31).

As these tumors extend laterally along the superior surface of the true cord, they tend to involve the lateralmost extremity of the laryngeal ventricle. Once the entire laryngeal ventricle is involved, they gain access to the paralaryngeal space. This type of deep infiltration can best be demonstrated with the modified Valsalva (blowing against the pursed lips) or the reverse phonation maneuver. Both of these maneuvers will distend the laryngeal ventricle. Phonation of E does show the undersurface of the true cords very well, but as the air passes cephalad between the true cords, it tends to displace contrast material into the laryngeal ventricle. The dense filling of the laryngeal ventricle during phonation of E may obscure small lesions of the mucosa.

As the true cord tumor becomes more bulky and infiltrates the paralaryngeal space, the vocal muscle becomes infiltrated. This is manifest on direct laryngoscopy and positive contrast laryngography as fixation of the vocal cord. CT examination will show the increase in density to the paralaryngeal space and the bulk of the tumor. If scanning times are prolonged to the range of 15–20 s, motion artifacts normally occur from the true vocal cords. An indirect sign of fixation on CT may be the lack of any motion artifacts in the involved fixed cord.

Infiltration into the cricoarytenoid joint is extremely important in patient management since it usually implies a much lower salvage rate by radiotherapy and represents a controversial area as to the feasibility of conservative surgery. On positive contrast laryngography, there is usually swelling of the involved postcricoid pad. This is manifest by distortion of the postcricoid line where the cricoid pad abuts the posterior pharyngeal wall (Fig. 2.32). The increased bulk of the tissues is also evident on oblique views with the patient performing the modified Valsalva. Phonation of E and quiet respiration generally will demonstrate the limited mobility of the posterior half of the involved cord. CT scanning is extremely helpful in that it will show displacement of the cricoid and at times local erosions of the cricoid cartilage if fast CT scans are available (2–3 s scanners). The indi-

rect signs of cricoarytenoid joint involvement are the increased bulk to the arytenoid area and thickening of the posterior portion of the aryepiglottic fold. Generally, the tumor mass can be followed extending into the paralaryngeal tissues. The thyroid cartilage on the involved side will be distorted by the increased bulk of tissues in the posterolateral larynx.

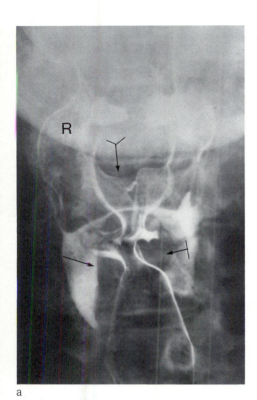

a

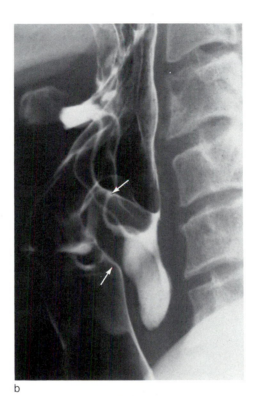

b

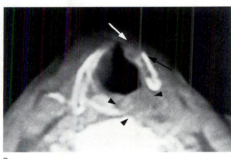

c

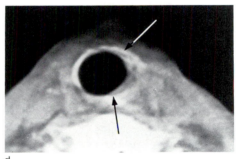

d

Fig. 2.**29**   Cricoid and Thyroid cartilage invasion.

a) Anteroposterior projection with phonation maneuver. The right true vocal cord (arrow) lies at a lower level than the normal left vocal cord (cross-hatched arrow). The asymmetry of the arytenoids (Y-shaped arrow) and the intra-arytenoid notch is highly significant, indicating that the arytenoid cartilage has rotated anteriorly. The subglottic space is asymmetric, but no bulky tumor mass can be identified.

b) Lateral projection during quiet respiration shows the forward subluxation of the arytenoid (upper arrow) and increase in soft tissue thickness at the level of the posterior commissure (lower arrow). Again, no bulky tumor mass can be identified.

c) CT scan at the level of the vocal cords shows that the right half of the top of the cricoid signet has been destroyed (arrowheads) and that there is tumor mass extending posterolaterally. Anteriorly, the thyroid cartilage is destroyed on the right (arrows), and the mass at the level of the anterior margin of the true cords is evident.

d) Inferiorly, at the level of the anterior ring of the cricoid the scan shows that there is no evidence of cartilage destruction; however, a soft tissue mass extends around the entire right half of the mucosal surface of the subglottic space (arrows).

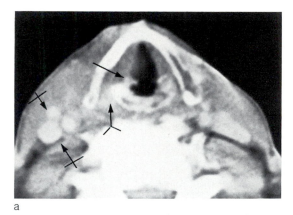

a

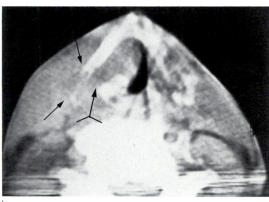

b

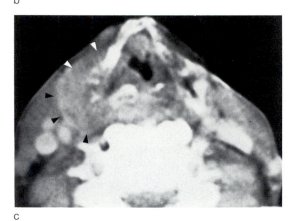

c

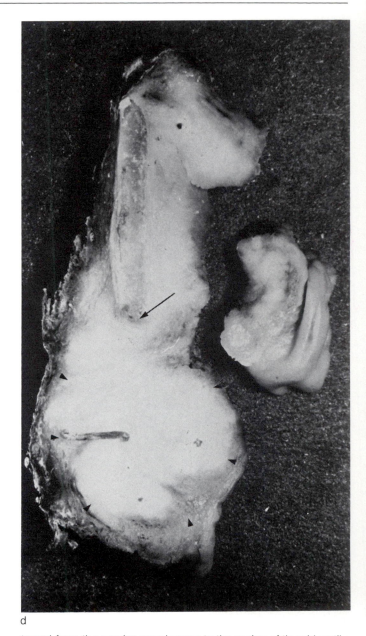

d

Fig. 2.**30** Thyroid cartilage invasion from tumor either arising in the appendix of the laryngeal ventricle or medial wall of the piriform sinus.

a) Scan at the level of the true cords shows marked thickening of the right true cord with widening of the space between the signet of the cricoid and the thyroid cartilage (Y-shaped arrow). The arytenoid cartilage (arrow) is displaced to the midline. This scan was taken with contrast infusion so that the carotid artery and jugular vessels are opacified (cross-hatched arrows). The mass is continuous from the true cord and paralaryngeal space through the space between the thyroid cartilage and cricoid cartilage (Y-shaped arrow) and extending into the vascular space posterior and lateral to the larynx.

b) Upper true cord level shows that the thyroid cartilage is destroyed in its posterior half (arrows). The tumor mass is again

traced from the paralaryngeal space to the region of thyroid cartilage destruction (Y-shaped arrow).

c) At the level of the aryepiglottic fold. The mass in the soft tissues of the neck can be outlined by some surface staining with contrast material (arrowheads). The preepiglottic space has lost its normal fat density, and there is a marked degree of thickening of the aryepiglottic fold region with the tumor mass crossing the midline posteriorly.

d) Vertical section through the thyroid cartilage showing the marked degree of destruction (arrow) and extension of the soft tissue mass outside the lumen of the larynx (arrowheads). Despite this extensive destruction, the pathologists could not feel the cartilage destruction at initial examination. Only after comparison to the CT scans were additional sections taken to confirm the invasion of the thyroid cartilage.

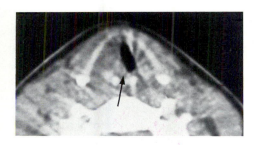

Fig. 2.**31**   Carcinoma of the left true cord involving the posterior commissure. The bulky tumor of the left true cord extends from the anterior commissure to the posterior commissure and crosses the midline posteriorly (arrow). There is involvement of the paralaryngeal space with some widening of the distance between the thyroid cartilage and cricoid cartilage. An indirect sign of cord fixation is present on this scan. The right true cord moves normally giving motion artifacts on the scan. The left true cord being fixed shows no evidence of motion artifacts.

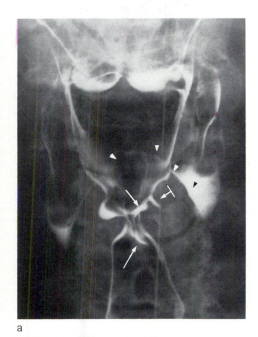

a

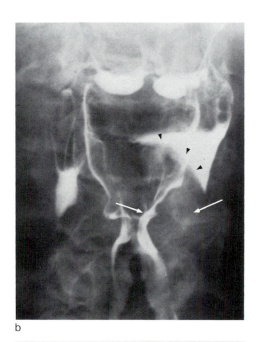

b

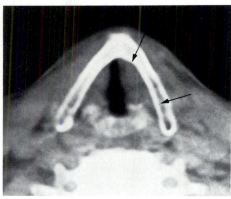

c

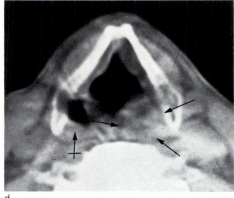

d

Fig. 2.**32**   Cricoarytenoid joint involvement.

a) AP laryngogram with phonation shows a bulky tumor mass of the right true cord (arrows). The tumor is distorting the false cord, but a slitlike laryngeal ventricle (cross-hatched arrows) separates the tumor mass from the false cord. The postcricoid line (arrowheads) is distorted on the side of the tumor indicating increased bulk of the cricoarytenoid region that is pressing against the posterior pharyngeal wall. The piriform sinuses are asymmetric.

b) Anteroposterior projection with quiet respiration shows the appearance of bulk to the mass of the right true cord, suggesting involvement of the paralaryngeal space (arrows). The postcricoid line is again distorted (arrowheads), and the inferior pole of the piriform sinus is elevated on the right by comparison to the normal left.

c) CT scan at the level of the true cord shows a marked degree of thickening of the right true cord with increase in density that extends into the paralaryngeal space. The space between the thyroid cartilage and the cricoid cartilage is not widened.

d) CT scan at the level of the upper false cord shows that the major portion of the tumor mass involves the cricoarytenoid joint region (arrows). The piriform sinus is obliterated on that side as compared to the normal piriform sinus on the left (cross-hatched arrow). The bulk of the tumor mass plus the midline position of the true cord indicates that the right vocal cord is fixed due to involvement of the cricoarytenoid joint.

Tumors that have extended inferiorly into the subglottic space are best demonstrated by the true Valsalva maneuver. As the true and false cords are brought forcefully together in adduction, the undersurface of the cords become straightened, and their anterior margins approximate a right angle to the lateral wall of the trachea. Posteriorly, there is still some retention of the normal dome-shaped undersurface of the true cords. In the lateral projection, both cords should superimpose at exactly the same level. Tumor masses infiltrating inferiorly either distort the contour of the true cord or cause the cords to lie at different levels on both the AP and lateral projections. During the reverse E maneuver, the true cords will not descend if infiltration has involved the vocal muscle and/or conus elasticus to any significant extent (Fig. 2.33). Rather than an exact measurement in millimeters of the size of the tumor, the clinician should be appraised of the inferior extent of the tumor and its relationship to the upper margin of the cricoid ring or the inferior margin of the thyroid cartilage. This measurement will allow surgical planning of the inferior extent of excision in any conservative surgery.

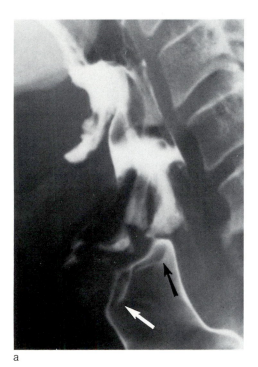

a

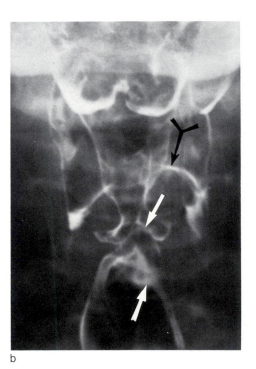

b

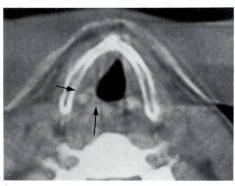

c

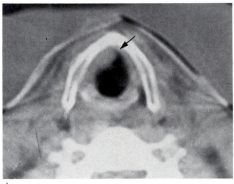

d

Fig. 2.33 Carcinoma of the left true cord involving the inferior surface.

a) Lateral view of the true Valsalva maneuver showing the distortion of the inferior surfaces of the true cords. The inferior surfaces of the true cords are not at the same level posteriorly nor anteriorly (arrows).

b) Reverse E maneuver shows that the true cords do not descend to any significant degree. The lateral wall of the laryngeal ventricle bulges relatively freely, and the piriform on the left descends. There is distortion of the postcricoid line, suggesting some posterior extension of the tumor (Y-shaped arrow).

c) CT scan at the level of the true cords shows increased bulk to the left true cord, which bulges at the midline but does not cross onto the right true cord. The thickening of tissues extends all the way to the arytenoid region, and there is a slight increase in bulk to the soft tissues between the cricoid signet and the thyroid cartilage (arrows).

d) Scan at the level of the inferior margin of the true cord shows the bulky tumor mass anteriorly that bulges and abuts the inferior surface of the right true cord. This close apposition of tumor to the normal tissues on the right explains the lack of contrast filling of the anterior commissure because the contrast material is unable to penetrate the tightly opposed surfaces (arrow).

A special situation exists as the tumor approaches the anterior ring of the cricoid cartilage. The lymphatics become much richer and communicate freely with the lymphatics in the mucosa of the trachea. Some tumors either have a propensity for rapid spread or originate from the undersurface of the true cord and will extend for great distances into the upper trachea. The tracheal extensions may be demonstrated by routine views and even on the preoperative chest x-ray (Fig. 2.34). The conus elasticus and tracheal rings usually retain these tumors to the confines of the trachea for long periods of time before they invade into the upper mediastinum and cervical tissues. CT scanning is of limited usefulness below the cricoid cartilage because of the artifacts imposed by the superimposed shoulders. Until these technical problems are resolved, information concerning the massive subglottic spreads are best obtained by positive contrast laryngography; however, some surveying is possible with routine views or xeroradiography.

False Cord and Aryepiglottic Fold Tumors

Tumors beginning primarily in the region of the false vocal cords or aryepiglottic folds are quite rare. Almost invariably, the false cords or aryepiglottic folds become secondarily involved from true cord tumors or deeply infiltrating lesions of the piriform sinuses. Because of their deeply infiltrating nature, CT scanning becomes the examination of choice. Plain views of the larynx are usually nonrevealing and may even give the false sense of security. Barium swallows will not demonstrate the tumors unless they have become quite bulky. The normal piriform sinuses will superimpose on the pathologic side in the lateral projection. On the anteroposterior projection, the major portion of the bolus usually passes along the lateral border of the pharynx and piriform sinuses. Small ulcerations are extremely difficult to see.

During positive contrast laryngography, quiet respiration will again show the bulk of the mass protruding into the laryngeal vestibule on the anteroposterior projection. Most helpful of all is the modified Valsalva maneuver. When the piriform sinuses are greatly distended and the laryngeal ventricle is distended, an accurate appraisal of the thickness of the lateral wall of the larynx can readily be made. The oblique views are excellent for showing the inferior poles of the piriform sinus. The oblique views will also show the integrity of the mucosa along the aryepiglottic fold and the thickness of the entire aryepiglottic fold. The thickness of this inferolateral portion of the aryepiglottic fold is difficult to obtain by any other maneuver in contrast laryngography.

CT scanning of the false cord and aryepiglottic fold lesions is excellent for showing the deep infiltration, but partial voluming of surrounding air structures becomes a problem. If the epiglottis is distorted by bulk of tumor, it is difficult to differentiate high false cord invasion from invasion lateral to the laryngeal ventricle. The aryepiglottic folds can be seen and any structural abnormalities noted. Unfortunately, the aryepiglottic folds tend to become edematous with deep false cord tumors, and whether the increase in thickness of the aryepiglottic fold is due to direct tumor invasion or edema may present difficulties. On CT scanning, the air in the laryngeal ventricle gives a somewhat diamond-shaped configuration to the total laryngeal airway. If the tumor has bulged inferiorly from the false cord, this diamond point becomes blunted. By the very nature of the false cords, the tumors have already gained access to the paralaryngeal space, and their extension posterolaterally and inferiorly can be accurately mapped by CT scanning (Fig. 2.35). Contrast infusion can be helpful under these circumstances as the tumor may be stained to a greater extent than the tissue planes of the strap muscles and about the carotid sheath.

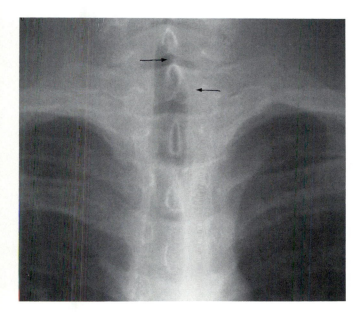

Fig. 2.**34**   Carcinoma of the left true vocal cord extending subglottically. Clinically, this lesion was felt to be a very early true vocal cord tumor. The preoperative chest film for direct laryngoscopy showed subglottic extension (arrow), which at the subsequent surgery required removal of five tracheal rings.

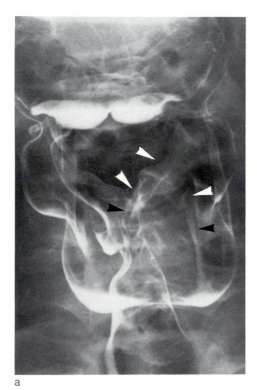

a

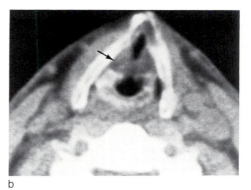

b

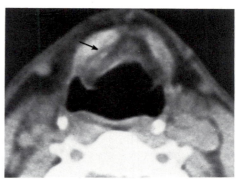

c

Fig. 2.**35**   Granuloma of the false cord.
a) PA view of the laryngogram in the modified Valsalva maneuver shows a bulky mass involving the false cord that extends posteriorly into the arytenoid region and aryepiglottic fold (white arrowhead). Laterally, the paralaryngeal space is involved (black arrowheads) with some thickening and lateral displacement of the medial wall of the piriform sinus. The laryngeal ventricle on the left does not fill due to the paralaryngeal and true cord involvement.

b) CT scan at the level of the false cords shows the marked degree of thickening (arrow). The increase in density extends posteriorly to the region of the top of the arytenoids.
c) Scan through the body of the epiglottis shows increase in density of the preepiglottic space on the left (arrow). The preepiglottic space on the right still shows normal fat density. The density of these infiltrations due to chronic granuloma are indistinguishable from the densities caused by a malignant lesion.

Suprahyoid Epiglottic Tumors

Epiglottic tumors may be divided into two groups by the level of the hyoid bone into suprahyoid and infrahyoid tumors. The suprahyoid tumors spread laterally along the pharyngoepiglottic fold gaining access to the lateral pharyngeal wall and superior hiatus of the piriform sinuses. They frequently fill the vallecula and extend anteriorly into the base of the tongue. The infrahyoid tumors penetrate the epiglottis to enter the preepiglottic space. They may spread along the mucosa to involve the false cords, true cords, and anterior commissure. The ulcerating and infiltrating tumors about the vallecula and base of the tongue are best evaluated by palpation and laryngoscopy. The bulky cauliflower types of growth are another matter, and visualization beyond the tumor may be considerably impaired. Positive contrast laryngography may be quite helpful to show mucosal spreads (Fig. 2.36). Tumor extensions along the laryngeal surface of the epiglottis or along the pharyngoepiglottic folds can be visualized in the lateral projection on quiet breathing and also by the modified Valsalva maneuver. Oblique projections of the modified Valsalva maneuver are most helpful in demonstrating extensions down the lateral pharyngeal wall and into the inferior poles of the piriform sinuses. Infiltrations anterior into the preepig-

lottic space will cause rigidity between the epiglottis and the hyoid bone. Positive contrast laryngography demonstrates the latter infiltration in an indirect manner. By comparing the true Valsalva in the lateral projection, lateral view of phonation, and quiet respiration, there should be changes in configuration of the epiglottis as well as distance between the hyoid bone and the epiglottis (Fig. 2.37). Tumor infiltrations will cause this configuration to maintain a constant relationship. CT scanning of the epiglottic lesions directly shows the change of density in the preepiglottic space. The normal low-density fat becomes replaced by high-density tumor infiltrations (Fig. 2.37). The epiglottis is frequently distorted by the tumor mass, and there may be changes in dimensions of the entrance into the piriform sinuses because of the tumor bulk. The angle formed by the two thyroid cartilages is generally spread. Extensions of these tumors into the base of the tongue present a diagnostic problem both from the point of view of positive contrast laryngography and CT scanning. The region is too variable in density and configuration to make an accurate appraisal by radiologic means. Since the base of the tongue can be readily palpated, this determination is left to clinical examination (38).

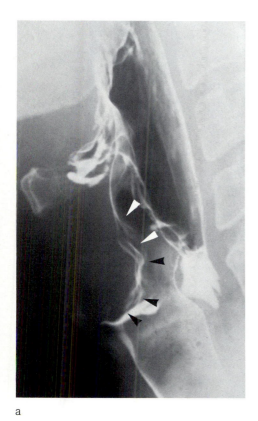

a

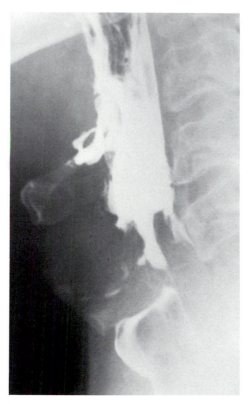

b

Fig. 2.**36**   Bulky epiglottic tumor.
a) Lateral projection during quiet respiration of the laryngogram. The bulky epiglottic tumor (arrowheads) involves the body and extends inferiorly to involve the petiolus of the epiglottis. A sharp margin of contrast material is retained at the level of the anterior commissure, indicating that this region is not involved.

b) Lateral projection during a true Valsalve maneuver. The thyroid cartilage has ascended and the hyoid bone descended to approximate each other (compare to Fig. 2.36a). The epiglottis has changed configuration, indicating that there is pliability of the preepiglottic space. The inferior surface of the true vocal cords is smooth and shows normal contours. This pliability of the preepiglottic space would tend to confirm that the lesion is exophytic and has not deeply infiltrated the preepiglottic space.

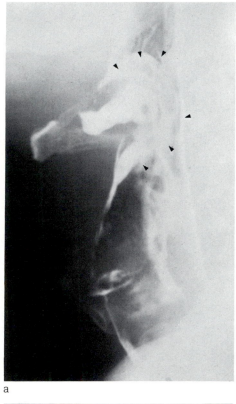

a

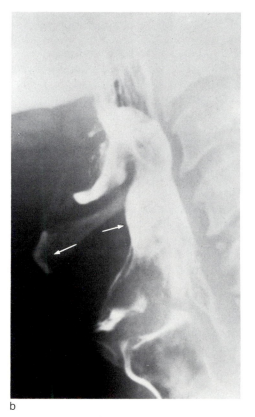

b

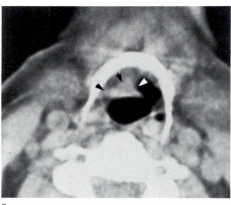

c

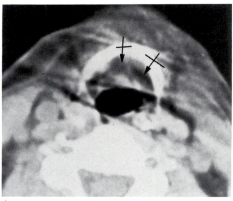

d

Fig. 2.**37** Epiglottic CA invading the upper preepiglottic space and vallecula region.

a) Lateral projection of the laryngogram with quiet breathing shows the bulky tumor mass involving the free margin of the epiglottis extending down toward the region of the body of the epiglottis (arrowheads). The space between the hyoid bone and the lateral surface of the epiglottis is increased.

b) With the true Valsalva maneuver, the thyroid cartilage should elevate to touch the region of the hyoid bone. Due to infiltration by

tumor, there is limited elevation of the larynx, and the space between the laryngeal surface of the epiglottis and the hyoid bone remain relatively constant (arrows).

c) CT scan at the level of the vallecula shows that there is extensive infiltration of the left vallecula by high-density tissue. Air remains in the vallecula on the right.

d) Tumor infiltration causes increase in density near the laryngeal surface of the epiglottis. Some normal fat is visible anteriorly in the mid to lower preepiglottic space (cross-hatched arrows).

Infrahyoid Epiglottis Tumors

Tumors of the infrahyoid epiglottis tend to present with a more flattened infiltrative type of growth. In general, they are less well differentiated tumors that spread widely. At times, the tumors will ulcerate through the body of the epiglottis and gain access to the preepiglottic space. The tumors spread inferiorly onto the anterior commissure or laterally in the paralaryngeal space. As the tumor spreads superficially along the mucosa, it goes posterolaterally onto the false cord and as a late manifestation into the region of the arytenoid.

The lateral views are exceedingly helpful to demonstrate the inferior extent of the tumor, especially if bulky. Knowledge of the status of the anterior commissure is mandatory clinical information because of the possibility of performing a horizontal supraglottic laryngectomy if the anterior commissure is clear of tumor (9, 10). The degree of pliability of the body of the epiglottis and mobility of the larynx can be appraised on the lateral projection during the changes that take place between quiet respiration, phonation of E, and the true Valsalva maneuver. On the PA projections during phonation and quiet breathing, mobility of the true cords, false cords,

and arytenoids is readily apparent. For the deeply infiltrating tumors that are extending laterally, the modified Valsalva PA will demonstrate any displacement of the medial wall of the piriform sinuses (Fig. 2.38).

CT scanning of infrahyoid epiglottic lesions shows the bulk of the tumor, the cartilage destruction, and the infiltration of the preepiglottic space. Spreads in the paralaryngeal space are readily apparent. As the tumor grows inferiorly along the petiolus, differentiation by CT scan of the anterior commissure invasion becomes difficult. This accurate type of appraisal is probably better obtained by positive contrast laryngography. Once these tumors have gained access to the preepiglottic space, they are very prone to invade into the thyroid cartilage. The bulky lesions will spread the thyroid cartilage, and there may even be buckling of the cartilage in the parasymphyseal region. Lymph node metastases to the carotid sheath can be suggested if contrast enhancement is used to accurately delineate the position of the carotid artery and jugular vein. Much of the work on lymph node spreads are still speculative since reactive lymph node hyperplasia may accompany carcinomas. CT will only show morphology and not histology.

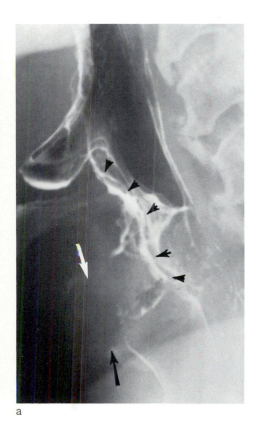

a

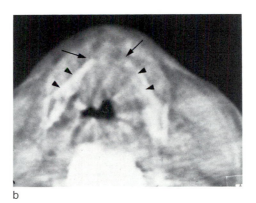

b

Fig. 2.**38** Infrahyoid epiglottic tumor infiltrating the preepiglottic space.
a) The exceedingly bulky tumor of the body of the epiglottis (arrowheads) has infiltrated the preepiglottic space and destroyed the symphysis of the thyroid cartilage (arrows). On this true Valsalva maneuver the larynx is not able to elevate to oppose the hyoid bone.
b) CT scan at the level of the body of the epiglottis shows total obliteration of the normal low-density fat areas and infiltration of the paralaryngeal space (arrowheads). The destruction of the symphysis of the two thyroid cartilages is evident (arrows). The angle formed by the two thyroid cartilages is widened due to the bulk of the tumor mass.

Piriform Sinus Tumors

Although not strictly laryngeal tumors, piriform sinus lesions and their extensions are well visualized by laryngography and CT scanning. Accurate appraisal of this area is extremely difficult by clinical means. The modified Valsalva maneuvers are ideally suited to show pliability of the wall and any filling defects within the lumina of the piriform sinuses during distension. Tumors of the medial wall of the piriform sinus will directly invade the lateral wall of the larynx producing impaired true and false vocal cord mobility that can be evaluated on phonation views. The lateral extremity of the laryngeal ventricles may show encroachment. Metastatic spread to the retropharyngeal area can be overlooked on clinical examination and is readily apparent on the lateral projections of quiet breathing, phonation, and the modified Valsalva maneuver. The reverse phonation in the PA projection will distend the laryngeal ventricles and show a disparity between the two sides (Fig. 2.39).

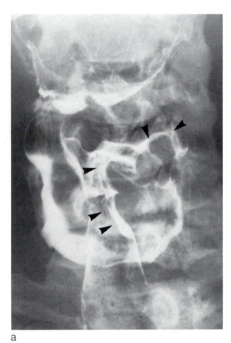

a

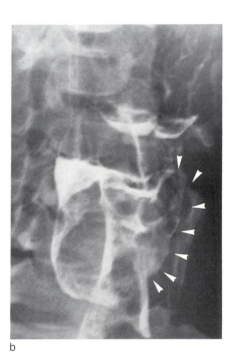

b

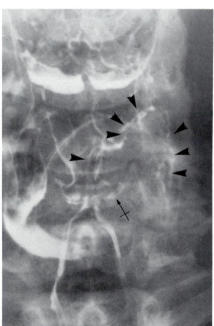

c

Fig. 2.**39**   CA of the anterior wall of the piriform sinus on the left.
a) The piriform sinus cancer displaces the true and false cord (arrowheads) from left to right and gives the impression of a very large bulky transglottic mass extending posteriorly to the aryepiglottic fold (upper arrowheads).
b) Right anterior oblique shows the irregularity of the anterior wall of the right piriform sinus (arrowheads) obliterating the inferior pole. The posterior wall of the pharynx and the right piriform sinus is shown to be entirely normal.
c) Reverse E maneuver shows that the left laryngeal ventricle fills very well (cross-hatched arrow), indicating that the major bulk of the tumor is extrinsic to the larynx and is only secondarily deforming the larynx. The tumor mass is principally in the piriform sinus and posterior paralaryngeal space (arrowheads).

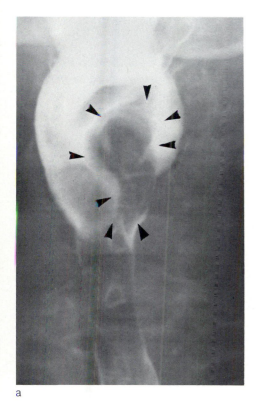

a

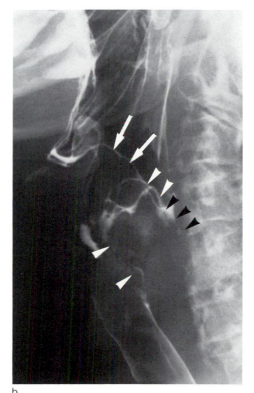

b

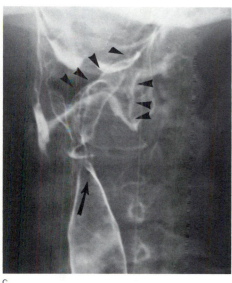

c

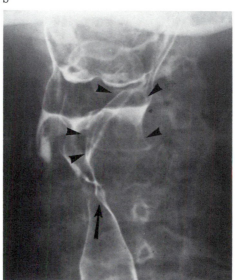

d

Fig. 2.40 Postcricoid carcinoma possibly arising in the medial wall of the piriform sinus and invading the aryepiglottic fold on the left.

a) Barium swallow shows the filling defect, creating an impression on the barium column due to the tumor of the postcricoid region extending into the aryepiglottic fold (arrowheads). The right piriform sinus fills out normally, and there is only slight distortion of the inferior pole of the left piriform sinus. The cervical esophagus is normal.

b) Lateral view in an attempted modified Valsalva maneuver. The patient is unable to distend the hypopharynx well due to the massive tumor. There is thickening of the aryepiglottic fold, and the tumor extends into the pharyngoepiglottic fold (arrows). The

superior border of the tumor in the postcricoid region is well outlined by contrast material (arrowheads); however, its inferior pole is not discernable. The anteriorly placed arrowheads show the invasion into the region of the posterior commissure.

c) True cords are in opposition (arrow), but the entire larynx is deviated from left to right. The interarytenoid notch is also displaced to the right, and thickening of the aryepiglottic fold and postcricoid line is clearly demonstrated (arrowheads).

d) During quiet respiration, the true vocal cord is retained in the paramedian position (arrow). The massive tumor in the paralaryngeal space extending inferiorly and into the soft tissue of the neck causes distortion of the laryngeal vestible (arrowheads).

Postcricoid and Esophageal Hiatus Tumors

Clinical examination of postcricoid tumors is extremely difficult. Generally, only the top of the tumor can be visualized. Postcricoid lesions are more apt to spread to the posterior pharyngeal wall and regional nodes but may go into the cervical esophagus. Undoubtedly, many of the so-called postcricoid tumors are, in reality, cervical esophagus lesions that have spread superiorly to the postcricoid region and posterior pharyngeal wall. The modified Valsalva maneuver in the lateral and oblique views is especially helpful in demonstrating mucosal irregularities and wall immobility. If deep infiltration of the postcricoid and arytenoid areas occur, fixation of the true or false cords may be evident on PA phonation studies. In general, barium swallow is indicated in this entire group to verify the status of the cervical esophagus (Fig. 2.40). CT scanning will show the tumor mass and the status of the cricoid cartilage. Extensions laterally and posteriorly into the carotid sheath region are well shown.

Summary

Laryngography is one of the methods for evaluating the extent of laryngeal tumors. Tomography and xeroradiography have proved useful in demonstrating subglottic extension of tumors and in some selected patients, deep infiltration of the lateral wall of the larynx. Patients with compromised airways or severe respiratory disease may not be able to tolerate laryngography. Limited studies, such as tomography or xeroradiography, can prove useful as an adjunct to the clinical examination. Occasionally, highly significant information can be obtained from a lateral soft tissue view of the neck in instances of thyroid cartilage invasion. This single film may dictate the necessity for laryngectomy without the need of more elaborate radiologic investigation. The accuracy of carefully performed laryngograms has proved to be comparable to direct laryngoscopy and at times superior for the evaluation of the "blind areas" as indicated above.

Laryngography has serious limitations in evaluating the base of the tongue, vallecula region, and deep infiltrations. Variations in volume and configuration of the lymphoid tissue is exceedingly difficult to evaluate. Laryngography should not be performed following direct laryngoscopy and biopsy. The edema and mucosal swelling caused by instrumentation will cause gross overestimation of the extent of disease processes. Similarly, edema following radiation therapy makes diagnoses of residual tumor difficult by any means including laryngography.

Cineradiography has been recommended as an adjunct to spot filming. In difficult patients, this modality has proved quite helpful. Cineradiography is also a valuable adjunct in confirming mobility and pliability in some of the patients where cooperation may be limited.

The future of laryngeal examination undoubtedly lies in CT scanning. As fast scanners and multiple projection reconstructions become available, tumor margins can be precisely calculated to provide the basis for precision radiation therapy or conservative surgery. Our surgical colleagues have compared CT scanning to performing direct laryngoscopy with the mucosa stripped away. This display of deep structures is precisely information needed by the clinician so that CT scanning becomes truly complementary to direct and indirect laryngoscopy rather than competitive.

References

1. Alonso WA, Pratt LL, Zollinger WK, Ogura JH: Complications of laryngotracheal disruption. Laryngoscope 84: 1276–1290, 1974
2. Baclese F: Carcinoma of the larynx. Br J Radiol (suppl) 3, 1949
3. Baily BJ, Calcaterra TC: Vertical, subtotal laryngectomy and laryngoplasty. Arch Otolaryngol 93: 232–237, 1971
4. Barnes EL, Tasneen Zatar: Laryngeal amyloidosis. Ann Otol 86: 856–863, 1977
5. Bassett LW, Hanafee WN, Canalis RF: The appendix of the ventricle of the larynx. Radiology 120: 571–574, 1976
6. Bienenstock H, Lanyl VF: Cricoarytenoid arthritis in a patient. Arch Otolaryngol 103: 738, 1977
7. Biller HF, Ogura JH, Pratt LL: Hemilaryngectomy for T$_2$ glottic cancers. Arch Otolarygol 93: 232–237, 1971
8. Bryce DP: The laryngeal subglottis. J Laryngol Otol 89: 667–684, 1975
9. Calcaterra TC: Laryngeal suspension after supraglottic laryngectomy. Arch Otol 94: 306–309, 1971
10. Calcaterra TC: Supraglottic laryngectomy with preservation of laryngeal function. Am Surgeon 37: 393–396, 1971
11. Cohn AM, Larson DL: Laryngeal injury – a critical review. Arch Otolaryngol 102: 166–170, 1976
12. Davies MRQ, Cywest S: The flaccid trachea and tracheoesophageal congenital anomalies. J Pediatr Surg 13: 363–367, 1978
13. Dedo HH, Izdebski K, Townsend JJ: Recurrent laryngeal nerve histopathology in spastic dysphonia. Ann Otol 86: 806–812, 1979
14. Doust BD, Ting YM: Xeroradiography of the larynx. Radiology 110: 727–730, 1974
15. Dunbar JS: Upper respiratory tract obstruction in infants and children. Am J Roentgenol Radium Ther Nucl Med 109: 277, 1970
16. Gendell HM, McCallum JE, Reigel DH: Cricopharyngeal achalasia associated with Arnold-Chiari malformation in childhood. Child & Brain 4: 65–73, 1978
17. Goodrich WA, Lenz M: Laryngeal chondronecrosis following roentgen therapy. Am J Roentgenol Radium Ther 60: 22–28, 1948
18. Harris HH, Tobin HA: Acute injuries of the larynx and trachea in 49 patients. Laryngoscope 80: 1376–1384, 1970
19. Hawkins DB: Glottic and subglottic stenosis from endotracheal intubation. Laryngscope 87: 339–346, 1977
20. Holinger LD, Barnes DR, Smid LJ: Laryngocele and saccular dysts. Ann Otol 87: 675–685, 1978
21. Holinger PH, Holinger LD, Reicher TJ, et al: Respiratory obstruction and apnea in infants with bilateral abductor vocal cord paralysis, meningomyelocele, hydrocephalus and Arnold-Chiari malformation. J Pediatr Surg 13: 368–373, 1978
23. Kilman WJ: Narrowing of the airway in relapsing polychondritis. Radiology 126: 373–376, 1976
24. Kirchner JA: One hundred laryngeal cancers studied by serial section. Ann Otol, Rhinol Laryngol 78: 689–709, 1969
25. Kirchner JA, Som ML: The anterior commissure technique of partial laryngectomy: clinical and laboratory observations. Laryngoscope 85: 1308–1317, 1975
26. Klein R, Fletcher GH: Evaluation of the clinical usefulness of roentgenologic findings in squamous cell carcinomas of the larynx. Am J Roentgenol Radium Ther Nucl Med 92: 43–54, 1964
27. Kushner DC, Harris BG: Obstructing lesions of the larynx and trachea in infants and children. Radiol Cl in North Am 16: 181–194, 1978
28. Lehmann QH: Reverse phonation: a new maneuver for examining the larynx. Radiology 84: 215–221, 1965
29. Lehmann QH, Gletcher GH: Contribution of the laryngogram to

the management of malignant laryngeal tumors. Radiology 83: 486–500, 1964

30. Mancuso AA, Calcaterra TC, Hanafee WN: Computed tomography of the larynx. Radiol Clin North Am 16: 195–207, 1978

31. Mancuso AA and Hanafee WN: Computed tomography of the injured larynx. Radiology 1979

32. Meine FJ, Lorenzo RL, Lynch PF, Capitanio MA, et al: Pharyngeal distension associated with upper airway obstruction. Radiology 111: 395, 1974

33. Merson RB, Ginsberg AP: Apasmodic dysphonia: abductor type. A clinical report of acoustic, aerodynamic and perceptual characteristics. Laryngoscope 89: 129–139, 1979

34. Metheny JA: Dermatomyositis: a vocal cord and swallowing disease. Laryngoscope 88: 147–161, 1978

35. Morgenstein KM: Treatment of the fractured larynx. Arch Otol 101: 157–159, 1975

36. Ogura JH, Biller HF: Reconstruction of the larynx following blunt trauma. Ann Otol. 80: 492–506, 1971

37. Ogura JH, Biller HF: Conservation surgery in cancer of the head and neck. Otolaryngol Clin North Am 1969

38. Ogura JH, Biller HF, Calcaterra TC, Davis WH: Surgical treatment of carcinomas of the larynx, pharynx, base of tongue and cervical esophagus. Int Surg 52: 29, 1969

39. Ogura JH, Heeneman H, Spector GJ: Laryngo-tracheal trauma diagnosis and treatment. Can J Otolaryngol 2: 112–118, 1973

40. Ogura JH, Powers WE: Functional restitution of traumatic stenosis of the larynx and pharynx. Laryngoscope 74: 1081–1110, 1964

41. Oliveira CA, Roth J, Adams G: Oncocytic lesions of the larynx. Laryngoscope 87: 1718–1725, 1977

42. Olofsson J: Growth and spread of laryngeal carcinoma. Can J Otolaryngol 3: 4, 1974

43. Olofsson J: Specific features of laryngeal carcinoma involving the anterior commissure and the subglottic region. Can J Otolaryngol 4: 618–632, 1975

44. Olofsson J, Freeland AP, Sokjer H, Renouf JH, et al: Radiologic-pathologic correlations in laryngeal carcinoma. Can J Otolaryngol 4: 86–97, 1975

45. Olofsson J, Renouf JHP, Van Nostrand AWP: Laryngeal carcinoma: correlation of roentgenography and histopathology. Am J Roentgenol Radium Ther Nucl Med 117: 526–538, 1973

46. Olofsson J, Van Nostrand AWP: Growth and spread of laryngeal and hypopharyngeal carcinoma with reflections on the effect of preoperative irradiation. Acta Otolaryngol (suppl) 308: 7–77, 1973

47. Parnes SM, Laborata AS, Myers E: Study of spastic dysphonia using videofiberoptic laryngoscopy. Ann Otol 87: 322–326, 1978

48. Powers W, McGeen H, Seaman W: Contrast examination of the larynx and pharynx. Radiology 68: 169–179

49. Pressman JJ, Simon MB, Monell C: Anatomical studies related to the dissemination of cancer of the larynx. Trans Am Acad Ophthalmol Otolaryngol 64: 628–638, 1960

50. Quick CA, Merwin GE: Arytenoid dislocation. Arch Otolaryngol 104: 267–270, 1978

51. Reed MH: Radiology of airway foreign bodies in children. J Can Assn Radiol 28: 111–118, 1977

52. Som PM, Nagel BD, Feuerstein SS, Strauss L: Benign pleomorphic adenoma of the larynx a case report. Ann Otol 88: 112–114, 1979

53. Taybi H: Congenital malformations of the larynx, trachea, bronchi and lungs. Prog Pediatr Radiol

54. Tucker GF: A histological method for the study of the spread of carcinoma within the larynx. Ann Otol Rhinol Laryngol 58: 910–921

55. Ward PH, Berci G, Calcaterra TC: New insights into the causes of postoperative aspiration following conservation surgery of the larynx. Ann Otol, Rhinol Laryngol 86: 724, 1977

56. Ward PH, Morledge D, Berci G, et al: Coccidioidomycosis of the larynx in infants and children. Ann Otol 86: 655–660, 1977

57. Watts FB, Slovis TL: The enlarged epiglottis. Pediatr Radiol 5: 133–136, 1977

58. Wesenberg RL: The Newborn Chest Harpor and Row, Hagerstown 1973 (chap 22)

59. Williams JL, Capitanio MA, Turtz MG: Vocal cord paralysis: radiologic observations in 21 infants and young children. A J R 128: 649–651, 1977

60. Wittenborg HM, Gyepes MT, Crocker D: Tracheal dynamics in infants with respiratory distress, stridor and collapsing trachea. Radiology 88: 653–662, 1967

61. Work WP, Coulthard SW: The injured larynx: a new surgical procedure for repair. Trans Am Acad Ophthalmol Otolaryngol 82: 460–465, 1967

Part V

Sialography

William N. Hanafee

Sialography has proved of use in the diagnosis of autoimmune disease, stones, and the management of tumors involving the parotid gland. Opinions as to its usefulness vary from worthless to indispensable. Close cooperation between the head and neck surgeon and radiologist will enhance the role of sialography in tumor management and place false negative information into a proper prospective. Some generalizations as to the clinical usefulness of sialography in tumors include location of the facial nerve with respect to the tumor, origin in deep lobe versus superficial lobe, growth characteristics of the tumor, and presence of tumor spread outside the gland.

Anatomy

The parotid gland, lying anterior to the ear, molds itself to adjacent skeletal structures and muscles in such a fashion that the ducts assume natural archlike configurations. The gland is divided into a deep lobe that curves around the posterior margin of the ramus of the mandible and extends to the carotid sheath and lateral wall of the pharynx. The deep lobe is connected to the superficial lobe by an isthmus. At the junction of the two lobes, a groove is formed for the passage of the five branches of the facial nerve and part of the anterior facial vein (Fig. 1.1). The superficial lobe of the parotid may be arbitrarily divided into a portion that extends superiorly to the region of the zygomatic arch, a posteroinferior region that encompasses the mastoid process, and an anteroinferior region or tail that curves around the angle of the mandible and ends in close proximity to the submandibular gland (Fig. 1.2). The main body of the parotid superficial to the main duct arches about the posterior margin of the masseter muscle. The main duct of the parotid gland (Stensen's duct) courses anterior with some of the branches of the facial nerve within the gland substance. The duct passes lateral in an archlike fashion over the masseter muscle and pierces the buccinator muscle to empty in the cheek opposite the second upper molar tooth.

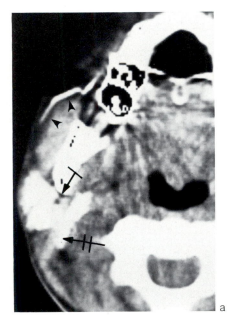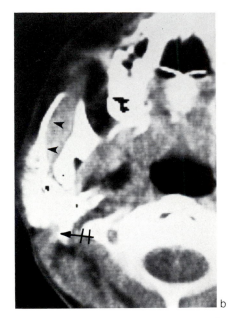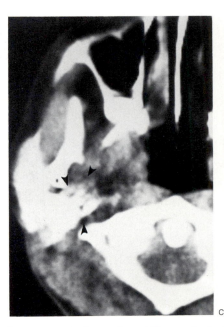

a   b   c

Fig. 1.1 Normal CT Sialogram

a) The patient was thought to have a tumor in the posterior inferior portion of the parotid which was shown by CT scan to merely represent a prominant indentation by the sternocleido mastoid muscle (↦). Parotidectomy showed no evidence of tumor in the specimen. The retromandibular vessels (↔) lie posterior to the angle of the mandible and should not be mistaken for tumors. Arrowheads show the anterior portion of the Stensen's duct.

b) Contrast outlines the more posterior portion of Stensen's duct in a scan taken 1 cm cephalad to 1.1 A. The posterior indentation by the sternocleido mastoid muscle is again noted (↦). The deep lobe of the parotid is projecting around the angle of the mandible.
c) 1 cm cephalad to figure 1.1 B shows the deep lobe of the parotid well outlined by contrast (▶). A portion of the deep lobe lies behind the styloid process and a greater portion anterior to the styloid process.

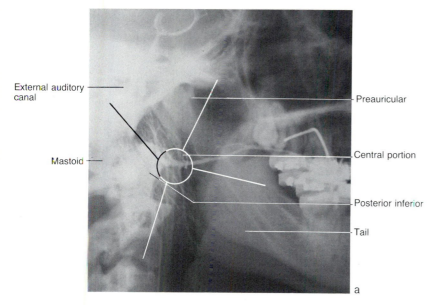

External auditory canal

Mastoid

Preauricular

Central portion

Posterior inferior

Tail

a

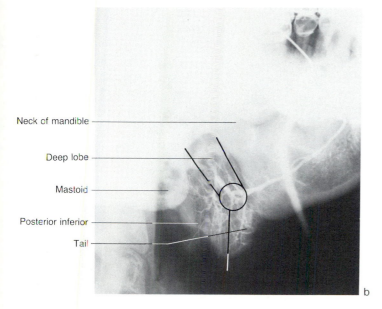

Neck of mandible

Deep lobe

Mastoid

Posterior inferior

Tail

b

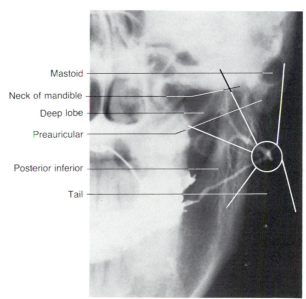

Mastoid

Neck of mandible

Deep lobe

Preauricular

Posterior inferior

Tail

c

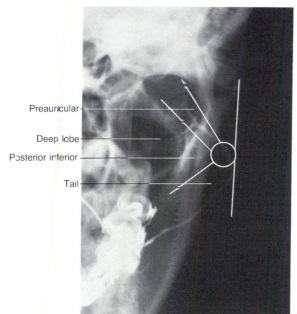

Preauricular

Deep lobe

Posterior inferior

Tail

d

Fig. 1.2   Normal parotid: same patient as Fig. 1.1.

a) Lateral projection. Stensen's duct gives off small branches to glandular tissue lying immediately above the main duct. The gland is not anatomically divided into lobes, but regions commonly designated for location are the preauricular, posteroinferior, tail, or anteroinferior, and the deep "lobes" of the parotid. The deep lobes superimpose on the preauricular region in the lateral projection.

b) Oblique projection. The patient's shoulders should be rotated to a 45-degree angle and the chin extended to open up the space between the angle of the mandible anteriorly and the superimposition of the mastoid process on the cervical spine posteriorly. A clear visualization of the deep lobe of the parotid is obtained in the space between the angle of the mandible and mastoid. The posteroinferior margin as well as the margins of the tail of the parotid are also well seen.

c) Anteroposterior projection of the parotid is helpful for visualizing the lateral surface of the gland, especially in the region of the tail and central portion of the gland. Lateral displacement of the central portion is readily visible in this projection. The deep portion of the gland superimposes on the mandibular structures.

d) Towne projection with the x-ray beam centered on the facial structures shows the deep lobe of the parotid through the antrum. The posteroinferior portion of the gland is partially cleared of superimposed bony structures.

The submandibular gland lies in the submandibular triangle and is divided into two parts. The upper portion lies in the submaxillary fossa in the medial side of the body of the mandible opposite the second and third molar teeth. The superficial portion of the gland arches from lateral to medial around the posterior margin of the mylohyoid muscle to lie above the anterior belly of the digastric. The mylohyoid muscle indents the anterior surface of the gland. The submandibular duct (Wharton's duct) runs between the mylohyoid and hyoglossus muscles to open in a small caruncula lying on either side of the frenulum of the tongue (Fig. 1.3). The sublingual glands lie in the floor of the mouth and empty through multiple openings that are not accessible to cannulation and sialography.

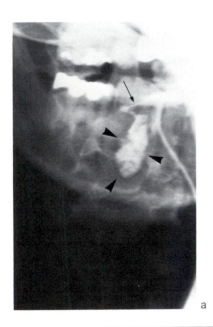

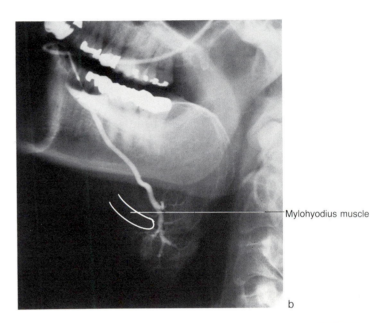

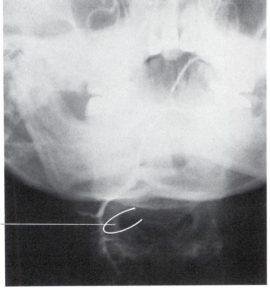

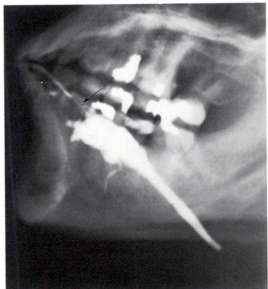

Fig. 1.3 Normal submandibular gland: cannulation technique.

a) Anteroposterior projection shows the cannula has been passed into a sublingual gland that opens into the submandibular duct near the ostium. A few drops of contrast material produce extreme staining of the gland. The cannula tip was removed and repositioned for the subsequent study.

b) Lateral projection of a normal submandibular gland. The mylohyoid muscle indents the anterior and medial margin of the submandibular gland at the junction of the upper third with the lower two thirds. The posterior margin of the submandibular gland is separated from the parotid gland by the cervical fascia.

c) On the antero posterior projection a bone free visualization of the submandibular gland may be obtained by superimposing the angle of the mandible on the occipital bone. The mylohyoid muscle indents the medial border of the submandibular gland. The inferior portion of the gland is also spoken of as the superficial portion of the submandibular gland.

d) Extravasation from the submandibular duct in another patient in whom the cannula had entered one of the ducts of the sublingual gland. The situation was not realized, and undue force was exerted on the cannula. The water-soluble contrast material resorbed without sequelae.

Technique of Sialography

Either water-soluble contrast material or oily-based media can be used for sialography. The oily-based media, such as ethiodized oil (Ethiodol) or isophendylate (Pantopaque), will give excellent visualization of the ductal system, but care must be exercised to prevent extravasation into the gland substance since these materials may cause granuloma formation. For tumor investigation, water-soluble media are preferred, and an attempt should be made to produce "staining of the gland" to better outline the margins of the expansive process. Renografin-76 or similar media have proved satisfactory for visualization of the gland parenchyma while still yielding acceptable densities of the ductal system.

Good light is essential for cannulation of the parotid or submandibular duct. The ostium is first sprayed with a local anesthesia such as lidocaine. The sphincter of the opening is usually contracted. A small amount of lemon juice on the tongue will relax the sphincter, allowing visualization of the red color of the epithelial lining of the duct. If the opening cannot be seen readily, the region of the opening should be dried with cotton swabs and the gland massaged. The flow of saliva from the duct will identify the opening. If difficulty is encountered cannulating the ostium with sialography catheters, gentle probing can be performed with lacrimal dilators. The Bowman probes are excellent for this purpose. They range from 0000 to #4. For the smallest submandibular cannula (Rabinov sialography needle, Cook Inc., Bloomington, Ind.), the operator can start with a 0000 probe and progress to 000 and then to 00, which will provide adequate dilatation. When performing parotid sialography using the tapered cannulas, dilatation to a number 1 or number 2 catheter may be needed.

Two diameters of cannulas are most helpful for parotid sialography (Fig. 1.4). If the opening of the duct is large, a tapered, side-hole needle is used (V. Mueller & Co.). For the smaller openings, the malleable "Lacrimal Cannula" (B-D & Co.) is most useful. This is a blunt cannula equivalent to a 23 gauge needle.

For the submandibular gland, the Rabinov sialography needle is excellent for duct cannulation and may not even require a preliminary dilatation. This same cannula can be used in extremely small parotid ducts in patients with parotid atrophy and sicca syndrome.

Anteroposterior, lateral, and oblique views are obtained in both parotid and submandibular sialography to obtain bone-free visualization of the various lobes of the glands. The oblique view should be obtained with the shoulders rotated 45 degrees and the chin well extended. This position will open the space between the angle of the mandible and the overlapping of mastoid process on the cervical spine (Fig. 1.2). The deep lobe of the parotid lies in this space and can be identified by the cephalad coursing of parallel ducts. For submandibular sialography, a base projection or submentotransorbital view is added to the armamentarium. Separate injections of contrast material are made for each roentgen exposure. This will insure adequate distension of the ductal system and a good parenchymal phase. The volume of contrast used will vary from 1.0 to 1.3 ml but at times may be less than 1 ml or more than 1.5 ml, depending on the diameters of the ductal systems and the amount of contrast material that is regurgitating from the duct opening into the patient's mouth. The end point of injection should be pain in the region of the gland, and the patient is given preliminary instructions to motion a signal with the hand when pain occurs. At this moment the injection is stopped and a roentgen exposure made. Bilateral studies should routinely be performed for the following reasons:

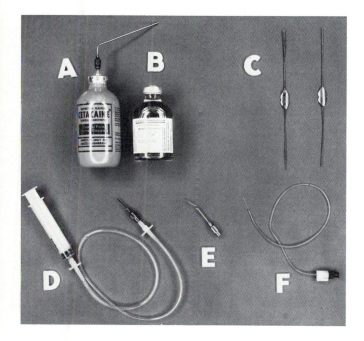

Fig. 1.4   Equipment for sialography.

a) Some type of topical anesthesia should be sprayed opposite the second upper molar for the opening of the parotid gland or to either side of the frenulum of the tongue (sublingual caruncle) for submandibular cannulization.

b) Water-soluble contrast agents, such as meglumine diatrizoate 76%, have proved most useful.

c) Bowman lacrimal dilators are helpful for submandibular cannulation starting with a 0000 size and increasing to a 00 size prior to cannulation of the submandibular duct. If necessary, the parotid ducts should be dilated to a number 1 size prior to cannulation.

d) The needle tip (V. Mueller & Co.) is a tapered tip with a side hole connected to a disposable syringe and polyethylene tubing. For each film of a series, small amounts of contrast material are injected until the patient experiences pain.

e) Lacrimal cannula (B-D Co.) with malleable tip equal in diameter to a 23 gauge needle. This diameter is intermediate in size between the tapered tip cannula and the Rabinov submandibular cannula. (Cook Inc., Bloomington, Ind.).

f) Rabinov submandibular sialographic cannula.

1. The same disease process may be occurring in the opposite gland only in a preclinical state.
2. Variations in normal size and configuration of the ductal system can better be appreciated.
3. Extrinsic masses may displace the gland in subtle fashion, which can be better appreciated when a normal size is available for comparison.
4. If the pathologic side is always examined first, the films taken of the normal side will serve as drainage films for the first side examined.

If the patient is hypersensitive, he may signal pain too soon before all the ducts are filled and give a false impression of gland atrophy. Repeat injections are indicated. In our hands, the use of subtraction techniques or xeroradiography have either been too cumbersome or have not materially influenced the diagnostic information.

CT sialography is conducted in exactly the same manner as conventional sialography except that CT scanning is used for recording the image (23). Present-day scanners require prolonged exposure times so that pressure must be maintained on the ductal system over a period of 20–40 s. The patient may be given the syringe filled with contrast material and told to continue the injection very slowly so as to maintain a minimum of pain within the gland. The same procedure can be followed with the radiologist merely retaining pressure on the syringe once the patient has signaled with the hand that he is experiencing pain. Regardless of who is performing the injection, the patient signals the start of the CT scan by waving the fingers when he experiences pain. CT scans are performed from the level of the external auditory canal to just below the angle of the mandible. Stensen's duct lies on a plane from just below the external auditory canal to the point the lips meet in the midline. Scans are performed at 1 cm intervals. Usually, four levels will include the entire gland, but additional levels may be obtained as needed. As with conventional sialography, bilateral studies prove helpful to compare normal anatomy and the amount of parenchyma in each gland.

Normal Sialography

Considerable variation exists in the size and configuration of the normal gland and its ducts. Ericson (14) gave an area of the parotid on the lateral view to vary from 10.1 to 21.1 cm^2 and a variation between the two sides of 2.5 cm^2. Thus, it would seem that the parotid gland can vary by a factor of 2 in area in normal individuals. The diameter of the duct also varied from 0.8 to 3.2 mm in diameter and a difference between right and left of 0.7 mm. Retention of contrast material after 5 min continues to be used as a reliable index of secretory ability (6, 30). On the other hand, in most clinical situations involving decreased secretory ability, other morphological alterations are sufficiently obvious to provide the diagnosis.

Contraindications to Sialography

The contraindications to sialography are few. Patients with known sensitivity to iodine should not be examined. Along a similar vein, people with a tendency to faint should be carefully questioned. Many of these reactions are related to a vagal reflex that can be alleviated by the administration of atropine intramuscularly (0.6–1.2 mg) 30 min prior to the study. The rather large dose is indicated since there has been some experimental evidence that small doses of atropine even exaggerate the vagal-vagal reflex.

Acute parotitis should represent another contraindication to sialography as the ductal epithelium is in a very fragile state and extravasation will occur throughout the gland. During the acute phase of parotitis, little diagnostic information can be expected from sialography. During the consolidation phase of acute parotitis, information regarding location of abscesses and relationships to the facial nerve may give very valuable information.

Iodinated compounds may be retained in the parotid gland for prolonged periods of time and interfere with thyroid function tests. If there is clinical suspicion of thyroid dysfunction, appropriate tests should be performed prior to sialography.

Technical Pitfalls

When cannulating the parotid duct, variations in course of the terminal portion of the duct may cause the tip of the cannula to lie against the wall of the duct. This is especially evident in patients with masseter muscle hypertrophy, which causes a right-angle bend in Stensen's duct as it courses around the muscle. Under these circumstances, the injected contrast material may regurgitate back through the opening of the duct into the oral cavity. Should poor visualization of the ductal system be evident on sialography, the tip of the cannula should be repositioned or manually bent to conform to the natural curvature of the duct. If the opening of the duct is unusually patulous, a tapered cannula may be required to prevent reflux of contrast material into the oral cavity.

Regardless of the type of cannula used, the operator must be extremely gentle and not exert undue force on the parotid or submandibular ducts. Perforations can occur, and injected contrast material will then pass into the subcutaneous tissue.

In submandibular sialography, the tip of cannula may pass into accessory sublingual ducts that empty near the natural opening of the submandibular gland (Fig. 1.3). The radiologist should be aware of the problem because during cannulation the tip of the cannula will start into the natural ostium and then pass for a distance of 2–3 mm only to meet resistance. At this point, undue force will perforate the duct (Fig. 1.3b). Contrast injections will then outline an exceedingly small amount of gland parenchyma in the sublingual region. This accessory gland will fill so promptly that the signal of the patient may be misinterpreted and extravasation will occur. If obstruction is met during cannulation, the tip of the cannula should be partially withdrawn and readvanced in a new direction (usually more superficially, laterally, and posteriorly). The cannula should pass freely for a distance of 12–14 mm when in the main submandibular duct.

With a little practice, it is suprising how easy cannulation of the natural opening of the submandibular duct can be accomplished. Adequate lighting and some form of magnification are essential. In the past five years, this author has only experienced two failures. One in a patient with Parkinson's disease with a rather coarse tremor and another in a patient with advanced carcinoma of the floor of the mouth in whom all of the anatomy was greatly distorted. At no time has any incision into the floor of the mouth or cutting on the sublingual duct been required (36).

Congenital Lesions

Sialography has little to offer in bronchial cleft remnants or in tumors that occur in the parotid region in the newborn or infant. The tumors are generally hemangiomas or lymphangiomas. The hemangiomas show characteris-

tic reddening and swelling (37). On the mucosal surface dilated veins may be identified along the lateral pharyngeal wall adjacent to the deep lobe of the parotid. The lymphangioma may extend into the neck or mediastinum presenting difficult problems of management. Sialography in this newborn period requires general anesthesia and offers little meaningful information. Tumors arising in children are another matter and will be discussed under benign and malignant lesions.

Functional Disorders

Bilateral chronic enlargement of the parotid glands may be found in chronic alcoholism, diabetes, starvation, obese alcholics, and occasionally lipomatous pseudohypertrophy of the parotid gland without specific etiology (21, 33). Biopsy of these glands is reported to show an increase in the number of zymogen granules, hypertrophy of the secretory cells, and a striking absence of inflammatory reaction. Sialography can be performed with ease and shows a normal appearing ductal system and parenchymal staining except that the glands are unusually large (Fig. 1.5). The gland bulges into the subcutaneous tissues without evidence of changes in the ratio of duct to glandular structures.

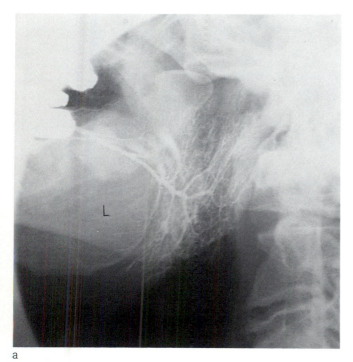

a

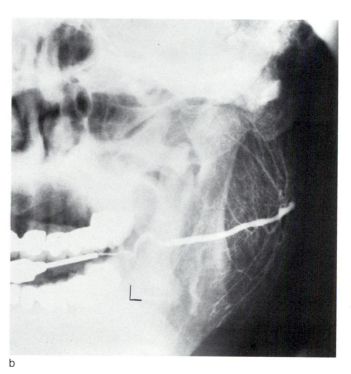

b

Fig. 1.5 a) and b)   Idiopathic hypertrophy. This 60-year-old physician was nondiabetic and denied history of alcoholism, endocrine disturbances, or medication. The parotid glands were bilaterally enlarged and nontender. The enlargement was not associated with any systemic disease.

Traumatic Lesions

Traumatic lesions of the parotid may be divided into early and late effects. The type of injury may be further divided into contusion injuries of the glandular elements, penetrating wounds, and ductal lacerations. Lesions of the parotid following radiation therapy are primarily those associated with secondary inflammatory change and general radiation fibrosis. Their radiologic appearance is not too dissimilar from other chronic inflammatory problems.

Acute traumatic lesions to the gland parenchyma are usually accompanied by hemorrhage within the gland substance. Edema and secondary infection are likely to follow. Sialography is generally contraindicated during the acute phase. If gland destruction leads to abscess formation, its relationship to the facial nerve may require sialography examination (Fig. 1.6).

Penetrating injuries may result in cutaneous salivary fistulas that are exceedingly difficult to manage clinically. Although sialography may confirm the site of the fistulous tract, management (26) is either by ligation of the main duct and irradiation of the gland, major glandular removal, or combinations of the above. Since attempts at local ligation of the offending duct within the gland parenchyma is too frequently associated with injury to the facial nerve or late stricture at the site of repair, obtaining sialography to identify a specific leak site is rarely required.

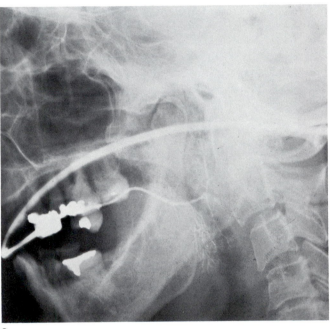

a

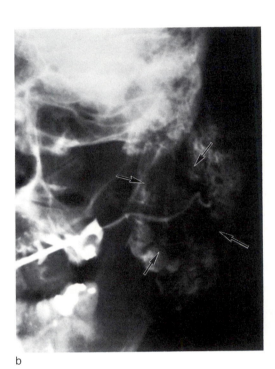

b

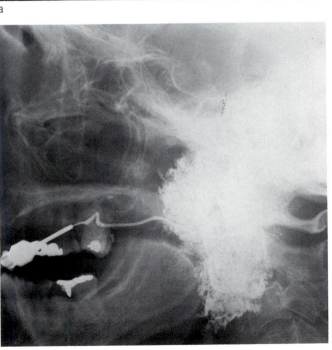

c

Fig. 1.**6** Post-traumatic parotid abscess. This elderly female was an assult victim and sustained trauma to the parotid gland approximately ten days prior to the study.

a) Parotid sialography was cautiously attempted to outline the extent of a parotid hematoma that was thought to be infected.

b) On the anteroposterior projection, a large central radiolucent zone was evident deep to the main portion of the parotid duct.

c) A second lateral projection was attempted to get better filling of the ducts. The tenuous state of the ductal epithelium is evident by the extensive extravasation of contrast material into the paraglandular tissue.

Injury to the main salivary duct will generally result in atrophy with fatty infiltration of the remaining gland unless duct reanastomosis was successfully carried out. When a mass lesion develops proximal to the obstructed duct, information is desired regarding the nature of the mass lesion (Fig. 1.7). Cyst formation is the usual result of duct obstructions; however, tumors can develop in the remaining functional salivary tissue. Sialography should be attempted to see if there are some accessory ducts that fill and aid in identifying the site of origin of the mass lesion.

Radiation injuries of the salivary glands are a well-known entity and rarely cause diagnostic problems. Following radiation of the nasopharynx or oral cavity lesions, radiation changes in the parotid gland are expected. The ductal system will usually fill, disclosing multiple areas of dilatation and narrowing with some irregular punctate collection of contrast material in the remaining glandular ductal system.

Infections

Much of the literature regarding inflammatory conditions of the parotid gland as seen by sialography is rather confusing if not contradictory. The problem is related to the natural reluctance of the clinician to perform biopsies of the parotid gland for relatively benign conditions. Many of the inflammatory lesions are self-limiting so that risk of injury to the facial nerve is unwarranted. Probably the most logical hypothesis was put forth by Hemenway (20) when he pointed out that the anatomy of the parotid gland is such that its response to a variety of inflammatory conditions may easily produce similar sialography appearances. He coined the phrase "chronic punctate parotitis" to explain many of the maladies of the salivary gland that may or may not be associated with systemic disease. The basic pathology is divided into three parts:

1. Hyperplasia of the epithelium and myoepithelial cells involving the intralobular ducts
2. Infiltration with lymphocytes
3. Disappearance of acini.

The disease may be seen early or late and secondary infection may be superimposed. Ductal obstruction due to mucous plugs and cellular debris contribute to the roentgen picture. One then needs only to add a few specific entities, and a classification of inflammatory diseases of the parotid gland becomes more rational as follows:

1. Acute infections bacterial, viral, postsurgical, and debilitative states
2. Chronic infections
   A. Ductal obstructions due to stones
   B. Recurrent pyogenic parotitis (25)
      1. Related to poor dental hygiene or ill-fitting dentures
      2. Drug-induced
      3. Granulomatous
      4. Idiopathic
   C. Chronic punctate sialadenitis (benign lymphoepithelial disease, Mikulicz's disease, Mikulicz's syndrome, Sjögren's syndrome, sicca syndrome, sialadenitis)
      1. Adult form
         a. With systemic disease
         b. Without systemic disease
      2. Childhood form
         a. Spontaneous remission at puberty
         b. Persistent chronic punctate sialadenitis.

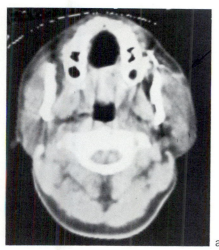

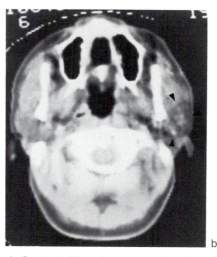

a   b

Fig. 1.7 Traumatic laceration of duct with cyst formation. This patient had received a laceration of the face ten years previously, following which he was totally asymtomatic until being struck in the face in an automobile accident six months prior to the CT sialogram. His chief complaint was recent swelling of the region of the parotid gland on the side of injury. The swelling was quite firm, and conventional sialogram showed that the duct did not fill beyond its midportion. The differentiation of tumor versus cyst was quite important.

a) Contrast filling the proximal portion of the duct and ending abruptly at an area of increased density that corresponds to the scar in the skin of the cheek. Beyond the scar, the gland is either of normal density or low density.

b) Section 1 cm cephalad to Fig. 1.7 a) showing an area of low density, which corresponded to fluid by CT numbers. The radiologic diagnosis of post-traumatic cyst was made and confirmed at surgery.

Acute Inflammatory Disease

Sialography is contraindicated during an acute attack of parotitis. The ductal and glandular epithelium are apparently in a very weakened state so that contrast material will extravasate freely into the interstitial tissues. Little information is to be gained, and contrast material will act very much like an interstitial injection into an area that is already inflamed. Attempts in the past have been made to outline abscesses, but the results are disappointing since parotid abscesses are usually more multilocular and require aggressive surgical management. At sialography one cannot be certain whether an area of nonfilling is due to abscess or to occlusion of one of the interlobular ducts. If sufficient pressure is exerted on the syringe to totally fill the ductal system, extravasation becomes widespread.

Stones

Twenty percent of stones are said to be radiolucent, and an additional 20% are probably not visualized due to superimposition of adjacent bony structures during routine filming (28). The incidence of radiolucent stones in the parotid may be much higher and has been quoted at 80%. They are more common in the submandibular gland or its ducts than in the parotid gland by a factor of eight to one. Multiple stones are said to occur in 25% of all patients (35). In the submandibular gland, they are frequently found either at the orifice of the submandibular duct or at the bifurcation of the main submandibular duct within the submandibular gland. In either the submandibular gland or the parotid gland, these stones usually do not cause total obstruction and aqueous contrast material will usually flow around the stone, outlining the status of the remaining ductal system. Small stones undoubtedly pass spontaneously and may leave areas of stricture. Chronic infection that occurs proximal to stones or strictures serves as an etiology of recurrent pyogenic parotitis (Fig. 1.8).

The roentgen pattern as seen by sialography is usually one of dilated ducts with multiple areas of strictures. There may be diminution in the number of secondary ductal branchings because of associated inflammatory changes, causing the ductal lumens to become obliterated, or multiple cystic spaces may be formed. The pattern may be identical to late stages of chronic punctate sialadenitis. Because of the overlap of the roentgen appearance in recurrent pyogenic parotitis due to stones with chronic punctate sialadenitis, multiple glands should be studied. If both parotids and submandibular glands are involved, one can be assured that this is not inflammatory disease due to stones and subsequent chronic infection.

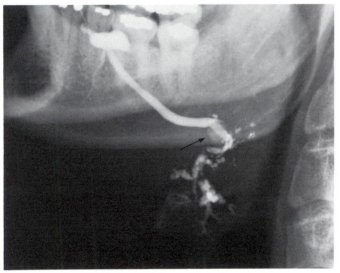

a

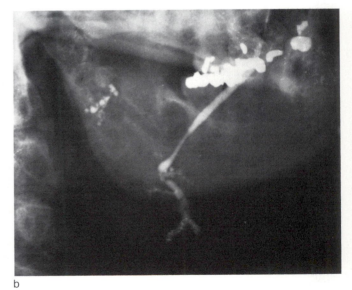

b

Fig. 1.8 Chronic sialadenitis secondary to stone formation. Bilateral swelling of the submandibular glands that seemed related to food.
a) A stone (→) is present in the submandibular duct near the junction of the duct with the gland. The entire ductal system is dilated, especially within the gland parenchyma. Contrast material flows slowly around the stone but fails to produce good filling of the parenchyma.

b) Sialography on the left side shows multiple areas of narrowing within the ductal system but no evidence of stones. The multiple areas of narrowing could be related to previously undiagnosed stones that pass spontaneously or to bilateral recurrent pyogenic sialadenitis that led to stone formation.

Recurrent Pyogenic Parotitis

Whether the entity of recurrent pyogenic parotitis truly exists or is in actuality a stage in chronic punctate sialadenitis may be open to question. The roentgen appearance is quite similar with cystic dilatation of the minor ducts and greatly enlarged major salivary ducts. The destruction of gland substance is the prominent feature that causes a diminution in the number of secondary branches from the major ducts. The major ducts may be only slightly enlarged and irregular in outline. One patient examined at approximately two-year intervals over a period of six years showed a changing roentgen pattern with some areas returning to near normal while other areas of the gland showed progression of disease (Fig. 1.9).

On clinical examination these patients show poor dental hygiene, which is believed to be the major etiologic factor. Others would contend that the chronically infected saliva predisposes to the dental caries. In some patients the etiology is obscure. The clinical and/or roentgen pattern is found following multiple episodes of stones so that autoimmune disease does not appear to be a major factor. The radiologic diagnosis cannot be made based on the sialographic appearance of the gland. Knowledge of the presence or absence of systemic disease and in particular rheumatoid arthritis is essential. The patient should also be examined for other stigmata of sicca syndrome. Multiple gland involvement is more characteristic of Sjögren's syndrome.

Chronic Punctate Sialadenitis

Chronic punctate sialadenitis is characteristically thought of as part of Sjögren's syndrome. Sjögren's monograph in 1933 pointed out the relationship between keratoconjunctivitis, xerostomia, and rheumatoid arthritis. The keratoconjunctivitis and xerostomia are directly related to the salivary dysfunction. When the mucosal manifestations occur without systemic disease, the entity is spoken of as sicca syndrome. Sialography in these patients takes on new meaning to establish a positive diagnosis because of the association of life-threatening illnesses in patients who do not have the full-blown Sjögren's triad. These patients are much more likely to develop Waldenström's macroglobulinemia, lymphoma,

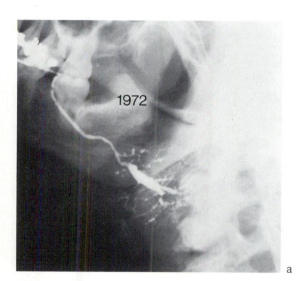
a

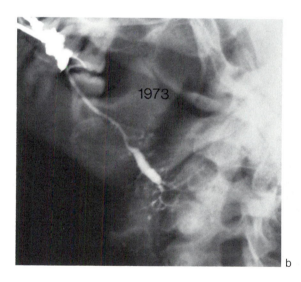
b

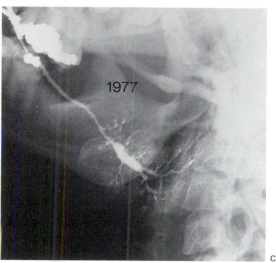
c

Fig. 1.9 a–c) Recurrent pyogenic sialadenitis. This 40-year-old woman without evidence of systemic disease had recurrent bouts of bilateral parotid swelling that were unremitting over a period of eight years of follow-up examination. The sialographic appearance fluctuated from minimal to moderate pruning of the duct but never normal. At all times, the disease process remained bilaterally symmetric. The main duct is dilated, and its primary branches show irregular margins. Some peripheral punctate dilatation are also evident. She showed no evidence of systemic disease or of sicca syndromes. Rheumatoid factors were negative.

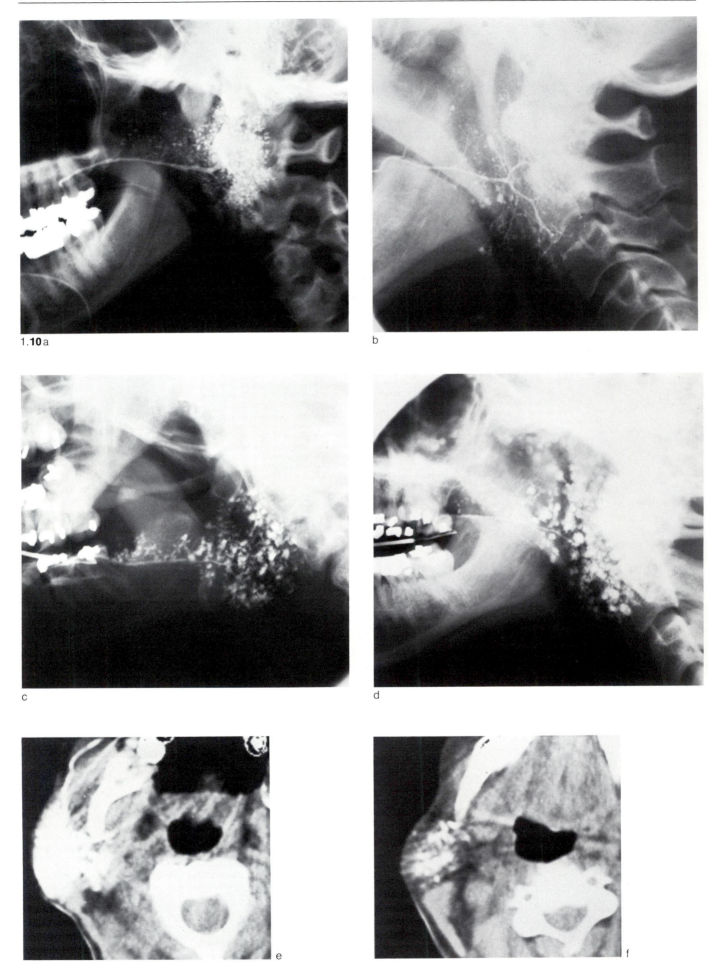

1.**10**a

b

c

d

e

f

and reticulum cell sarcoma (11). At times the lymphomatous expressions are more benign and have been designated as pseudolymphoma based on whether or not the lymph proliferations are extraglandular or involve multiple organ systems. Some patients after 15 years or more of benign disease may show extraglandular spread to organs consistent with malignant forms of lymphoma. The patterns of change as seen by sialography may be divided into four stages (28, 30) Stage I is punctate sialectasia in which globules of contrast material are evenly spaced throughout the gland and measure less than 1 mm in diameter (Fig. 1.10). Stage II is globular sialectasia in which the contrast material collections measure 1–2 mm in diameter. Stage III is cavitary sialectasia in which the globules are larger and irregular in size and distribution. Stage IV is destructive sialectasia with bizzare patterns of contrast collection and irregular puddling with diminution in number of ducts and local duct dilatations.

Patients with Sjögren's syndrome and arthritis are less likely to develop life-threatening illnesses. Most often the sicca complex develops insidiously in patients who already have rheumatoid arthritis (11). In about 10% of the patients the eye and mouth symptoms precede the arthritis. The severity of the salivary disease does not necessarily parallel the degree of involvement by arthritis.

Regardless of whether the disease occurs with or without systemic disease, the sialographic appearance is identical. Early in the disease, the punctate form of globules will be found on sialography with normal appearing ducts. Twenty percent of the patients will have unilateral disease. Bilateral studies are indicated when searching for evidence of sicca syndromes. As the disease progresses, sialography will demonstrate a diminution in the number of secondary and tertiary radicals within the parotid gland. In the late stages, some of the larger cavitary areas may resemble extravasation as seen in malignant diseases of the parotid. Late in the disease, atrophy will be the dominant factor, and the ductal system has been compared to a "pruned tree." The main duct may be normal caliber or dilated, and the branches become slender and terminate abruptly. Care must be taken during sialography to insure that the ducts are completely filled since the pruned tree appearance is mimicked by incomplete filling (Fig. 1.11).

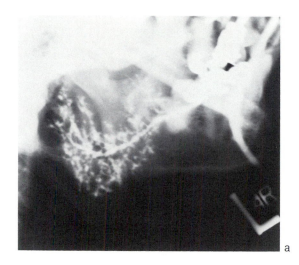

a

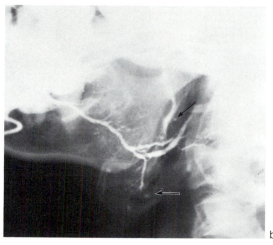

b

Fig. 1.10 Stages of chronic punctate sialadenitis.
a) Early punctate sialadenitis in a young physician whose only symptoms were slight parotid swelling of three weeks duration. Following the sialogram, additional laboratory studies showed a positive Schirmer's test and positive rheumatoid factors. The 1 or 2 mm collection of contrast material presumably represent dilatation terminal ducts related to glandular atrophy.
b) Globular form of chronic punctate sialadenitis with slightly larger collections of contrast material consistent with more advanced atrophy. Near the periphery of the gland, the ducts are quite sparse consistent with a lymphocytic infiltration.
c and d) Views in the advanced stages of chronic punctate sialadenitis with cyst formation.
c) Oblique projection taken with the patient erect and prior to the true lateral projection in Fig. 1.10d. Distinct contrast fluid levels can be identified in this early film of the series, whereas the later films of the series show that the cystic spaces are almost completely filled with contrast material.
e and f) Views from the same patient as illustrated in Fig. 1.10b). CT sialography shows a relatively homogeneous staining of the gland in the midportion as illustrated by Fig. 1.10e). Near the periphery of the gland (Fig. 1.10f), the more punctate collections of contrast material become evident and are separated by spaces of low-density material consistent with lymphocytic infiltrations that occur in chronic punctate sialadenitis.

Fig. 1.11a and b) Technical cause of poor filling in late Sjögren's syndrome. This 60-year-old female with Sjögren's syndrome was not entirely cooperative. Injection of the parotid system on the left showed dilatation of the terminal ducts consistent with chronic punctate sialadenitis. She was reluctant to undergo complete examination so that the study of the right system was conducted with a Rabinov submandibular cannula without dilatation of the parotid duct opening. No pressure could be exerted, and the contrast material refluxed freely into the mouth. The ductal system gave the pruned tree appearance with only minimal filling of the dilated terminal ducts characteristic of chronic punctate sialadenitis (arrows).

Secretory studies, whether performed by radionuclides or by obtaining delayed films during roentgen examination, have been proposed as being helpful in differentiating the sicca syndromes from recurrent pyogenic parotitis. The rate of secretion is markedly reduced in the sicca syndromes, whereas there may be a relatively good flow of saliva in the recurrent pyogenic parotitis. Cultures may also demonstrate the secondary infection in the inflammatory lesions, but of more significance is the clinical picture and evidence of multiple gland involvement in the sicca syndrome.

CT scanning with simultaneous sialography will show large ducts with irregular areas of contrast collections within the gland. The lobular pattern of the parotid gland becomes accentuated, presumably related to atrophy, myoepithelial hyperplasia, and lymphocytic infiltrations (Fig. 1.10).

Another form of chronic punctate sialadenitis may occur with specific disease entities, such as leukemia, lymphosarcoma, TB, syphillis, and to a lesser extent sarcoidosis (31) (Fig. 1.12). Some have referred to the entity as Mikulicz's syndrome; however, the distinction does not appear to be entirely justified. The roentgen pattern is identical with the previously described four stages of chronic punctate sialadenitis unless there has been involvement of the lymphatics within the parotid gland by extensive cellular infiltrations and/or granuloma formation. When the patient has been severly debilitated or in uveoparotid fever (sarcoid), the roentgen pattern may approximate that of the acute patterns of inflammation of the parotid gland or show multiple rounded areas of non-filling due to gland displacement.

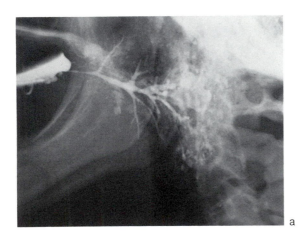

a

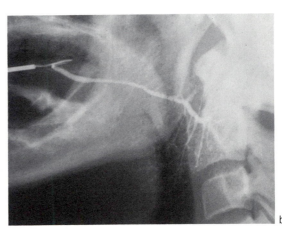

b

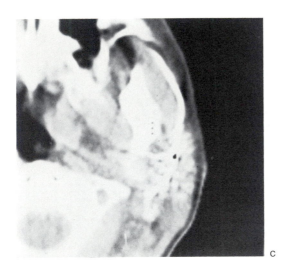

c

Fig. 1.12   Comparison of sarcoid and late Sjögren's syndrome.
a) Bilateral parotid swelling in a patient with sarcoidosis and positive lip biopsy. The major ducts are dilated, and the secondary branches show pruning with diminution in the amount of gland parenchyma. Some terminal ducts show puddling of contrast material not unlike the globular form of chronic punctate sialadenitis.
b) The roentgen pattern of this patient with Sjögren's syndrome is strikingly similar with pruning of the secondary ducts and some punctate collections of contrast material in the terminal ducts. There is also diminution in the amount of glandular tissue.
c) CT sialogram of the same patient with Sjögren's syndrome shows the collections of contrast material in the ductal system with multiple spaces throughout the gland, presumably representing the lymphocytic infiltrations that occur in advanced chronic punctate sialadenitis. It is not surprising that the roentgen appearance of the two diseases would be similar since both are based on cellular infiltrations that follow the lymphatics in both sarcoid and Sjögren's disease. Presumably, these cellular infiltrations lead to atrophy in sarcoid in a manner similar to Sjögren's syndrome.

Chronic Punctate Sialadenitis of Childhood

In children and occasionally in infants, the disease tends to occur in the form of repeated attacks lasting for 24–36 h up to several days. The parotid glands become swollen and are frequently mistaken for recurrent mumps. The condition is more likely to affect males around five to eight years of age in contradistinction to the adult form, which is more common in women. Systemic systems are quite mild, and compression of the gland may disclose turbid saliva extruding from the opening of Stensen's duct.

Sialography should be performed during a period of quiescence. Contrast injections will show the characteristic chronic punctate sialadenitis pattern. Rarely are the globules more than 1–2 mm in diameter, and there is generally no real evidence of major duct dilatation. No large series has been followed into adult life, but generally these patients become asymptomatic at puberty, and presumably the ductal system returns to normal. On occasion, their bouts of recurrent parotitis may cause them to lose an inordinate amount of school time under the mistaken belief that the condition is contagious. Under unusual circumstances, parotidectomy has been performed to relieve the symptoms of recurrent acute parotitis (Fig. 1.13).

Salivary Gland Tumors

The importance of sialography as a routine diagnostic test in parotid tumors is controversial. Some feel that the information yield is highly accurate and valuable (12, 17, 25, 36), while others claim that the method yields no essential information (15, 16, 29). The goal of sialography should be to differentiate benign from malignant tumors, to locate the tumor with respect to the facial nerve, and to differentiate extrinsic from intrinsic tumors and the status of the deep lobe of the parotid. There will always be the strange and unusual case that will present

with swellings or postoperative changes that require differentiation of inflammatory expansions from true new growth. CT scanning during contrast injection offers considerable advantage over conventional sialography because the tumor mass can be seen as a positive shadow and correlated to the remaining salivary tissue. The mode of presentation (axial plane) is ideal for locating tumors and their relationships to the facial nerve.

Benign Tumors

Pleomorphic Adenoma

Approximately 80% of parotid tumors are benign, whereas the ratio drops to 50%–60% in the submandibular gland. The most common benign tumor is the mixed tumor (pleomorphic adenoma), accounting for 65% of all tumors of the parotid gland (4). The tumor is solitary and composed of multiple nodules that with growth compress the adjacent tissue, creating a capsule of varying thickness. The surface of the tumor contains outgrowths from the main mass that penetrate the capsule for varying distances. The small outpouchings are not visible on roentgen examinations but are responsible for recurrences when surgical extirpation is attempted by mere enucleation of the tumor by extirpation through the capsule.

Microscopically, the mixed tumors may present a variety of mixtures of epithelial mesenchymal elements. At times, one or the other component tissues are quite sparse, and the lesions have been referred to as monomorphic adenomas. The difference in density of cellular pleomorphic adenomas versus predominantly mesenchymal pleomorphic adenomas is not sufficiently great to be distinguished by CT scanning or other roentgen techniques. The internal architecture of pleomorphic adenomas is well developed to cast shadows on the CT scans and also to be reflective at ultrasound (Fig. 1.14).

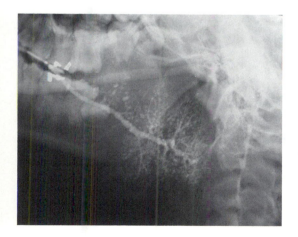

Fig. 1.**13**   Childhood chronic punctate sialadenitis. Eight-year-old child with recurrent bouts of parotitis for the past two years. Bilateral sialogram shows multiple areas of dilatation of the terminal ducts and dilatation of the main duct. There was no evidence of stones within the parotid gland or ductal system. There was no evidence of systemic disease, and rheumatoid factor studies were normal.

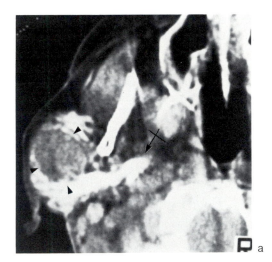

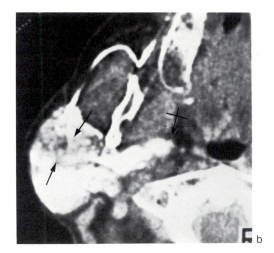

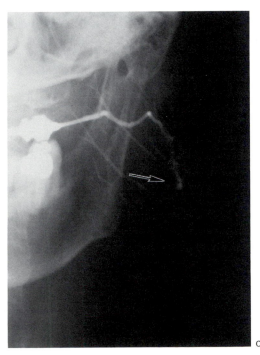

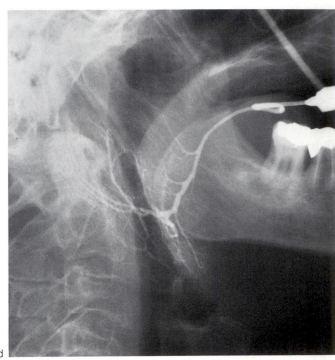

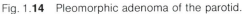

Fig. 1.**14** Pleomorphic adenoma of the parotid.

a) Sharply circumscribed intrinsic mass (arrowheads) in the parotid lying rather high in the superficial lobe. The deep lobe is extremely large and extends well medial into the parapharyngeal space (cross-hatched arrow).

b) Section 1 cm more caudad shows the entire Stensen's duct and the inferior pole of the tumor mass (arrowheads). The tumor is superficial to the major portion of the ducts, indicating that the facial nerve would lie deep to the tumor. There is no evidence of adenopathy in the space beneath the sternocleidomastoid muscle.

c) Anteroposterior view of the sialogram shows that the major ducts are displaced laterally, causing some stretching as the ducts pass to the deep lobe around the neck of the mandible.

d) Only some attenuation of the duct is visible but no definite tumor masses could be identified. From the conventional sialogram, one cannot be certain whether the tumor was intrinsic or extrinsic to the parotid gland.

The ability of sialography to demonstrate pleomorphic adenomas is related to the size and location of the tumor mass. Their size varies from a few millimeters to massive lesions that interfere with patient mobility. Small lesions are prone to arise from the periphery of the gland. As these small lesions grow, there is very little disturbance of the architecture until the tumor mass is above 1 cm in diameter. Localization of benign tumors is discussed on p. 328–330.

Warthin's tumor or papillary adenocystoma lymphomatosum accounts for approximately 6%–7% of all parotid tumors. The tumor is more commonly found in males with the male to female ratio being approximately 5:1. Between 2%–6% of the tumors are bilateral, but synchronous bilaterality is rare (18).

The cellular components of Warthin's tumor have considerable bearing on the sialographic diagnosis of this lesion. As the name papillary adenocystoma lymphomatosum implies, there is a cellular component and a lymphatic component to the tumor. The accepted theory of pathogenesis is an origin from heterotrophic salivary gland tissue within lymph nodes. The lymph nodes may be within the parotid gland or external to the parotid gland (9). The salivary oncocyte is the epithelial mutation that contributes the glandular element to this tumor. When the oncocyte forms a tumor mass in the absence of lymphoid tissue, the tumor is no longer called Warthin's tumor but merely an oncocytoma. When the oncocytes form the tumor in lymphatics, the lesions may be located superficial to the parotid or deep within the parotid sub-

stance and totally surrounded by gland parenchyma. The lymphatics are richer in the posteroinferior portion of the parotid gland; hence, there is a propensity for Warthin's tumor to form deep within the parotid gland along its posteroinferior margin (Fig. 1.15). In addition, the oncocytes are rarely found in salivary tissue before the host is 50 years of age; hence, most cases of Warthin's tumor are found in males 40–70 years of age. The tumors are grossly encapsulated and contain a central cystic space filled with mucus or brownish-tinged fluid. On cut sections, multiple papillary projections are noted, alternating with areas of lymphoid stroma.

The oncocytoma is a nodular circumscribed but unencapsulated collection of swollen eosinophilic granular cells. They are usually quite small and have no characteristics that permit their recognition by radiologic means other than a circumscribed expansive process. Malignant transformations of the oncocytoma to an oncocytic carcinoma has been reported on occasion (22).

Miscellaneous Tumors

Neurofibroma, lipoma, hemangioma, and benign lymphoid hyperplasia have all been described within the parotid gland. The hemangioma is the more common of the above lesions and found predominantly in children. The few sialographic descriptions of these lesions are unusual, varying from total obstruction of the main ducts to irregular expansive processes within the gland parenchyma. Their patterns of growth are not sufficiently characteristic to permit a roentgen diagnosis.

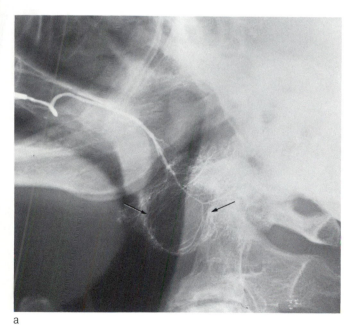

a

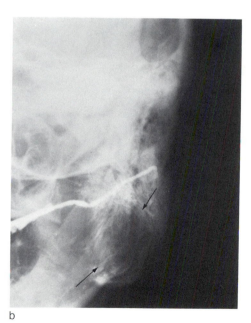

b

Fig. 1.15a and b) Warthin's tumor in a 51-year-old male. The parenchymal staining of the gland clearly outlines a radiolucent tumor completely surrounded by glandular elements in both the anterior and lateral projections. The location of this expansion in the posteroinferior portion of the parotid is characteristic of Warthin's tumor.

Localization by Roentgen Technique

Tumors 1 cm in diameter or less are exceedingly difficult to demonstrate by sialography, especially if they are peripherally located. The indentation of the gland parenchyma cannot be demonstrated by routine sialography; however, on CT scans small mass lesions can be seen as positive densities, and the stained parenchyma of the remaining normal gland will outline the tumor mass. More experience is needed with this modality; however, early results are highly encouraging, regardless of the location of the mass lesion (Fig. 1.16).

Tumors greater than 1 cm in diameter that are located near the periphery of the gland will cause a "beaking" of the stained gland parenchyma around the margins of the tumor due to the distension of the capsule of the parotid gland. A filling defect shaped like a half-moon within the gland parenchyma can readily be seen. The margins of the filling defect should be quite smooth, and there should be no evidence of extravasation of contrast material into adjacent gland parenchyma in benign lesions (Fig. 1.17). If the tumor is located posteriorly near the mastoid tip, the relationship of the tumor to the mastoid tip and styloid process of the mastoid should be carefully noted (Fig. 1.18). The facial nerve exits from the stylomastoid foramen, which is immediately lateral to the styloid process. If the tumor is adherent to bone or poorly movable near the exit of the facial nerve, the surgeon will encounter difficulties in his dissection. In performing a superficial parotidectomy, the surgeon routinely identifies the facial nerve posteriorly and then elevates the superficial lobe of the parotid off of the facial nerve by sharp dissection. When the tumor is adherent posteriorly, the surgical procedure is usually reversed, and the facial nerve is first identified near the anterior border of the parotid gland and the dissection directed posteriorly. Prior knowledge of the altered anatomy allows a more orderly planning of the surgical procedure. Benign tumors arising in the deep lobe show rather characteristic findings on sialography. Surgical management of deep lobe tumors carries a greater risk of injury to the facial nerve. The ducts to the deep lobe of the parotid sweep around the posterior margin of the neck of the mandible just below the condyle. On the anteroposterior projections during sialography, these ducts can be seen medial to the neck of the mandible and in the normal patient have a parallel course passing obliquely from inferolaterally to superomedially. With deep lobe tumors, their orderly parallel arrangement is disrupted (Fig. 1.17). On the true lateral projection, these ducts will superimpose on the preauricular portion of the gland so that demonstration of small tumors is difficult. An oblique view is most helpful for the deep lobe to open up the space between the ascending ramus and neck of the mandible and the cervical spine. In the oblique projection, the ducts should be parallel to each other and have an intimate relationship to the neck of the mandible. Distortion of the ducts or displacement away from the mandible are readily apparent signs of deep lobe neoplasm.

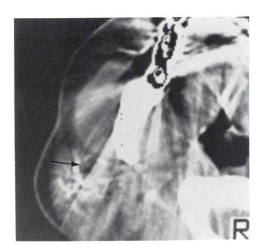

Fig. 1.16 Small parenchymal mass. A small 5 mm mass could be palpated adjacent to the parotid duct when the patient would fully open the mouth. Conventional sialography was entirely within normal limits; however, the CT scan shows an area of lucency in exactly the position of the palpable mass. The patient has refused surgery so that this lesion is as yet unproved.

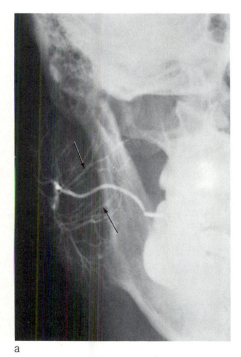

a

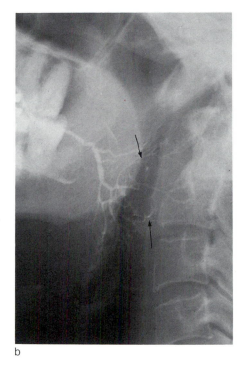

b

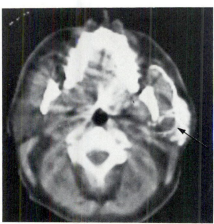

c

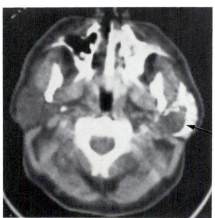

d

Fig. 1.17 Pleomorphic adenoma involving deep lobe.
a) Anteroposterior projections and b) lateral projection showing displacement and arching of the ductal system about the mass that extends from the central area into the deep lobe of the parotid. The main duct is in a somewhat lateral position. Ducts can be seen extending around the neck of the mandible in a relatively normal fashion that would give one the impression that the deep lobe was relatively spared.

c) On the CT sialogram, the lower border of the tumor is visualized when the main duct is in the plane of the scan. The lesion is sharply circumscribed from the surrounding gland tissue.
d) Section taken 1 cm superior to Fig. 1.17c) shows the tumor is much larger and more extensive with a major involvement of the deep lobe of the parotid. From the scan, it was suggested that the tumor is intimately involved with the facial nerve, which proved to be the case. The facial nerve was displaced medial to the tumor.

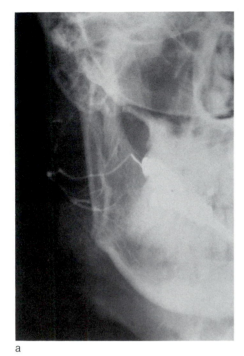

a

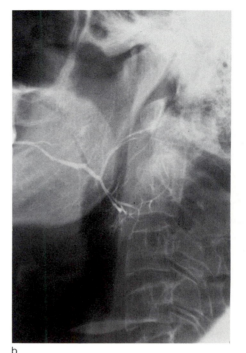

b

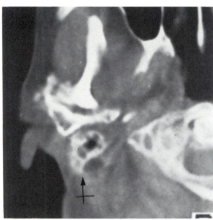

c

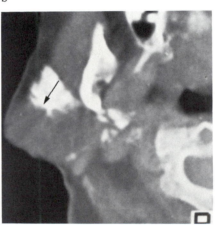

d

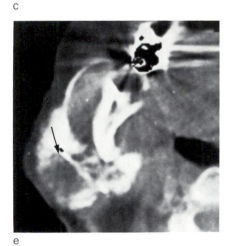

e

Fig. 1.**18** Pleomorphic adenoma that was immediately adjacent to the mastoid process requiring tracing of the facial nerve in a reverse direction.

a) Anteroposterior view of the sialogram shows the arching displacement of the parotid ducts. The ducts to the deep lobe are seen in a relatively normal position arching posterior to the neck of the mandible.

b) In the lateral projection, ductal displacement by the tumor mass is quite obvious.

c) CT sialogram through the mastoid tip (cross-hatched arrow) and condylar process of the mandible show the preauricular portion of the gland.

d) The rather irregular outline of the anterior border of the tumor (arrow) and the bulging of the tumor beneath the skin surface can be visualized.

e) At the level of the major duct, the tumor is slightly more rounded in appearance. The deep lobe of the parotid is clearly identified and is normal. The facial nerve could be predicted to be deep to the tumor mass, but the lobulated pattern of the tumor (→) was not characteristic of the usual pleomorphic adenoma and indicated aggressive behavior.

CT scanning of deep lobe lesions is quite simple since in the axial projection the gland parenchyma can be seen staining with contrast material and lying posterior to the neck of the mandible. The deep lobe is characteristically triangular in shape, and a lucent zone is seen posterior to the mandible that narrows the gland to an isthmus connecting the deep lobe to the superficial lobe. The lucency is made up of digastric muscle and facial nerve, external carotid artery, and some facial veins and lymphatics. The relationships of the deep lobe of the parotid to the carotid sheath and styloid process makes accurate localization of tumor quite simple.

Papillary adenocystoma lymphomatosum or Warthin's tumor is felt to arise from parotid ductal tissue included in lymph nodes located in or near the parotid gland (26). This may well explain why Warthin's tumor tends to be more centrally located within the parotid gland rather than on the extreme periphery (Fig. 1.19). With water-soluble contrast agents, a rim of parotid parenchyma can usually be seen staining the gland surrounding the periphery of the Warthin's tumor. These tumors may be bilateral, which gives another clue to their possible histologic diagnosis.

Warthin's tumor may take up radionucleotides to a greater degree than the surrounding normal parotid tissue. This may be used as a differential diagnostic point but is not infallible (24). Some malignant tumors as well as inflammatory lesions concentrate technetium. Ultrasound of the parotid may also demonstrate the cystic nature of Warthin's tumor and aid in patient management.

Unfortunately, sialography does not give the final histologic diagnosis, and the occasional malignant neoplasm will masquerade as a sharply circumscribed expansive process within the parotid gland. Malignant tumors may even begin in benign tumors, or there may be malignant transformation of long-standing benign tumors that will defy sialographic diagnosis.

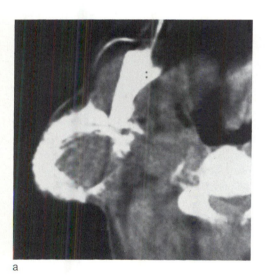

a

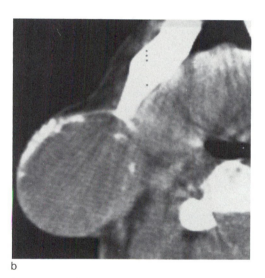

b

Fig. 1.19   Warthin's tumor in a 60-year-old male. CT sialogram.
a) Intraglandular location of the tumor mass.
b) View through the inferior portion of the parotid gland shows that only a rim of glandular tissue surrounds the tumor mass. The tumor mass itself is relatively homogeneous and no cystic elements could be delineated on the CT scan. The CT sialographic diagnosis was a benign expansive process with no histologic diagnosis attempted.

Malignant Tumors

The terminology of parotid tumors will vary depending on whether the classification is based on growth, morphological characteristics, or the histogenesis of the tumor. The diversity of growth patterns expressed by salivary gland tumors is exceedingly varied and approaches that of the female reproductive system. The uniqueness may be explained by the presence of the myoepithelial cell, which is not found in other exocrine glands (2). Some appraisal of the relative incidence of tumors can be taken from the report by Skolnik (34) with the following classification:

Adenocarcinoma	24%
Mucoepidermoid	22%
Squamous cell	20%
Undifferentiated	13%
Adenocystic	7%
Malignant mixed	7%
Miscellaneous	7%

Depending on the referral patterns and the individual pathologist, the relative incidence of specific tumors in different cities will vary considerably. Some mucoepidermoid carcinomas and acinic cell carcinomas are of low-grade malignancy so that they are frequently well managed at the first surgical intervention and are not referred to major centers from which most of the statistics are derived. On the other hand, adenocystic carcinomas, although slow growing, tend to invade nerves and require major surgical resections to extirpate the tumor. In some series, the incidence of adenocystic carcinomas have been reported as high as 14% (10). The vast majority of the tumors fall into the category of glandular-forming epithelial tumor of varying degrees of differentiation. The tumors spread by direct extension and metastases to the regional lymph nodes. Distant (hematogenous) metastases may occur with any of the tumors but are more likely to occur from the adenocystic variety. The general growth characteristics of the various tumors are such that no statement can be made as to the histologic variety from sialography or CT examinations of the parotid gland. The tumor that is known for its propensity to invade the facial nerve and travel in perineurolymphatics for great distances is the adenocystic carcinoma. The incidence of facial nerve dysfunction approximates 25% in this tumor (5, 13). At times, demineralization about the stylomastoid foramen or demineralization about the facial nerve can be demonstrated by mastoid tomography. This bone invasion and demineralization is only present in advanced lesions after widespread tumor involvement has occurred.

The manner of clinical presentation can be extremely helpful in the diagnosis of malignant lesions. Facial pain, areas of numbness or tingling, and evidence of rapid growth are all highly suggestive of a malignant neoplasm. The malignant tumors tend to be much firmer in consistency and may show fixation to osseous structures. Tumors of the deep lobe may be deceiving in size unless a bimanual examination is performed. Externally, only the tip of the tumor will be palpable.

The overall incidence of salivary gland tumors in childhood is quite low, representing only about 3.2% of all salivary tumors. However, if a tumor of the salivary gland is present in a child, the incidence of malignancy is over 50% (32). The majority of the tumors in children are mucoepidermoid carcinomas followed by acinic cell carcinomas and undifferentiated carcinomas.

The sialographic diagnosis of malignant tumors depends on their growth characteristics and consists of the following:

1. Encasement of major ducts producing an irregular outline of the lumen (Fig. 1.20)
2. Destruction of duct walls allowing extravasation of contrast material (Fig. 1.20)
3. Grossly irregular outlines of the tumor masses (Fig. 1.21)
4. Cystic cavities within the parotid tissue that fill with contrast material (Fig. 1.22)
5. Total obstruction of major ducts due to pressure and invasion of the malignant growth.

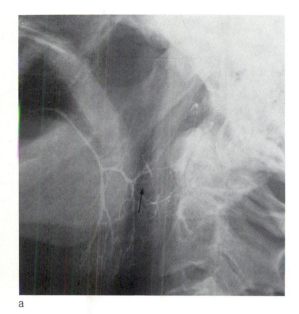

a

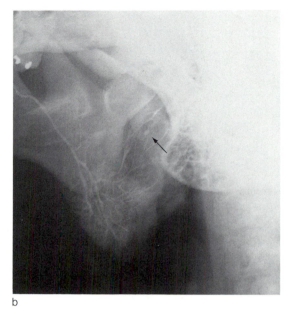

b

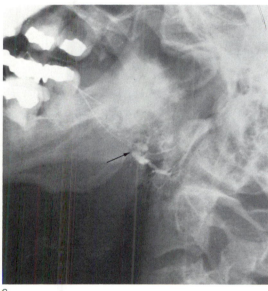

c

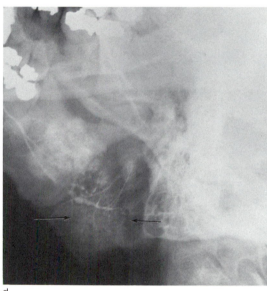

d

Fig. 1.20 Malignant tumors showing duct irregularity, leaking of contrast, and duct encasement.

a) Lateral projection of an adenocystic carcinoma involving the deep lobe of the parotid. Ducts that are going to the deep lobes show areas of narrowing followed by areas of widening, while the more superficial portions of the parotid ducts appear normal.

b) In the oblique projection, the ducts that lie between the tip of the mastoid and angle of the mandible show displacement and distortions. Several small areas of puddling of contrast material within tumor spaces can be identified (arrow).

c) Another patient with mucoepidermoid carcinoma of the posterior inferior portion of the parotid. The main duct is encased (arrow), causing localized constriction with proximal dilatation.

d) Same patient with mucoepidermoid carcinoma shows that in the area of the tumor multiple ducts are almost totally occluded by encasement, and the glandular patterns of staining are quite irregular (arrows). The patterns of ductal distortions are not specific for any particular type of malignancy.

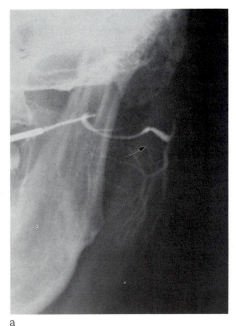

a

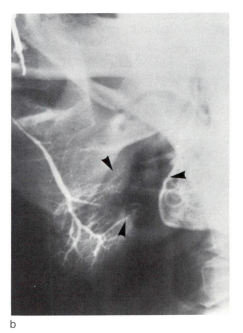

b

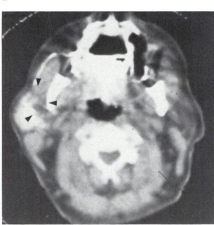

c

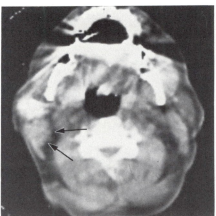

d

Fig. 1.**21** Adenocystic carcinoma of the deep portions of the parotid and invasion of the sternocleidomastoid muscle.

a) Anteroposterior projection shows the entire gland is displaced laterally, and none of the ducts pass deep to the neck of the mandible.

b) Oblique projection shows many of the ducts leading to the deep lobe of the parotid, and the preauricular portions are amputated. There is no filling of the deep lobe of the parotid. The tumor mass is irregular in outline.

c) At the level of the main duct, the tumor mass extends anteriorly to the masseter muscle and widens the space between the deep portions of the parotid gland and the angle of the mandible (arrowheads).

d) Section 1 cm caudad to Fig. 1.21 c) shows that the deep lobe of the parotid does not fill out well, and there is a tumor mass lying posterior to the main portion of the parotid. The mass is irregular in outline and has invaded the sternocleidomastoid muscle (arrows).

As noted in the above criteria, one would only find changes in a tumor of significant size. Exactly what dimensions are necessary to show evidence of duct encasement or central necrosis is not clear. Certainly the lesion under 1 cm in diameter would not as yet have overgrown its blood supply to such an extent as to undergo central necrosis. Many benign lesions may show characteristics similar to malignant tumors. Cystic cavities and contrast extravasation can be found in inflammatory lesions. Lipomas and hemangiomas occasionally cause total ductal obstruction. Irregular outline of the duct is common with intermittent obstruction and secondary infection.

In a recent review by Calcaterra (7), an assessment of the accuracy of sialography in the diagnosis of malignant parotid tumors was attempted. In a series of 37 tumors, 7 were found to be malignant at surgical extirpation. Five of the 7 tumors were diagnosed as malignant at sialography; however, in the remaining 30 benign tumors, 6 lesions were also diagnosed as malignant. He concluded that sialography can at times be highly suspicious of malignancy but should be interpreted in light of clinical findings.

Although the precision diagnosis by sialography does not approach that of many roentgen techniques, it can play a vital role in the psychological preparation of the patient prior to surgery. The patient may be told of the likelihood of facial paralysis prior to his surgical procedure so that he will be much more capable of adjusting to the deformity. All patients should be consulted for a true cancer operation prior to excision of any parotid mass; however, many times the emphasis is placed on the likelihood of the lesion being benign. The surgeon's attitude as well as the patient's response is vastly different when both are appraised of a high probability of malignancy in the preoperative discussions.

The place of CT scanning with sialography has not been thoroughly evaluated, and information available is preliminary (8, 23). In the UCLA experience, 2 of 12 mass lesions were proved to be malignant, and both were correctly diagnosed as malignant from the CT sialographic findings. In one instance of a patient with a nasopharyngeal tumor, a metastasis was found in a parotid gland by CT sialography that could not be palpated clinically. Approximately three weeks after the sialogram, the lesions became clinically palpable (Fig. 1.23). In another instance, the examining surgeon thought he felt a very small tumor although CT sialogram was interpreted as normal. On pathologic examination of the excised parotid gland, no tumor was found. The presence of an irregularly outlined mass that can be seen arising from within the parotid gland is taken as strong evidence of the invasive nature of the tumor. The real problem of diagnosis is going to come with the very small lesions under 1 cm in diameter that are at the very limits of visibility by scanning and palpation. Whether high resolution CT scanning will solve the problem of the small lesion remains to be seen. Regardless of the outcome of malignant versus benign diagnosis in the small lesion by CT sialography, the information available concerning the relationship of the tumor mass to the facial nerve, stylomastoid foramen, and deep lobe of the parotid will all confirm that CT sialography has a permanent place in the armamentarium of parotid tumor management.

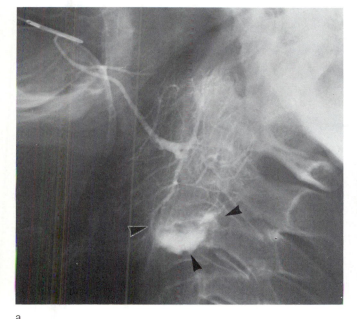

a

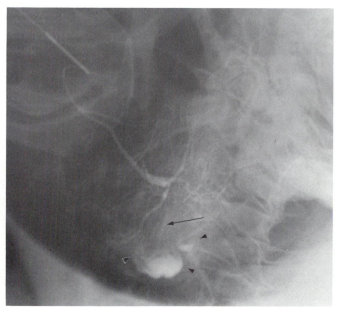

b

Fig. 1.22   Adenocarcinoma with central necrosis. Lateral projection (a) and the oblique view (b) show that contrast material has extravasated into a central necrotic area in this adenocarcinoma. The ducts are displaced about the mass, and one of the ducts (arrow) shows irregularity in outline with leakage of contrast material into the necrotic area of the tumor (arrowheads).

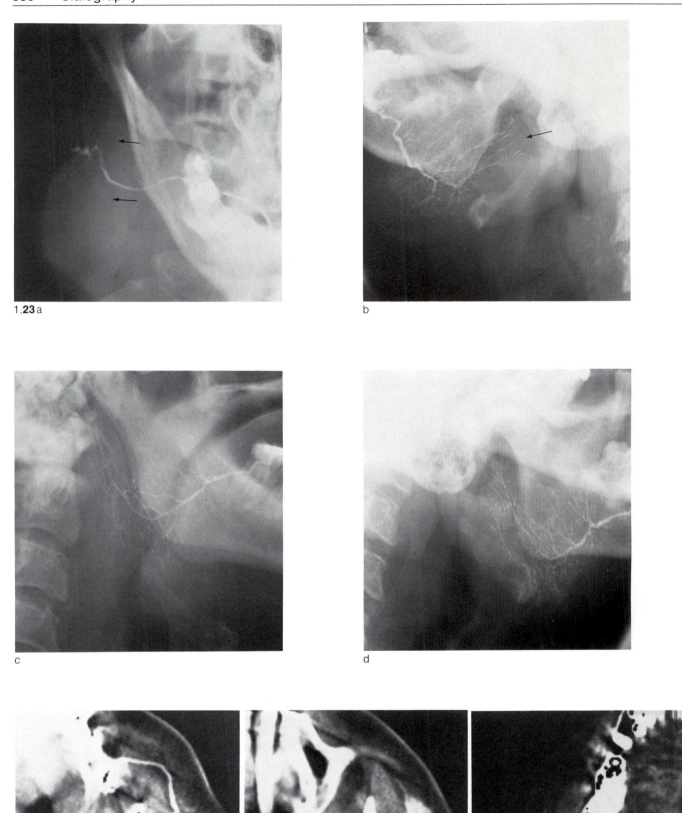

1.23 a

b

c

d

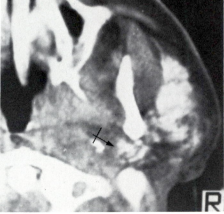

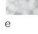

e   f

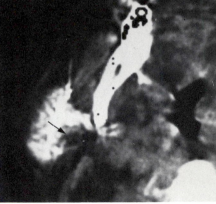

g

The differentiation of extrinsic mass versus intrinsic parotid tumor should be a relatively simple matter by CT scanning, whereas this problem can be extremely difficult to resolve by conventional sialography. In Calcaterra's report, seven patients with extrinsic lesions were not diagnosed on sialography (Fig. 1.24). By comparing CT with sialography, the complete outline of the parotid would be available, and extrinsic masses should be identifiable as a soft tissue mass. When extrinsic masses are immediately adjacent to the gland, there should be evidence of pressure defect without a sharp margin to the gland parenchyma that one might see with a tumor arising in the margin of the gland. Since many of these extrinsic lesions are lymph nodes that contain tumor, CT scanning also provides the opportunity of scanning the nasopharynx for the site of a primary lesion.

In summary, it would seem that the role of sialography is changing under the impact of CT scanning. Tumor masses will undoubtedly be evaluated in the future by CT sialography to answer the vital questions of intrinsic versus extrinsic, position of the facial nerve, location within the parotid gland, and if possible malignant versus benign tumor. The detail of ductal anatomy and glandular patterns is more readily available by conventional sialography. The classification of autoimmune diseases and inflammatory lesions of the parotid or submandibular gland can be more readily accomplished with conventional filming techniques.

Fig. 1.23 Squamous cell carcinoma of the tonsilar fossa invading the parotid gland bilaterally. This 61-year-old male complained of a one-year history of right parotid swelling. On clinical examination, it was not certain whether the tumor had originated in the pharynx and invaded the parotid gland or whether the tumor had originated in the deep lobe of the parotid and extended into the parapharyngeal space.

a and b) Anteroposterior and lateral projections of the right parotid sialography showing distortion of the ducts to the deep lobe and lateral displacement of the entire parotid gland.

c and d) Rather sparse filling of the left parotid ductal system is visible but no discreet masses can be identified. The pharyngeal soft tissue swelling is evident on the lateral projection (c).

e) CT sialography through the level of the parotid duct shows that the entire duct is accordion-shaped due to anterior displacement of the gland. The infiltrations in the posterior portion of the gland are very irregular (arrowheads).

f) Some contrast material is present in deep lobes of the parotid immediately posterior to the ramus of the mandible (cross-hatched arrow). The soft tissue changes in the oropharynx are evident consistent with the massive tumor.

g) The opposite parotid gland shows a filling defect. At the time of the CT scan, tumor could not be felt in the left parotid by multiple observers. Three weeks post scanning, the tumor in the left parotid became palpable.

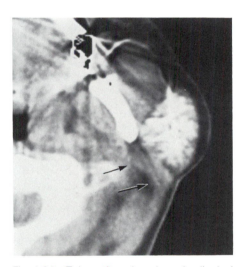

Fig. 1.24 Tuberculous lymph node displacing the parotid gland. This 20-year-old female had a recent conversion of a tuberculin skin test to positive accompanied by swelling of the right parotid gland. CT sialography shows that the swelling is outside the parotid gland, and at least two lymph nodes can be identified deep to the parotid gland and anterior border of the sternocleidomastoid muscle (arrows). The entire gland stains almost homogeneously and is displaced laterally and anteriorly. Although not surgically proved, the presumptive diagnosis is tuberculosis adenitis.

References

1. Batsakis JG, Chinn E, Regezi JA, Repola DA: The pathology od head and neck tumors: salivary glands, part 2. Head Neck Surg 1:167–180, 1978
2. Batsakis JG, Regezi JA: The pathology of head and neck tumors: salivary glands, part 1. Head Neck Surg 1:59–68, 1978
3. Batsakis JG, Regezi JA: The pathology of head and neck tumors: salivary glands, part 4. Head Neck Surg 1:340–349, 1979
4. Batsakis JG, Regezi JA, Bloch D: The pathology of head and neck tumors: salivary glands, part 3. Head Neck Surg 1:260–274, 1979
5. Beahrs OH, Chong GC: Management of the facial nerve in parotid gland surgery. Am J Surg 124:473–476, 1972
6. Blatt IM, Magielski JE, Maxwell JH, et al: Secretory sialography in diseases external to major salivary glands. Ann Otol Rhinol Laryngol 68:175–186, 1959
7. Clacaterra TC, Hemenway G, Hansen GC, Hanafee WN: The value of sialography in the diagnosis of parotid tumors. Arch Otolaryngol 103:727–729, 1977
8. Carter BL, Karmody CS: Computed tomography of the head and neck. Semin Roentgenol 13: 257–266, 1978
9. Cohen MA, Batsakis JG: Warthin's tumor revisited. Mich Med 67:1341–1345, 1968
10. Conway J, Dingman DL: Adenocystic carcinoma in the head and neck (cylindroma). Arch Otolaryngol 100:81–90, 1974
11. Cummings NA: Sjogren's syndrome newer aspects of research, diagnosis, and therapy. An Int Med 75: 937–950, 1971
12. Einstein RAJ: Sialography in the differential diagnosis of parotid masses. Surg Gynecol Obstet 122:1079–1083, 1966
13. Eneroth CM, Andreasson L, Beran M, et al: Preoperative facial paralysis in malignant parotid tumors. ORL 39:272–277, 1977
14. Ericson S: Sialographic appearances of the normal parotid gland. Acta Radiol 14:593–612, 1973
15. Farr HW: Tumors of the parotid gland in Conley (ed): Cancer of the Head and Neck: International workshop on cancer of the head and neck. Butterworths Washington 1967, pp 542–549
16. Frazell EL: Observations on the management of salivary gland tumors. Cancer 18:235–240, 1968
17. Gates GA: Current status of radiosialography in tumor diagnosis. Trans Am Acad Ophthalmol Otolaryngol 74:1183–1195, 1970
18. Hales B, Hansen JE: Bilateral simultaneous warthin's tumor in a woman. South Med J 70:257–258, 1977
19. Hausler RJ, N'Guyen VT, Ritschard J, Montandon PB: Differential diagnosis of xerostomia by quantitative salivary gland scintigraphy. Ann Otol 86:333–341, 1977
20. Hemenway W: Chronic punctate parotitis. Laryngoscope 81:485–509, 1971
21. Hemenway WG, Allen GW: Chronic enlargement of the parotid gland: hypertrophy and fatty infiltration. Laryngoscope 69:1508–1523, 1959
22. Johns ME, Regezi JA, Batsakis JG: Oncocytic neoplasms of salivary glands: an ultrastructural study. Laryngoscope 87:862–871, 1977
23. Mancuso AA, Rice D, Hanafee WN: CT scanning of the parotid with contrast sialography. Works in progress. Radiology: 1979
24. McGurt WF, McCabe BF: Limitations of parotid scans. Ann Otol 86:247–250, 1977
25. Meine FJ, Woloshin HJ: Radiologic diagnosis of salivary gland tumors. Radiol Clin North Am 8:475–485, 1979
26. Olson NR: Traumatic lesions of the salivary glands. Otolaryngol Clin North Am 10:345–350, 1977
27. Pane RT: Proc R Soc Med 31: 1937
28. Potter G: Sialography and the salivary glands. Otolaryngol Clin North Am 6:509–522, 1973
29. Quinn HJ: Diagnosis of parotid swelling. Laryngoscope 86:22–25, 1976
30. Rubin P, Holt JF: Secretory sialography in diseases of the major salivary glands. Am J Roentgenol 77:575–579, 1957
31. Schaeffer, Jacobsen: Am J Dis Child 34: 1927
32. Schuller VE, McCabe B: The firm salivary mass in children. Laryngoscope 82:1891–1898, 1977
33. Simonetta B: The lipomatous pseudohypertrophy of the parotid gland. Otorhinolaryngol 20:106, 1952
34. Skolnik EM, Friedman M, Becker S, Sisson FA, Keyes GR: Tumors of the major salivary glands. Laryngoscope 87:843–861, 1977
35. Suzuki S, Kawashima K: Sialographic study of diseaes of the major salivary glands. Acta Radiol Diagn 8:465–478, 1969
36. White IL: Sialoangiography: x-ray visualization of major salivary glands. Laryngoscope 82:2032–2048, 1972
37. Work WP: Cysts and congenital lesions of the parotid gland. Otolaryngol Clin North Am 10:339–343, 1977

Index

Acoustic neuroma 95–107
  cerebellopontine cisternography 100
  CT 100
  opaque cisternography, CT 105
  pantopaque cisternography 102
  pneumocisternography, CT 102
  radiographic visualization 100
  selection of diagnostic procedure 106
  vertebral arteriography 105
Adenoids 243, 245
  CT 252
  enlargement, CT 248
Ala of vomer 153
Ameloblastoma 202
Angiofibroma 233
Anterior cranial
  fossa and frontal sinus 145
Anterior cranial
  fossa and ethmoid sinus 148
Antrum, mastoid, pneumatization 3
Antrum, see Maxillary Sinus
Arytenoid, post traumatic dislocation
  284

Basal (submental vertex) view 11, 137
  diagnostic curvilinear line 138
  ear 139
Blowout fractures 136
  generation 170
  radiographic findings 170
  tomography 172

Carotid artery 163
Carotid artery, ectopic 43–45
Carotid body tumors 258, 259
Cerebellopontine cisterns 100
  cisternography 102, 105, 106
  CT pneumocisternography 107
  Cerebrospinal fluid otorrhea,
    congenital 41
Chausse III projection 7
Choanal atresia 249
Choanal polyps 254
Cholesteatoma 61–79
  aditus 67
  antrum 68
  classification of radiographic findings
    62
  clinical and otoscopic findins 61
  combined pars flaccida and pars tensa
    67
  complications 68
  CT 73
  conventional 62
  diagnosis, erosion of bony structures
    62
  evaluation of extent 67

external auditory canal 74
fistulae 69
limitations of conventional
  radiography 62
mastoid 68
middle ear 71
middle ear and mastoid 61
pars flaccida 63
pars tensa 65
patterns of radiographic findings 63
petrous extension 70
petrous pyramid 72
radiographic technique 62
recurrent 77
soft tissue lesion 62
tegmen and sinus plate erosion 69
tomography 62
total perforation 67
Chronic punctate sialenitis 321
  in children 325
Cisternography, cerebellopontine 100,
  102, 103, 104, 105
  extra canalicular tumor 105
  intracanalicular filling defects 105
  lesions extending into the cistern 105
  pathology 105
Cleft larynx 280
Cleft palate 249
Cochlear aqueduct anomalies 40
Computerized tomography, CT
  angiofibroma 233
  artifacts 215
  centering and window setting 215
  cholesteatoma 73
  cisternography 102, 105, 107
  contrast material 214
  cribriform plate 230
  encephalocele 230
  equipment 214
  ethmoiditis 219
  eustachian tube 227
  Vth nerve, Schwannoma 225
  fossa of Rosenmüller 227
  glomus tumors 85, 89
  infratemporal fossa 222
    abnormal 225
    anatomy 222
    boundaries 222
    contents 222
  juvenile angiofibroma 245, 256
  larynx radiologic techniques 278
  maxillary sinus 231, 232, 235
  meningioma 82
  mucocele 229, 232
  nasal cavity 227, 235
  nasopharyngeal examination 227,
    246

nasopharynx 227, 246
  adenoids 247
  anatomy normal 247
  indications for examination 246
  malignant tumors 221, 234, 263
  neurogenic tumors 258
  pitfalls in examination 246
nasopharynx, nasal cavity and
  paranasal sinus 227–235
  abnormal 229
  benign tumor 229
  development 229
  infection 229
  trauma 229
  tumors 223
orbit 216–219
  anatomy, abnormal 218
  anatomy, normal 216
  fractures 218
oropharynx and mandible 236–240
  anatomy, abnormal 237
  anatomy, normal 236
otosclerosis 108
paranasal sinuses 227
radiation exposure 215
sialography 316
sinusitis 232
skull base 220
  sphenoid sinus, myeloma 235
  temporal bone 26–29
  tomographic plane 213
  torus tubarius 227
Conus elasticus 278
Cranial nerve neuromas 82, 95–107,
  225, 228
Craniometaphyseal dysplasia 116
Cricoarytenoid joint, tumor involvement
  299
Cricoid cartilage 267
  fracture 287
  tumor invasion 297

Dentigerous cysts, multiple 202
Dermatomyositis 282

Ectopic carotid artery 43
  arteriographic findings 44
Encephalocele, cribriform plate CT 230
Epiglottitis, acute 289
Epiglottis, tumors 303–305
Esophageal hiatus, malignant tumor 308
Ethmoid air cells 143
Ethmoid canal 150
Ethmoid sinus 132, 135, 139, 142, 159
  anterior and posterior cells in
    infection 183

evaluation 183
mucocele 188
mucocele, CT 233
reticulum cell sarcoma 199
spurious opacification 183
squamous cell carcinoma 200
Ethmoid sinus fractures 178
    clouding 178
    entrapment of medial rectus muscle
        179
    orbital emphysems 178
Ethmoiditis, proptosis, CT 219
Ethmomaxillary plate 133, 150
Eustachian tube, disturbed physiology by
    tumor 265
External auditory canal
    agenesis 34
    atresia 37
    carcinoma 91
    cholesteatoma 74
    postoperative stenosis 76
    stenosis 36

Face, categories of fractures 168
Facial nerve
    anomalies 37
    in cholesteatoma 70
    neuromas 122
    trauma
        bullet wounds 120
        classification of radiographic
            findings 120
        iatrogenic lesions 120
Facial nerve canal
        cholesteatoma 119
    chronic otitis media with
        cholesteatoma 119
    congenital anomalies 118
    congenital atresia 119
    inflammatory conditions 119
    in malignant external otitis 119
    in skull fractures 120
    petrous pyramid cholesteatoma 119
Vth nerve, schwannoma CT 225
Foramen rotundum 157
Frontal sinus 131, 135, 139, 156
    asymmetry 182
    asymmetrical thickness of walls 141
    carcinoma 201
    fractures 179
    margin 131
    mucocele 188
    orbital border 135
    retention cyst 186
    spurious opacification 182
    thick wall 141
    thick anterior wall 182

Glomus jugulare 86
Glomus tumors 85, 258, 259
    arteriography 87
    CT 85, 89
    jugular venography 87
    retrograde venography 85
Glomus tympanicum 86

Hard palate 141, 164
    destruction 206
    plasmacytoma 206
    reticulum cell sarcoma 207
Hiatus semilunaris 146

Incus and malleus anomalies 36
Incus dislocation post operative 76
Inferior orbital fissure 156
Inferior turbinate 139, 163
Infraorbital canal 146, 156
Infraorbital sulcus 150
Infratemporal fossa 222
    CT 222
    metastatic carcinoma 226
    sarcoma 226
    tumors, classified 225
Inner ear anomalies 38
Innominate line 160
Internal auditory canal 95–107
    abnormal 98
    anomalies 40
    conventional radiography 96
    cortical outline 98
    crista falciformis 98
    diameter 98
    length 98
    normal 96
    radiographic techniques 96
    shape 98
    tomography 96
Intravagale tumors 258

Jugular fossa 83, 87, 164
Jugular vein anomalies 42
Jugular venogram 43
Juvenile angiofibroma 254, 256
    CT 256
    embolization 257

Labyrinthine windows
    anomalies 36
    in otosclerosis 109
Labyrinthitis
    obliterative, congenital 41
Lacrimal apparatus 158, 160
Lamina papyraciea 132, 139
Laryngocele 290
Laryngography 270
    contraindications 277
    radiologic anatomy 273
    technique 271
Laryngotracheobronchitis 288
Larynx
    acute infection 288
    adenoma 290
    anatomy 267
    amyloid 290
    anesthesia levels 272
    benign cyst 290
    benign tumor 290
    blunt trauma 286
        late effects 287
    carcinoma 269, 294, 299–301
        laryngogram 270–277

cartilagenous invasion 296
choice of Roentgen examination 268
chondronecrosis 285
chronic infections 289
    blastomycosis 289
    coccidiomycosis 289
    granuloma 289
    rhinosclerma 289
    tuberculosis 289
congenital defects 280
    dermatomyositis 282
    multiple sclerosis 282
    myasthenia gravis 282
functional disorders 282
granuloma false cord 302
hemangioma 281, 290
inflammatory lesions 288
intubation injuries 283
laryngocele 292
laryngeal ventricle in carcinoma 292
laryngography 270
malignant tumors 293
    false cord and aryepiglottic folds
        301
    infrahyoid epiglottic 305
    subglottic extension 300
    suprahyoid epiglottic 303
    tumor grouping 293
oncocytoma 290
papilloma 281
paralytic states 282
plain views 269
polyp, laryngogram 291
radiation injuries 283, 285
radiologic techniques 269
spastic dysphonia 282
subglottic stenosis 284
subglottic web 270
tomography 270
trauma 282
trauma, classifications 282
true cord tumors 294
tumors 290
    ventricle (saccule) 290
Law projection 4
LeFort fractures 174
    associated nasopharyngeal mass 176
    bilateral vs unilateral 175
    classification 178
    mobility of the face 174
    pterygopalatine fossa 174
    types
        LeFort I fracture 177
        LeFort II fracture 178
        LeFort III fracture 178

Malar eminence 142
    displacement 173
Malignant external otitis 55, 119, 253
Malleus fixation 37
Mastoid
    diploic 57
    pneumatization 3, 34
    pneumatization variation 58
    postoperative radiology 75–77

Mastoidectomy
　radical and modified radical 75
　simple 75
Mastoiditis acute 54
Mastoiditis and otitis media acute 54–56
　differential diagnosis 54
　radiographic findings 54
　radiographic technique 54
Mastoiditis and otitis media, chronic
　57–60
　clinical findings 57
　otoscopic findings 57
　radiographic findings 57
Maxillary hiatus 146
Maxillary nerve 153
Maxillary sinus (antrum) 132, 134, 139,
　142, 164
　ameloblastoma 202
　calcified hematoma, CT 231
　chronic sinusitis, CT 232
　cylindroma (adenocystic carcinoma)
　　198, 205
　fracture
　　air fluid level 169
　　bright lines 169
　　opacification 169
　　superior orbital fissure 170
　histiocytic lymphoma, CT 235
　hypoplasia, unilateral and bilateral
　　181
　lateral wall 136, 138
　leiomyosarcoma 196
　malignant tumors 193–199
　medial wall 136
　mucocele 188
　ostium 146
　roof 135
　squamous cell carcinoma 193–199,
　　200, 204
　spurious opacification 181
Maxillofacial trauma 166–180
　general consideration 166
　importance of previous trauma 167
Meniere's disease
　vestibular aqueduct, tomography 124
Meningioma, CT 82
Meningocele 76, 249
Meningoencephalocele 76
Michel anomaly 38
Microtia 34
Middle ear anomalies 36
Middle ear in chronic otitis media and
　mastoiditis 59
Mikulicz's disease 319, 324
Modini anomaly 39
Mucorales in nasopharynx and pharynx
　251
Mucormycosis 253
　maxillary sinus 191
Multiple sclerosis 282
Myesthemia gravis 282

Nasal cavity, carcinoma, CT 235
Nasal fossa, lateral wall 133
Nasal septum, lateral crest 146
Nasofrontal canal 158
Nasolacrimal canal 143, 163

Nasolacrimal apparatus, abnormal 143
Nasopharyngogram 244
Nasopharynx 141
　anaplastic carcinoma 262
　benign tumors 254
　carcinoma 207, 260, 263
　carcinoma, CT 221, 234
　contrast nasopharyngography 262
　CT 263
　granulomatous infections 253
　inflammatory polyps 256
　lateral projection 141, 242
　malignant tumors 234, 260
　　CT 253
　　contrast nasopharygography 262
　　direct extension 261
　　otitis media in 264
　　roentgen findings 261
　　site of origin 264
　　spread to neck nodes 265
　obstruction, functional 250
　sarcoid 253
Neuroma, parapharyngeal area 259
Neuromas, VIII cranial nerve, see
　Acoustic neuromas
Neuromas V, VII, IX, X, XI XII cranial
　nerves 82, 122, 225, 258, 259

Odontogenic cyst 202
Olfactory plate 146
Oncocytoma 327
Optic canal (Rhese)view 142
Orbit 136, 160
　CT 216–219
　fractures 169
　fractures, CT 218
　floor, posterior portion, fracture 172
　lateral floor 160
　lateral wall 138
　medial wall 132, 135, 143, 146, 149,
　　150
　metastatic carcinoma, CT 219
　roof 150
　tumors, classification 219
Oropharynx, paresis, CT 231
Oropharynx and mandible 236–238
Ossicular dislocation 52
Ossicles, postoperative 76
Osteogenesis imperfecta 116
Osteopetrosis 116
Otosclerosis 108–113
　cochlear, tomography 111
　clinical course 108
　CT 108
　fenestral 109
　labyrinthine windows, pre and
　　post operative 109
　post stapedectomy tomography 109
　tomography in labyrinthine
　　windows 108
Owen projection 6

Paget's disease 114
Paranasal sinuses
　axial tomographic projection 159
　Caldwell view 130
　carcinoma 194

coronal tomographic projection 143
　granulomatous sinusitides 191
　　fungus diseases 191
　　other granulomatous lesions 192
　　rhinoscleroma 191
　　Wegener's granulomatosis 192
　inflammatory diseases 181–192
　inflammatory masses 185
　　choanal polyp 186
　　nonsecretory cyst 186
　　polyp 186
　　retention cyst 186
　lateral view 140
　lateral view in diagnosing opacifi-
　　cation 183
　lateral tomographic projection 153
　normal tomographic anatomy
　　143–165
Paranasal sinuses, tumors 193–209
　alveolar recesses 206
　differential diagnosis of bone
　　destruction 202
　ethmoid sinus, anterior lamina
　　papyracea destruction 199
　ethmoid sinus destruction 199
　frontal sinus destruction 201
　hard palate destruction 206
　maxillary sinuses 193–199
　　ethmomaxillary plate destruction
　　　195
　　lateral wall destruction 193
　　maxillary alveolar ridge
　　　destruction 198
　　medial wall destruction 194
　　roof destruction 195
　　sphenoid sinus destruction 201
Parotid gland 312–338
　adenocarcinoma 335
　adenocystic carcinoma 334
　carcinoma extension into temporal
　　bone 92
　classification of inflammatory
　　diseases 319
　displacement by tuberculosis node
　　337
　idiopathic hypertrophy, sialogram
　　317
　invasion by squamous cell carcinoma
　　of tonsil fossa 337
　laceration of duct, CT 319
　post traumatic abscess 318
　pseudohypertrophy 317
　recurrent carcinoma in temporal bone
　　93
　recurrent pyogenic sialadenitis 321
　sialography 312
Parotitis, chronic punctate 319
Parotitis, recurrent pyogenic 321
Passavant's ridge 249
Petrous pyramid 50, 51, 53, 57, 114,
　115, 117, 155, 157
　projections 8
Pharyngeal recess (foss of Rosenmüller)
　228, 246
Pharynx 242–266
　airway in infants, normal 281
　angiography 245

base projection 243
carcinoma, CT 265
functional disorders 250
infections 251
neurogenic tumors 258
neurophysiology disturbances 250
plain views 242
radiographic anatomy, normal 245
thorium necrosis 252
tomography, projections 244
trauma 251
xeroradiography 244
Phonation, "E" in laryngography 274
Pickwickian syndrome 250
Piriform sinus, malignant tumors 306
Pleomorphic adenoma 325
Postcricoid malignant tumors 307, 308
Proptosis 156
Pterygoid plate 163
    lateral 138
    medial 138
    medial and lateral 164
Pterygopalatine fossa 138, 141, 153, 157,
    160, 164
    abnormalities 158
    five connections 160
    fracture 162, 175

Retraction pickets, epitympanic 65
Reverse "E" maneuver in laryngography
    277
Rhinoscleroma 253
Rhinorrhea, post traumatic 179
Riley-Day syndrome 282
Rosenmüller fossa, asymmetry, CT 244

Salivary gland tumors 325
Schüller projection 5
Schwannoma, Vth nerve, CT 225
Sella turcica 133, 141
Semicircular canal anomalies 40
Sialadenitis 319
Sialadenitis, chronic 321
Sialography 312
    accuracy of diagnosis in malignant
        parotid tumors 335
    acute inflammatory diseases 320
    anatomy 312
    benign tumors 325
    chronic punctate parotitis 319
    chronic punctate sialadenitis 321
    chronic punctate sialadenitis in chil-
        dren 325
    CT 224, 312, 316, 335
    congenital lesions 317
    contraindications 316
    equipment 315
    functional disorders 317
    infections 319
    malignant tumors 332
    miscellaneous tumors 327
    normal 316
    oncocytoma 327
    parotid gland normal 312, 313
    pleomorphic adenoma 325
    stones 320
    submaxillary gland 314

technical pitfalls 316
technique 315
traumatic lesions 318
tumors 325
    localization by Roentgen tech-
        nique 328
Warthin's tumor 327
Sicca syndrome 319, 321, 324
Sinusitis 181–192
    acute and chronic 184
    air fluid level 184
    radiographic diagnosis 181
    sclerotic wall 185
Sinusitis, complications 190
    brain abscess 191
    orbital cellulitis 190
Sjögren's syndrome 319, 321
Skull base 137
    CT 220
    sclerosis in carcinoma of the naso-
        pharynx 207
Spastic dysphonia 282
Sphenoid, greater wing 160
Sphenoid sinus 133, 136, 139, 142, 153
    accessory septum 160
    fractures 179
        air fluid level 180
        bilateral rectus paralysis 180
        loss of vision 180
    mucocele 188
    myeloma, CT 235
    retention cyst 185
    squamous cell carcinoma 201
    unilateral opacification 183
Sphenoid spine 164
Stenvers projection 9
Submaxillary gland 314
    sialography 314
    chronic sialadenitis 320
Superior orbital fissure 133, 152, 156,
    170

Temporal bone
    adenoma 78
    anomalies 31, 34
    benign tumors 78
    carcinoma 90
    CT 26–29
    conventional radiography 3
    direct mastoid fracture 50
    eosinophilic granuloma 84
    embryology 32
    exostoses 78
    extension, parotid gland carcinoma
        92, 93
    fibrous dysplasia 116
    fractures 46–53
    hemangioma 78
    longitudinal fractures 48
    malignant tumors 90
    meningioma 80
    meningioma CT 82
    osteoma 78
    postoperative pathology 76
    postoperative soft tissue changes 76
    projectile missiles 53
    sarcoma 90

secondary malignancies, direct exten-
    sion 92
secondary malignancies, metastatic
    extension 93
vascular anomalies 42
Temporal bone, tomography 12
    axial projection 20
    coronal projection 16
    horizontal projection 14
    longitudinal projection 24
    multidirectional tomography, normal
        13
    sagittal projection 22
    semiaxial projection 18
    transverse fracture 50
Temporal bone trauma 46–53
    classification 46
    clinical findings 46
    radiographic techniques 47
    tomography 47
Thornwadt's bursa 249
Thorium necrosis, pharynx 252
Thyroid cartilage 267
    fracture 287
    radiation injury 283, 284
    tumor invasion 297, 298
Towne projection 10
Tracheomalacia 280
Transorbital projection 8
Trimalar fracture 167, 173, 174
    anatomy 173
    base view 173
    lateral view 173
    radiographic representation 173
    Water's view 174
Tympanic bone, anomalies 34
Tympanoplasty 75
    lateralization of graft 77
Tuberculosis in the middle ear and
    mastoid 60
Tympanosclerosis 60

Uveoparotid fever (sarcoid) 324

Valsalva maneuver in laryngography
    273, 275
Vascular anomalies, temporal bone 42
Vestibular aqueduct 124
    abnormalities 124
    anomalies 40
    obliteration 125
Vertebrobasilar vascular insufficiency,
    CT 126
Vocal cord paralysis 280

Waardenburg syndrome 40
Warthin's, papillary adenocystoma lym-
    phomatosum 327, 331
Water's view 134

Zygomatic arch 136, 169
Zygomatic arch fracture 168
    change of contour 168
    depression 167, 168
    linear lucency 168
    oval density 168